Ultrasound and the Ovary

Dedication

To Professor Erik Hauptmann who taught me how to write my first scientific paper

PROGRESS IN OBSTETRIC AND GYNECOLOGICAL SONOGRAPHY SERIES

SERIES EDITOR: ASIM KURJAK

Ultrasound and the Ovary

ASIM KURJAK

The Parthenon Publishing Group
International Publishers in Medicine, Science & Technology
NEW YORK LONDON

British Library Cataloguing in Publication Data
Ultrasound and the Ovary. – (Progress in Obstetric & Gynecological Sonography, ISSN 1352–9528)
I. Kurjak, Asim II. Series
618.1

ISBN 1-85070-508-9

Library of Congress Cataloging-in-Publication Data
Ultrasound and the ovary / edited by Asim Kurjak.
p. cm. – (Progress in obstetric and gynecological sonography series, ISSN 1352–9528; v. 1)
Includes bibliographical references and index.
ISBN 1-85070-508-9
1. Ovaries–Ultrasonic imaging. 2. Ovaries–Diseases. 3. Ovaries–Physiology. I. Kurjak, Asim. II. Series. [DNLM. 1. Ovary–ultrasonography. 2. Ovarian Cysts–ultrasonography. 3. Ovarian Neoplasms–ultrasonography. WP 320 U465 1994]
RG441.U48 1994
618.1'107543–dc20
DNLM/DLC.
For Library of Congress 94-2029
CIP

Published in the UK and Europe by
The Parthenon Publishing Group Limited
Casterton Hall, Carnforth
Lancs. LA6 2LA

Published in North America by
The Parthenon Publishing Group Inc.
One Blue Hill Plaza
Pearl River
New York 10965, USA

First published 1994

Composed by Servis Filmsetting Ltd, Longsight, Manchester
Printed and bound in Spain by T.G. Hostench, S.A.

Progress in Obstetric and Gynecological Sonography Series

An ongoing series documenting recent advances in key subject areas, with a new volume scheduled for publication approximately every 3 months.

Titles currently planned in the Series include:

Ultrasound and the Ovary	A. Kurjak (Croatia)
Ultrasound and the Fetal Brain	F. A. Chervenak (USA) and A. Kurjak (Croatia)
Ultrasound and the Uterus	A. Kurjak (Croatia) and R. Osmers (Germany)
Ultrasound and Early Pregnancy	D. Jurković (UK) and E. Jauniaux (Belgium)
Ultrasound and the Fallopian Tubes	I. E. Timor-Tritsch (USA) and A. Kurjak (Croatia)
Ultrasound and Fetal Heart	J. W. Wladimiroff (The Netherlands) and G. Pilu (Italy)
Ultrasound and Fetal Growth	J. M. Carrera (Spain) and S. Uzan (France)
Three-dimensional Ultrasound	K. Baba (Japan) and D. Jurković (UK)
Ultrasound and Infertility	A. Kurjak (Croatia) and W. Feichtinger (Austria)
Ultrasound and Endoscopic Surgery	S. Kupešić (Croatia) and M. Goldenberg (Israel)
Ultrasound and Prenatal Diagnosis	W. Holzgreve (Germany) and D. A. Nyberg (USA)
Doppler in Gynecology	A. Kurjak (Croatia) and H. Shulman (USA)
Doppler in Obstetrics	K. Maršál (Sweden) and B. Trudinger (Australia)
Safety of Diagnostic Ultrasound	G. Kossoff (Australia) and S. Barnett (Australia)

From an exciting novelty, ultrasound has now become the best single diagnostic technique available in obstetrics and gynecology. The original excitement is, of course, still felt by many of us. One cannot stop wondering how many applications of this relatively simple invention the future will hold. On the other hand, the wave of interest created by the present possibilities is spreading rapidly through almost all major journals. Any interested individual will find it difficult to read or even scan all of these articles, although he might wish to do so. The purpose of this newly conceived series of books is to overcome the problem by providing expert, up-to-date analyses of current advances in each specialized topic.

This new series is dedicated to the in-depth evaluation of the latest developments and advances in an area where progress is on a wide front and where diagnostic potential changes so rapidly. Each book contains critical reviews by leading experts, backed up by the best bibliographical information available. Unique and contemporary in concept, design and content, the new series provides a timely and continuing resource of expert information in a highly readable, consistent format.

It is hoped that this unique series will promote current awareness and help clinicians and research workers to keep abreast of today's most significant research and current developments.

Therefore titles in this series will be produced accurately, concisely and rapidly over a short time period. The chapters provide not only essential new data, but also serve as guides for interpretation of the literature and to the repercussions for clinical practice. In other words, the objective of each book is to inform our colleagues of the evidence and data available on the topic concerned, how reliable this information appears to be and what conclusions may be drawn from it. It should be a tool for distinguishing facts from fiction.

We believe that these new volumes will prove to be major sources of innovative ideas and effective solutions for the practice of obstetric and gynecological sonography.

Asim Kurjak
Series Editor

Contents

List of principal contributors

A. H. Balen
Department of Reproductive Endocrinology
The Middlesex Hospital
Mortimer Street
London W1N 8AA
UK

F. G. Balen
Department of Radiology
The Middlesex Hospital
Mortimer Street
London W1N 8AA
UK

H. R. K. Barber
Department of Obstetrics and Gynecology
Lenox Hill Hospital
100 East 77th Street
and Department of Clinical Obstetrics and Gynecology
Cornell University Medical College
New York, New York 10021
USA

J. Beires
Department of Gynecology
Hospital S. João
Faculty of Medicine
Porto
Portugal

I. Brosens
Department of Obstetrics and Gynecology
University Hospital Gasthuisberg
B3000 Leuven
Belgium

F. A. Chervenak
Department of Obstetrics and Gynecology
The New York Hospital–Cornell Medical Center
525 East 68th Street
New York, New York 10021
USA

V. Dramusic
Department of Obstetrics and Gynaecology
National University of Singapore
National University Hospital
5 Lower Kent Ridge Road
Singapore 0511

Lj. Kostović-Knežević
Department of Histology and Embryology
School of Medicine
University of Zagreb
41000 Zagreb
Croatia

S. Kupesic
Ultrasonic Institute
University of Zagreb
Sveti Duh 64
41000 Zagreb
Croatia

A. Kurjak
Ultrasonic Institute
University of Zagreb
Sveti Duh 64
41000 Zagreb
Croatia

J. P. Lerner
Department of Obstetrics and Gynecology
Columbia Presbyterian Medical Center
Sloane Hospital for Women
622 W. 168 Street
New York, New York 10032
USA

I. R. McFadyen
Department of Obstetrics and Gynaecology
Royal Liverpool University Hospital
Prescot Street
Liverpool 7
UK

J. Menczer
Department of Obstetrics and Gynecology
Gynecologic Oncology Service
Sheba Medical Center, Tel Hashomer
Sackler School of Medicine
Tel Aviv University
Tel Aviv
Israel

D. W. Pilling
Department of Radiology and Ultrasound
Liverpool Maternity Hospital
Oxford Street
Liverpool 7
UK

A. Prys Davies
Department of Obstetrics and Gynaecology
University Hospital of Wales
Cardiff
UK

S.-L. Tan
Department of Obstetrics and Gynaecology
King's College Hospital School of Medicine and Dentistry
London SE5 8RS
UK

M. Toth
The New York Hospital–Cornell Medical Center
Department of Obstetrics and Gynecology
525 East 68th Street
New York, New York 10021
USA

G. Volpe
Department of Obstetrics and Gynecology
'Ospedale Di Venere'
Bari-Carbonara 70012
Italy

I. Zalud
Department of Obstetrics and Gynecology
Winthrop University Hospital
State University of New York at Stony Brook
Mineola, New York 11501
USA

L. Zergollern
Ultrasonic Institute
University of Zagreb
Sveti Duh 64
41000 Zagreb
Croatia

Foreword

The ovary is one of the most active organs in the female body. It progresses through many changes, including puberty, pregnancy and menopause. It is complex in its embryology, histology and steroidogenesis. Furthermore, it is made up of germinal epithelium, germ cells of gonadal stroma, and mesenchymal cells – each with their own potential to form a tumor. The ovary is the site of origin for a larger variety of primary cancers than any other organ. In addition, the ovary is unique in that it not only gives rise to a great variety of malignancies but is also a favorite site for metastasis from other organs. Furthermore, there are many clinical entities in human medicine linked with ovarian changes, etiologically connected with abnormal quantity and quality of the human genome.

Ultrasound, more than any other modern technique, has enabled the direct assessment of many of the ovarian functions. Transvaginal sonography has revolutionized the morphological evaluation of the ovary and its conditions, both benign and malignant. The advancement and wider availability of therapies of assisted conception have occurred to a large extent as a result of developments in ultrasonography.

Transvaginal color Doppler has opened up exciting new possibilities for the better understanding of the physiology and pathophysiology of ovarian blood flow, resulting in a number of completely new diagnostic parameters.

Most of these exciting developments are described in this book. We all hope that readers will find our contributions useful and stimulating. For me as an editor, it has been a real pleasure to work again with The Parthenon Publishing Group and, in particular, David Bloomer, Jean Wright and Julia Tissington.

Asim Kurjak

The development and structure of the ovary

1

Lj. Kostović-Knežević and Đ. D. Grbeša

Our knowledge of ovarian development is based on investigations of human embryos by 'static' morphological and morphometric methods and on investigations of experimental animals.

We used the criteria of the Carnegie staging system to categorize the early periods of ovarian development. It is based on groups of morphological characteristics for determined stages of embryonic development. Other common criteria for estimating developmental stages, crown–rump length (CRL) and embryonal age, are shown in Table 1. There is no systematic classification system for fetal development and we used fetal age in weeks and lunar months.

The genetic sex of human embryos is determined at the time of fertilization. Until the 6th week of development the embryonic gonads of either sex are morphologically indistinguishable. Morphological sex differentiation begins in the 6th week of development when the gonad begins to differentiate into either a testis or an ovary. The gonadal anlage appears at the 4th week and differentiation is complete at the end of the 9th week of human development[1]. Morphological sexual differentiation can be divided into three periods:

(1) Indifferent stage – from 4–6 weeks (Carnegie stages 14–19) when the gonads and external genitalia are morphologically indistinguishable;

(2) Gonadal differentiation – from 7–8 weeks (Carnegie stages 20–23) when the gonads begin to differentiate, while the external genitalia remain sexually indistinguishable; and

(3) Gonadal and external genitalia differentiation – after the 9th week, when both the gonads and the external genitalia become sexually differentiated.

Three overlapping stages have been recognized in the morphogenesis of the human ovary[2]:

(1) The first stage (from the 4th to the 8th week of development) when the gonadal anlage is colonized by the primordial germ cells;

(2) The second stage (from the 8th to the 18th week) when sex cords develop; and

(3) The third stage, when the ovarian cortex and medulla differentiate and a massive formation of primordial follicles (folliculogenesis) takes place.

In all mammalian species, including the human, gonads develop in intimate contact with mesonephric tissue[3]. In the 4th week of development (stage 14), longitudinal swellings develop on the dorsal celomic wall lateral to the aorta and dorsal mesentery – the urogenital ridges. The lateral part of the urogenital ridge is the mesonephros, the second of the three nephric structures which develop during fetal life[4].

PRIMORDIAL GERM CELLS

The nephrogenic cells that differentiate into the mesonephros arise in the mesenchyme between the primitive aorta and the somites, near the celomic epithelium. The celomic epithelium proliferates towards the mesonephros, the mesenchyme condenses and the gonadal ridge develops in the medial area of the urogenital ridge[5]. At the same time the first primordial germ cells appear in the endodermal wall of the yolk sac, near the allantois. Some of these separate and migrate into the surrounding mesenchyme. The formation of the hind-gut is started and a few primordial germ cells are located in the gut epithelium.

At the end of the 4th week the primitive gut is

Table 1 Criteria for estimating developmental stages in the human embryo

Carnegie stage	*Crown–rump length* (mm)	*Number of somites*	*Age* (days)	*Age* (weeks)
1				
2			1.5–3	1
3			4–4.6	
4			5–6	2
5	0.1–0.2		7–12	
6	0.15–0.2		13–15	
7	0.4		16	
8	1–1.5		18	3
9	1.5–2.5	1–4	20	
10	2–3.5	7–10	22	
11	2.5–4.5	13–17	24	
12	3–5	20–23	26	4
13	4–6	28–30	28	
14	5–7		32	5
15	7–9		33	
16	8–11		37	6
17	11–14		41	
18	13–17		44	7
19	17–20		47–48	
20	21–23		50–51	
21	22–24		52	8
22	25–27		54	
23	28–31		56–57	

formed by invagination of the yolk-sac wall. The primordial germ cells are settled in the gut epithelium or in the mesenchyme. Some separate from the gut epithelium, and its basal lamina is broken. Primordial germ cells located in the gut mesenchyme are irregular in shape and have irregular cytoplasmic processes, the pseudopodia[6].

Migrating primordial germ cells also have an irregular shape, pseudopodia and a spherical nucleus with 2–3 nucleoli. Glycogen and lipids are decreased in their cytoplasm in the early stages of development. The rough endoplasmic reticulum is abundant but it decreases later. There are many free ribosomes and mitochondria with lamellar cristae and small membrane-bound bodies with electron-dense contents. Their number changes in germ cells before, during and after meiosis, and their nature and significance are still obscure. They may play a role in the meiotic process.

The mechanisms by which the primordial germ cells are translocated from extragonadal sites to the gonadal ridges are poorly understood. The primordial germ cells migrate actively[7], attracted by chemotactic substances or teloferon, produced by the developing gonadal ridge[8]. During migration there is a close association between these cells and fibronectin from the intercellular matrix[6].

The origin of the primordial germ cells is still uncertain. Goette (1875) and Nussbaum (1880) were the first to recognize that primordial germ cells arise from undifferentiated cells located some distance away from, and appearing before the formation of, the genital ridges[9]. Some authors claim that primordial germ cells may be derived from the extraembryonic endoderm, the primitive streak material[10], the mesoderm[11] or the yolk sac[12–14]. Ultrastructural studies of the human primordial germ cells appeared in 1977[6,15], and studies by immunological methods appeared in 1978[16].

They have been recognized in the 4.5-day-old human blastocyst[17]. At the beginning of the 4th

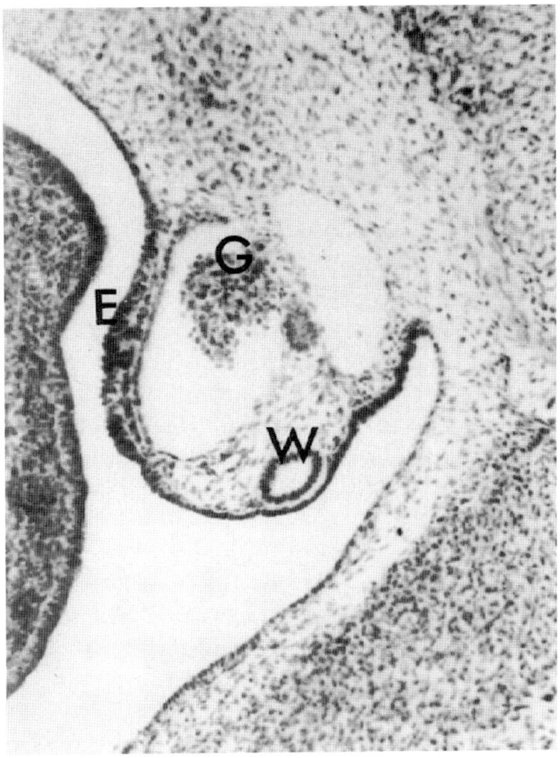

Figure 1 Urogenital ridge at the beginning of the 5th week of human development (crown–rump length 6.5 mm). E, gonadal epithelium; G, mesonephric glomerulus; W, Wolffian duct. (×202)

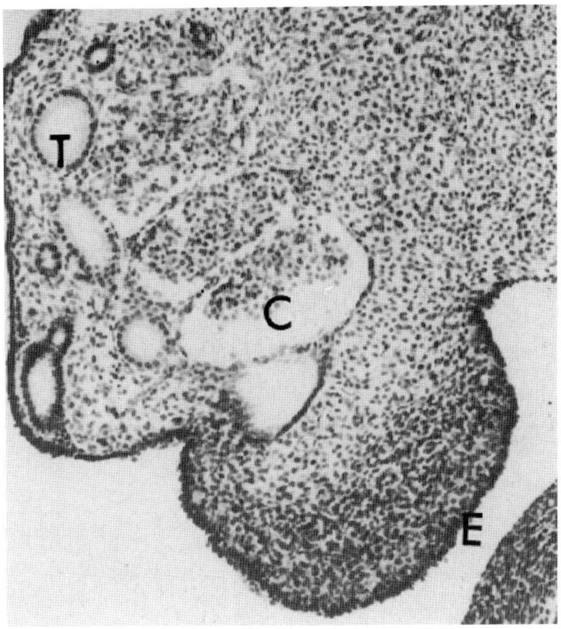

Figure 2 Gonadal anlage and mesonephros in the 5th week of human development (crown–rump length 7.6 mm). C, mesonephric corpuscle; E, gonadal epithelium; T, mesonephric tubule. (×152)

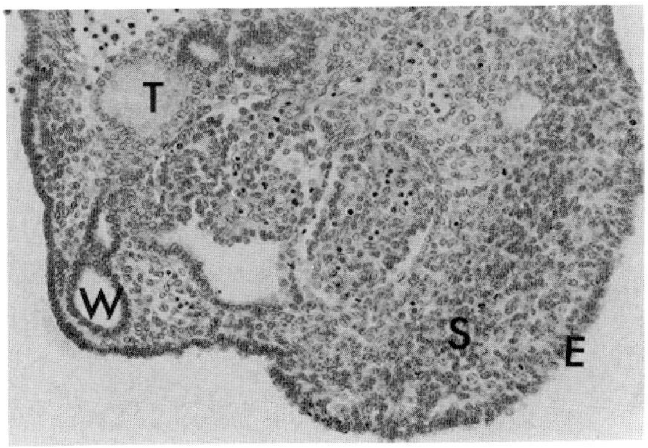

Figure 3 Gonadal anlage at the end of the 5th week of human development. E, celomic epithelium; S, gonadal stroma; T, mesonephric tubule; W, Wolffian duct. (×99)

week of development the germ cells migrate by ameboid movement to the genital ridge. In the 5th week of development they are settled in the mesenchyme of the gonadal ridge, a small bulge on the dorsal celomic wall[5,18]. Laterally to the gonadal ridge, in the mesonephros, mesonephric cells differentiate into the Wolffian duct, the mesonephric tubules and Malpighian bodies with the mesonephric glomeruli (Figure 1).

The mesenchyme of the gonadal ridge is concentrated and connected to the mesonephric glomeruli. The mesenchyme between the mesonephric tissue and the celomic epithelium changes from loose tissue to a compact mass of cells. The surface celomic epithelium proliferates and becomes stratified, forming a gonadal protrusion[5].

The migration of the primordial germ cells into the gonadal ridge induces its differentiation into the gonadal anlage (Figure 2), which is situated at the ventral cranial area of the mesonephros. It consists of mesonephritic tissue, mesenchyme, primordial germ cells scattered among them, and the celomic epithelium on the surface (Figure 3). At very early stages the gonadal anlage is invaded by capillaries, followed by an ingrowth of nerves. The gonad develops by inductive interactions of these different cells. If primordial germ cells do not migrate to the gonadal ridge, the gonadal

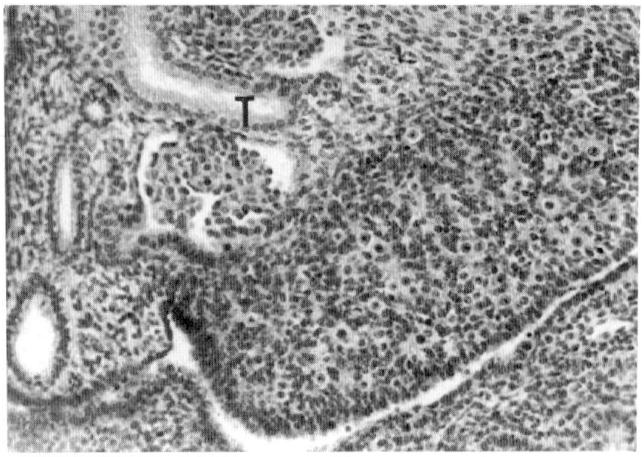

Figure 4 Gonadal anlage with primordial germ cells of the 6-week-old human embryo (crown–rump length 13 mm). T, mesonephric tubule. (× 117)

differentiation ceases[5]. The formation of the gonadal anlage is completed by week 5–6 of gestation[19].

During migration to the gonad, primordial germ cells divide mitotically and their number increases rapidly. In the 5-week-old human embryo the number of migrating germ cells is about 700–1300[13] and in the 8th week their number increases to 600 000[20]. When they reach the gonads, they transform to germ cells whose proliferation and differentiation are regulated by the surrounding somatic cells[5] (Figure 4).

Extragonadal germ cells that did not reach the gonads by the time of sex differentiation, disappear rapidly. However, primordial germ cells persist occasionally in extragonadal sites. They may produce teratomas because of uncontrolled pluripotentiality.

The epithelium that covers the gonad has been falsely termed 'the germinal epithelium', but the germ cells do not derive from the epithelium; they pass through it.

SEX CORDS

The stratified celomic epithelium proliferates into gonadal mesenchyme and develops into short, cord-like structures, the 'primary sex cords'. Some of the primordial germ cells which migrated into the gonadal ridge are in contact with the mesonephric tubules. The basal lamina has not been observed between the primordial germ cells and mesonephric cells[5,18].

Cells derived from the mesonephros also proliferate and form cord-like structures, the so-called 'primordial sex cords'. Each primordial sex cord is contiguous with the mesonephros and branches from the mesonephros towards the celomic epithelium. The cells of the primordial sex cord possess epithelial, not mesenchymal characteristics. Basal lamina has been observed around the primordial sex cord, but it gradually disappears. Vesicles containing basal lamina-like material have been seen in the cells of the primordial sex cords[18].

The primary sex cords (those which developed from the celomic epithelium in the ovarian mesenchyme) are flattened and do not branch. These cords display no continuity with the mesonephros or the primordial sex cords at any stage or site.

The gonadal anlage protrudes into the celomic cavity rapidly (Figure 5). In the 6th week of development, the migration of the primordial germ cells into the gonadal ridge ends, although some of the cells still remain in the dorsal mesentery.

The mesonephric cells invade the central part of the gonadal anlage and push the germ cells towards the periphery (Figure 6). An ovarian cortex and a medulla are formed. The cortex consists of germ cells distributed into clusters, and the medulla consists mainly of the mesonephric cells. The germ cells proliferate in the distal portion of the primordial sex cords. Those cords, situated in the basal portion of the ovary, are stretched and still contiguous with the mesonephros. The celomic epithelium at the surface of the ovarian anlage is stretched to form a single layer.

In the 13th week of development the ovary grows laterally. Because of the intensive proliferation of the germ cells the primordial sex cords enlarge. In the medulla, newly-formed interstitial tissue and the primordial sex cords displace toward the peripheral regions to form the 'folliculogenous sex cords'[18]. These cords branch from the centre towards the periphery of the ovary. Near the celomic epithelium they run parallel to the epithelium. They are flatter than those at the central portion of the ovary. It seems that the folliculogenous sex cords are formed from primordial sex cords.

The celomic epithelium is completely sur-

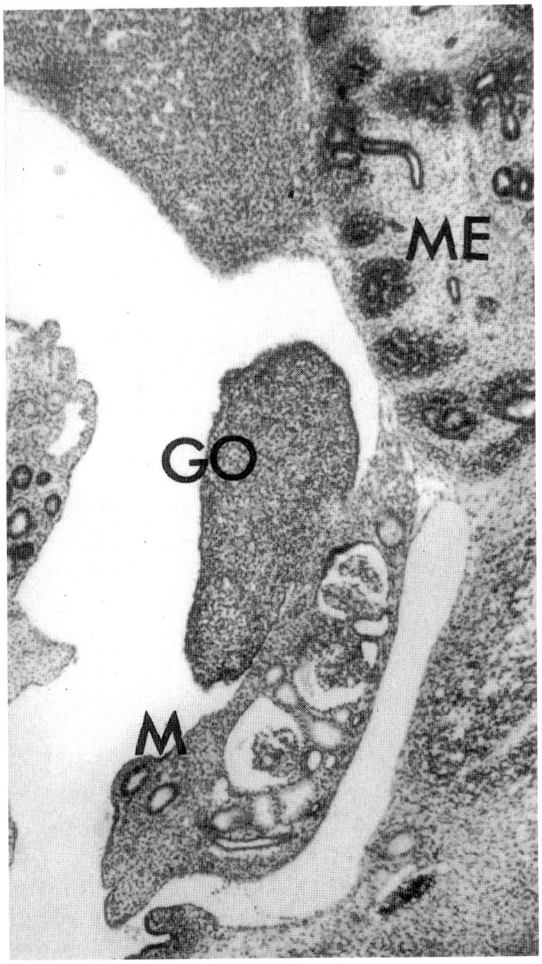

Figure 5 The gonad–mesonephric complex of the 7-week-old human embryo (crown–rump length 18 mm). GO, gonad; M, mesonephros; ME, metanephros. (× 59)

rounded by basal lamina. There is no sign of degeneration or disappearance of the primordial sex cords, especially in the ovarian medulla.

In the 18th week of development the folliculogenous sex cords have many proliferating germ cells and oogonia[18]. The adjacent interstitium is compressed due to enlargement of the folliculogenous sex cords. The ovarian medulla has clusters and islets of previous primordial sex cords, 'rete ovarii'. Fusion of the celomic epithelium and folliculogenous sex cords occurs at sites where the basal lamina has partially disappeared. The primordial germ cells, especially those situated between the celomic epithelium and sex cords,

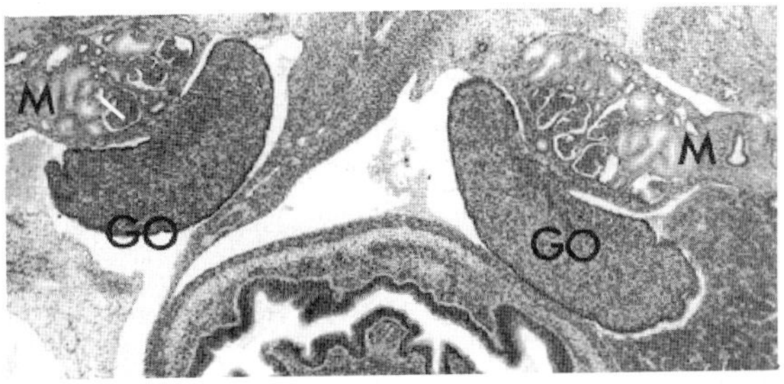

Figure 6 Human gonads during the 8th week of development (crown–rump length 25 mm). GO, gonad; M, mesonephros. (× 27)

possess some capability for dissolving the basal lamina. These cells therefore form sites of contact between the celomic epithelium and sex cords.

OOGENESIS

In mammals, oogenesis begins early in fetal development and ends in a sexually mature adult. Oogenesis begins with primordial germ cells, continues to oogonia (in the fetus), to oocytes (in the fetus) and to eggs (in the adult). Three important events occur during the early stages of oogenesis[5]:

(1) The initiation of meiosis (meiotic prophase);

(2) The formation of follicles (the diplotene oocyte is enclosed within granulosa cells); and

(3) The differentiation of steroid-producing cells.

Initiation of meiosis

When migration of primordial germ cells into the gonad has ended, their differentiation in the ovary begins. The life cycle of a normal female germ cell includes a series of mitotic divisions before meiosis is initiated. Groups of germ cells divide synchronously. The mitotically dividing germ cells, termed oogonia, continue to divide mitotically until they enter meiosis. The oogonia retain a positive reaction to alkaline phosphatase at least until they begin meiosis. The ultrastructure of oogonia resembles that of primordial germ cells. When multiplication ceases, the cells enter meiosis and are termed oocytes.

Meiosis is controlled by a series of factors that interact, such as the formation of a specific milieu around the germ cells, the secretion of steroids and specific meiosis-regulating substances[7]. The mesonephric cells secrete substances that influence the onset of meiosis: a meiosis-inducing substance (a small molecule, less than 2000 Da, with hydrophilic and hydrophobic characteristics[21]) and a meiosis-preventing substance (a polypeptide possessing a molecular weight of more than 5000 Da).

The meiosis-inducing substance is isolated in the follicular fluid of preovular follicles in the human fetal ovary, in the human fetal adrenal glands at the time when meiosis starts, and in the human fetal testis[7]. Secretion of this substance by the mesonephric cells is associated with the mesonephric influence on gonadal steroid production. The onset of meiosis in the ovary is correlated with cessation of mesonephric excretion and regression[22].

Around the third month, the first germ cells entering the first meiotic prophase are situated at the inner part of the ovarian cortex. Intercellular bridges develop between oogonia and oocytes in the early stages of meiosis. These intercellular bridges facilitate the exchange of parental gene products or substances such as hormones. In this way, germ cells undergo synchronous division. Gradually, more peripherally situated oogonia enter meiosis, even during the eighth lunar month[7].

The initiated meiosis is arrested in the last phase of the meiotic prophase, the diplotene stage. This stage lasts for a long time, possibly more than 50 years. A large percentage of oocytes that enter meiosis will not reach the diplotene stage, but will become pyknotic and degenerate. Only about 5% of germ cells reach the diplotene stage.

The number of germ cells reaches its maximum (7 000 000 in each ovary) during the 15th to the 20th week of development.

At the end of fetal development a majority of oocytes have entered the diplotene stage and a few days later nearly all oocytes have reached the diplotene stage, where they will remain until the time of ovulation.

In the postnatal period the number of oocytes decreases to 2 000 000, and by puberty it has fallen to 400 000.

Folliculogenesis

Early folliculogenesis depends on migration of mitotically dividing mesonephric cells, i.e. it depends on whether a sufficient number of mesonephric cells has invaded the developing ovary. The mesonephros-derived cells are in fact the granulosa cell precursors[7]. Some of these surround the diplotene oocytes to become granulosa cells, while others become the first interstitial cells. When the oocyte reaches the diplotene stage it must become enclosed in a follicle. Single oocytes are surrounded by granulosa cells, delineated by a basal lamina. If the oocyte in the diplotene stage fails to be enclosed into a follicle, it degenerates. The mechanisms that trigger follicular growth are unknown. Follicles begin to form in the inner part of the ovarian cortex. Initially the granulosa cells of these developing follicles are connected with the mesonephros-derived cells (rete cords).

Many oocytes degenerate at different stages of meiosis and they are eliminated via phagocytosis by the surrounding mesenchymal cells.

Light- and electron-microscopic studies of human gonadal development have produced controversial results. In paraffin-embedded sections, the primordial sex cords were not recognized but the primary sex cords and folliculogenous sex cords were observed. This was the reason for the erroneous view that the primary sex cords separate from the celomic epithelium and that the secondary sex cords are formed by the proliferation of celomic epithelium.

The use of the electron microscope has supported the thesis that during the early stages of ovarian development three types of sex cords occur, in regard to structure, location and origin[18]:

(1) Primary sex cords – peduncular structures from the celomic epithelium;

(2) Primordial sex cords – ramified structures contiguous with the mesonephros; and

(3) Folliculogenous sex cords – the structures formed by enlargement and relocation of the primordial sex cords at the peripheral portion of the ovary.

The ovarian medulla derives from the mesonephric mesenchyme in contact with proximal tubules.

Mesenchymal cells derive from the mesonephros in the early stages of embryogenesis and differentiate into epithelial cells possessing cell junctions and basal lamina.

Folliculogenous sex cords later give rise to follicular cells. These cords split into clusters whose cells enclose one or more primordial germ cells. In about the 6th month primitive granulosa cells organize around the dividing oocytes to form a single layer of follicular cells, establishing the primordial follicle.

Steroid-producing cells

The enclosure of germ cells in germ cell cords or follicles seems to play a major role in differentiation of the steroid-producing cells[7]. In the human fetal ovary the first steroid-producing cells differentiate concomitantly with the formation of small follicles. The origin of the early steroid-producing cells in the human ovary is still uncertain. In the mouse and rabbit, they differentiate from mesonephric cells. Although the aromatizing system functions from the 8th week, the fetal human ovary produces minimal amounts of sex steroid hormones before follicles start to develop[3]. The interstitial cells are localized in the medulla, and exhibit activity of 3β-hydroxysteroid dehydrogenase[3]. Ovarian steroidogenesis will not take place until follicles are formed. When follicles appear, interstitial cells contain mitochondria with tubular cristae, smooth endoplasmic reticulum and lipid droplets. These cells appear after the 12th week in the inner part of the cortex, close to follicles. The fetal ovary contains 'interstitial hilar cells' that also exhibit 3β-hydroxysteroid dehydrogenase activity. They are present in the human ovary from the 13th week onward. For a long time it has been assumed that the fetal ovary was incapable of the synthesis of steroids. The appearance and the position of the interstitial cells and the developing follicles within the ovary suggest that the closing up of the follicle may interact with early differentiation of the extrafollicular steroid-producing cells[3].

The neonatal period represents a stage in the development of the human ovary when oocytes and differentiating and maturing follicles coexist (Figures 7 and 8).

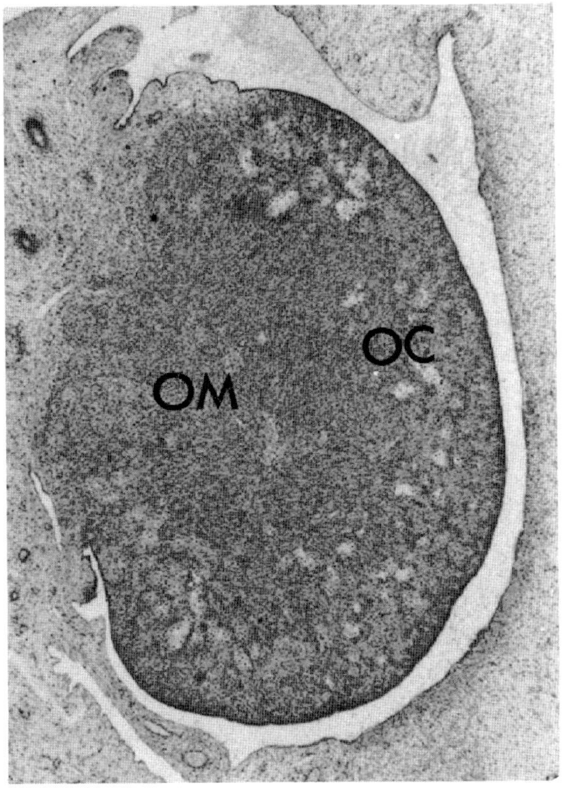

Figure 7 Human neonatal ovary. OC, ovarian cortex; OM, ovarian medulla. (× 35)

The mean volume of the neonatal ovary is 126 mm^3 and the cortex forms 4/5 of the organ. Follicles account for 10–25%, the interstitium for 35–45% and the medulla with blood vessels and nerves for 10–30% of the neonatal ovarian volume. The mean number of follicles is 266 000. Most are primordial follicles (95%); primary follicles account for 5% and secondary follicles are very rare, but there are a few Graafian follicles[4].

The organogenesis of the mammalian ovary is completed when the cortex disappears due to its cells being involved in folliculogenesis[4]. The clusters of naked oocytes gradually give way to follicles in various stages of maturation and they extend to the limit of the medulla.

This stage of development has not been clearly defined in the human ovary. Shortly after birth follicular growth is still in progress. Ovarian organogenesis proceeds throughout the prepubertal period.

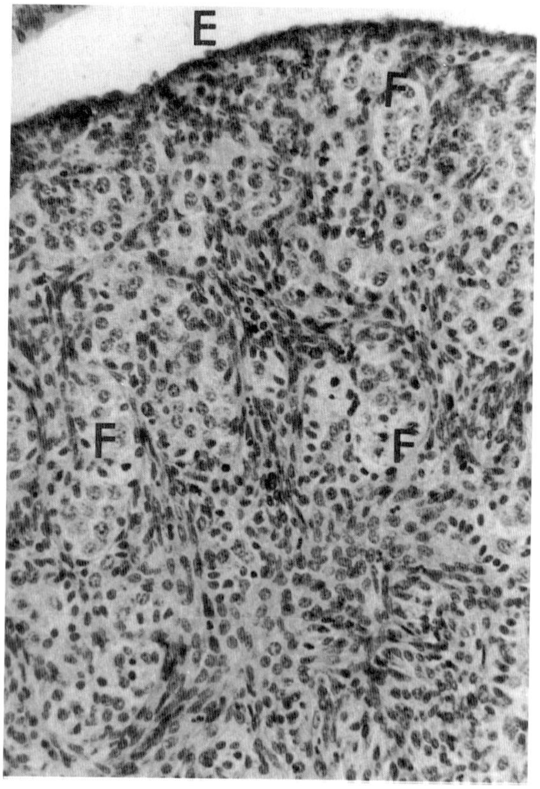

Figure 8 Cortex of human neonatal ovary. E, surface epithelium; F, folliculogenous sex cords. (× 194)

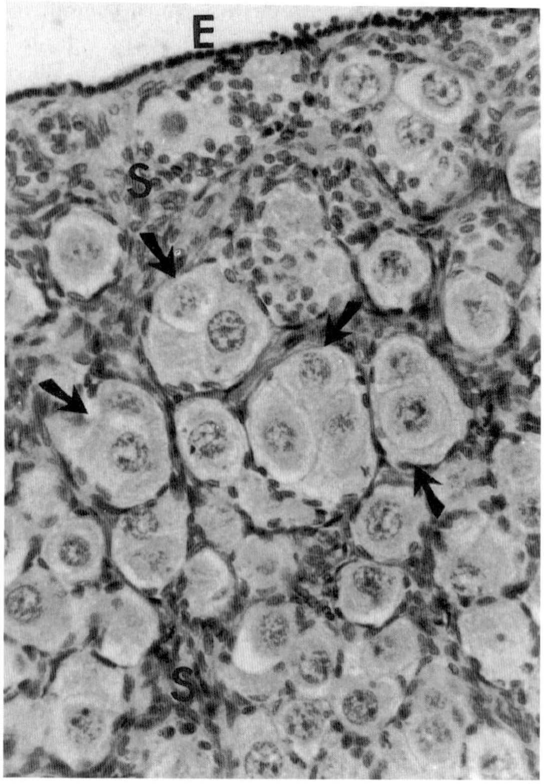

Figure 9 Primordial follicles in the cortex of a young girl. Four polyovular follicles are seen (arrows). The oocytes are surrounded by a single layer of flattened follicular cells. E, surface epithelium; S, stroma. (× 243)

STRUCTURE OF THE OVARY

The human ovaries are flattened, paired organs, 2–5 cm in length, 1.5–3 cm in width and 0.6–1.5 cm in depth. The size of the active ovary varies considerably from week to week during the menstrual cycle and pregnancy. More than any other organ, the ovary undergoes continuous morphologic changes which are necessary for its physiologic functions. The ovary consists of two major regions: the outer cortex, where ovarian follicles containing oocytes are located, and the inner medulla, where connective tissue with blood and lymphatic vessels dominate.

The stroma of the cortical region is composed of spindle-shaped fibroblasts and smooth muscle cells that respond in a different way to hormonal stimuli than do these cells of other organs.

The surface connective tissue (tunica albuginea) of the adult ovary is covered by a single-layered, cuboidal or low columnar epithelium[23–25] (Figure 9). The epithelium is supported on a distinct basal lamina. It is only disrupted where follicles ovulate. Repair occurs over the stigma within 2–4 days. Ultrastructural studies of the human ovary have shown that the surface epithelium has two types of epithelial cells (called A and B) situated in their own zones (A and B zones)[26–28]. Type A cells are cuboidal and sometimes tall with a density of apical microvilli. Type B cells are flat squamous cells with broader and flatter apices. The A and B zones are common to all surfaces of the ovary including the distending follicle. The relationship of the B zones to the surface bridges on the ovarian surface, and the association of these with ovulation sites, suggest that the B cells are metaplastic cells derived in response to chronic surface injury with ovulation[28].

Table 2 Morphological characteristics of developing ovarian follicles

Category of follicles	*Size*	*Follicular cells (granulosa cells)*	*Theca cells*	*Intercellular junctions*	*Basal lamina*
Non-growing follicles					
Primordial follicle (unilaminar)	25 μm	< 25 cells single layer of flattened cells		desmosomes between follicular cells	underlies follicular cells
Growing follicles					
Primary follicle (preantral)	50–200 μm	26–100 cells cuboidal or low columnar cells; synthesis of zona pellucida	differentiation of theca interna and theca externa	large gap junctions between granulosa cells	(1) between granulosa and theca interna; (2) between theca interna and theca externa
Secondary follicle (early antral)	200–500 μm	101–300 cells 6–12 layers irregular, small cavities with liquor			
Antral follicle	500–6000 μm	300–1000 cells formation of antrum folliculi; cumulus oophorus		gap junctions between theca cells; gap junctions between granulosa cells and oocyte	
Tertiary follicle (mature, Graafian, preovulatory)	> 6000 μm 1.5–2.5 cm	decrease of mitotic activity of granulosa cells; corona radiata formation			

OVARIAN FOLLICLES

The follicles are embedded in the stroma of the cortex. A follicle consists of an oocyte surrounded by one or more layers of follicular cells called the granulosa cells. The follicle represents the principal steroidogenic unit of the ovaries. Its biosynthetic activities change greatly depending on its progressive stage of differentiation. Follicular growth may be divided into several stages according to its appearance, size, rate of growth and other morphological and functional characteristics[29–31] (Table 2).

In the human female at birth, the number of follicles is about 1 million per ovary, and by puberty it has decreased to 250 000–300 000 oocytes. This decrease is brought about through the process of naturally occurring cell death, called atresia of the follicle. The follicular regression will continue during the reproductive years. After menopause only a small number of follicles remains. Atresia can affect any type of follicle, from the primordial to those of the preovulatory stage.

Non-growing follicles

Primordial follicle (unilaminar)

Primordial follicles are found in the periphery of the cortex, beneath the tunica albuginea. They are most numerous before birth. Each consists of a single layer of flattened follicular cells, which are joined together by intercellular contacts called desmosomes. A basal lamina underlies the follicular cells, forming the boundary between the basal part of the follicular cells and the surrounding stroma. A primordial follicle may contain more than one oocyte. Polyovular follicles are more common in fetal and immature ovaries, and have been described in mammals including the human[32] (Figure 9).

The oocyte in the primordial follicle is a spherical cell about 25 μm in diameter. It has a large eccentrically-placed nucleus with a prominent nucleolus.

Growing follicles

Primary follicle (preantral)

Development and growth of follicles occurs as a continuous process throughout approximately 30 years of ovarian function. The initial growth of the inactive primordial follicles to the early preantral stage is independent of gonadotropins. The transition from primordial to developing follicle involves cytological changes in the oocyte, as well as in the follicular cells and adjacent stromal cells[33].

Follicular cells become cuboidal or low columnar (Figure 10). They proliferate intensively by mitosis and form stratified epithelium called the granulosa layer. Ultrastructurally, mitochondria, rough endoplasmic reticulum and free ribosomes abound. The Golgi complex becomes prominent. These cells have the ultrastructural characteristics of protein-secreting cells. Intercellular contacts, called gap junctions, appear between granulosa cells. A thick basal lamina separates the granulosa cells from surrounding stromal cells. At the same time, interstitial cells (stroma), adjacent to the follicle, become arranged concentrically around the follicle to form the theca folliculi (Figure 10).

By further increase of the growing follicles, the stromal theca folliculi differentiates into the theca interna and the theca externa. Numerous small vessels penetrate the theca externa and give rise to a rich capillary plexus in the theca interna. The cells of the theca interna, when completely differentiated, have the same ultrastructural characteristics of steroid-secreting endocrine cells.

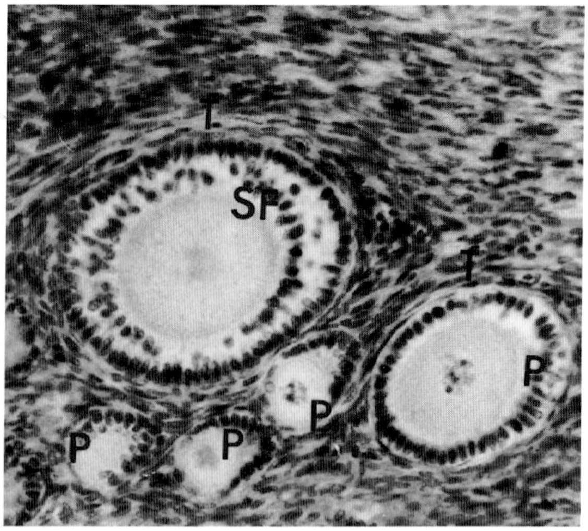

Figure 10 Human growing follicles. P, primary follicles; SF, secondary follicle; T, theca folliculi. (×213)

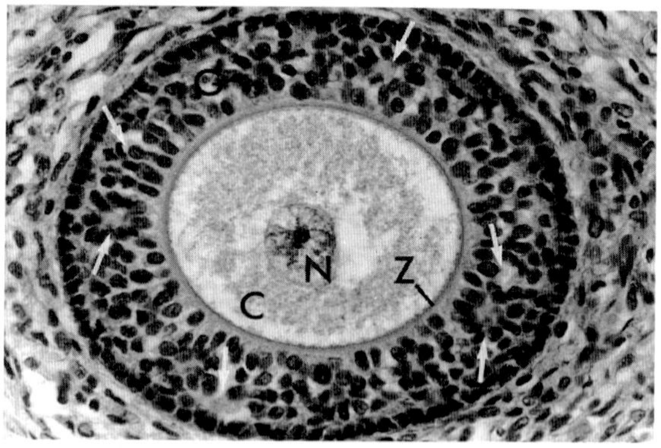

Figure 11 Human secondary follicle. C, cytoplasm of the oocyte; G, granulosa cells and small cavities between them (arrows); N, nucleus with a nucleolus; Z, zona pellucida. (×205)

The boundary between theca interna and theca externa is formed by a well developed basal lamina. No capillaries penetrate the granulosa.

The oocyte is surrounded by a thick coat, named the zona pellucida, composed of a jelly-like substance formed by three different glycoproteins. It is mildly eosinophilic in routine histological preparations, and gives a positive reaction with the periodic acid Schiff treatment[34]. Both the oocyte and granulosa cells contribute to the synthesis of the zona pellucida (Figure 11). Long, apical processes of follicular cells and short microvilli of the oocyte penetrate the zona pellucida and make intercellular contacts by gap junctions. The zona pellucida has an essential role at the time of fertilization and during the preimplantation period (in the cleavage process). *In vitro* experiments with the removal of the zona pellucida from human embryos at 2- and 4-cell stage have shown that isolated blastomeres undergo cleavage with abnormal blastocyst formation as a result of disaggregation[35,36]. These results suggest that diagnostic biopsy by disaggregation may eventually be possible in the human after the embryonic 8-cell stage.

Secondary follicle (antral)

Under endocrine stimulation during each ovarian cycle after puberty, 6–12 primary follicles develop into secondary follicles. The follicular growth and further development of the secondary follicle is related to the selection of a 'dominant' single follicle destined to mature. The maturation and ovulation of the dominant follicle is related to its capacity for estrogen biosynthesis, as well as to oocyte maturation[37]. These complex events are associated with complex endocrine, paracrine and autocrine mechanisms. The growth process involves an increase in the size of the oocyte and in the number of layers of granulosa cells that surround the oocyte (Figures 10 and 11).

When the follicle reaches a diameter of approximately 0.2 mm by further proliferation of granulosa cells, an accumulation of clear fluid (liquor folliculi) appears between the cells. As the follicle enlarges, irregular spaces filled with fluid between the granulosa cells become confluent, and small cavities fuse and form the antrum folliculi (Figure 12).

The granulosa cells are more numerous at one part of the follicle, forming a hillock of cells called the 'cumulus oophorus' with the oocyte in the middle. The cumulus protrudes into the antrum folliculi. Follicular fluid contains transudates of plasma and products secreted by follicular cells.

At this stage of the growing follicle, the granulosa cells make special intercellular contacts called gap junctions (nexus or communicating junctions) with surrounding theca as well as with the oocyte. The first cell communications by gap junctions are found among granulosa cells in the preantral follicle. Junctional units are formed in the opposing cell membranes from protein hexamers with a hydrophilic pore[38]. It has been shown experimentally that gap junctions permit the interchange between cells of molecules with a molecular weight below 1500[39]. Substances such as hormones, cyclic AMP and ions transport information between granulosa cells and their neighbouring theca cells and oocytes, causing them to act in a co-ordinated manner. In this way, heterocellular communication is established between genetically different cells.

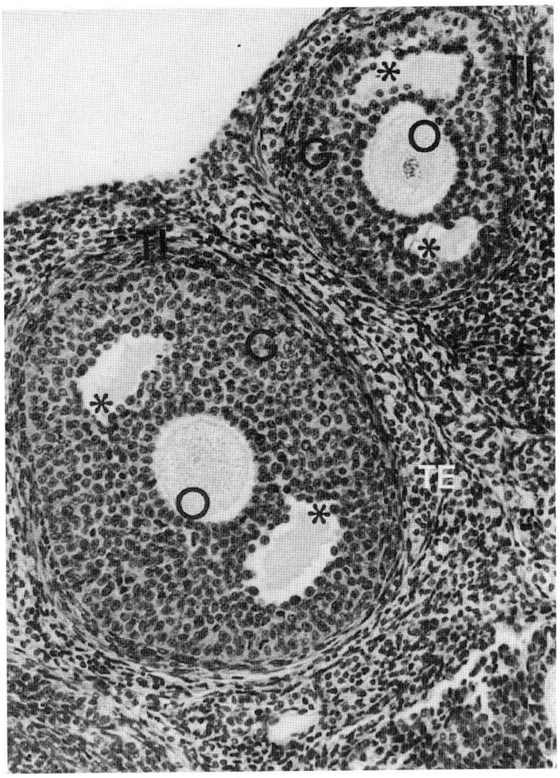

Figure 12 Two human secondary follicles of antral type; large irregular spaces in the follicular walls contain amorphous material, the liquor folliculi (asterisk). G, granulosa cells; O, oocyte; TI, theca interna; TE, theca externa. (× 144)

Mature follicle (tertiary, Graafian follicle)

During each menstrual cycle only one secondary follicle is usually destined to develop into a mature follicle. This follicle, as mentioned before, is called the dominant follicle.

A mature follicle is 1.2–2.5 cm in diameter. It protrudes from the surface of the ovary. The follicular cavity is maximally increased. At this stage of follicular growth, mitotic activity of the granulosa cells decreases. The granulosa cells around the zona pellucida and oocyte lengthen and form the corona radiata. As ovulation approaches, the cumulus separates from the follicular wall so that the oocyte with the corona radiata floats free in the antrum. The corona radiata is present after ovulation, during the process of fertilization. Further enlargement of the antrum results in the attenuation of both the granulosa and theca layers.

Ovulation

Ovulation depends on a complex sequence of endocrine events of the hypothalamus–hypophysis–ovary axis associated with local vascular and chemical changes of the preovulatory follicle[40] Ovulation is followed by some morphologically specific features:

(1) Follicular fluid seems to accumulate;

(2) The oocyte with corona radiata detaches from the wall of the follicle;

(3) A locally changed oval area called a stigma appears on the outer surface of the ovary;

(4) Part of the follicular wall protrudes through a small opening of the stroma on the ovarian surface and becomes progressively thinner[40,41]; and

(5) The surface epithelium and underlying tunica albuginea of the ovary become discontinuous.

The mechanism of rupture of the follicle is still controversial. The presence of smooth muscle in both the stroma and the follicular wall initiated the idea that ovulation is mediated by contractions[42]. The conclusion at present is that smooth muscle cells facilitate evacuation of follicular contents. The rupture of the follicle occurs under intrafollicular pressure of 15–20 mmHg.

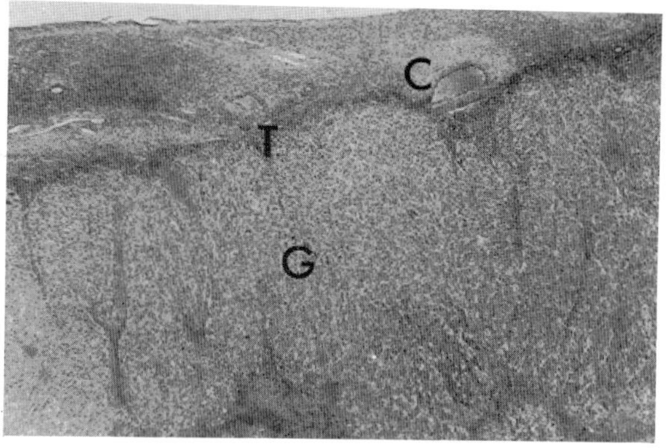

Figure 13 Portion of human corpus luteum. C, capsule with blood vessels; G, granulosa lutein cells; T, theca lutein cells. (× 15)

Corpus luteum (yellow body)

After rupture of the mature follicle followed by ovulation, the empty antrum fills up temporarily with blood, forming the corpus rubrum (hemorrhagicum). The granulosa cells lining the follicular wall form folds. Soon after, a loose connective tissue develops in the antral space (Figure 13).

Formation of the corpus luteum is initiated by a series of morphological and biochemical changes in the cells of the theca interna and granulosa cells of the preovulatory follicle. This process is termed luteinization. Both granulosa and theca interna cells transform into lutein cells. This transformation process has been shown *in vitro*[43,44].

During the process of luteinization, granulosa lutein cells become structurally specific and show features of steroid-secreting cells:

(1) The cells multiply and enlarge by hyperplasia and hypertrophy into polyhedral cells filled with cholesterol-rich lipid droplets;

(2) Smooth endoplasmic reticulum becomes prominent; and

(3) The number of mitochondria with developing tubular cristae increases.

Theca lutein cells are smaller than granulosa lutein cells and resemble steroid-secreting cells. The ultrastructural characteristics of lutein cells are correlated with the synthesis of progesterone. The basement membrane of the granulosa disap-

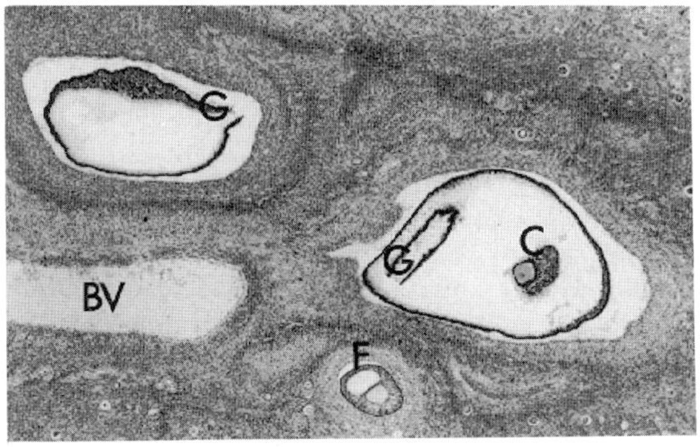

Figure 14 Two atretic follicles, showing detachment of follicular wall and degenerated granular cells. BV, blood vessel; C, remnant of cumulus oophorus with dead oocyte; F, normal growing follicle; G, detached follicular wall. (× 18)

pears and capillaries of the theca interna invade and sprout avascular granulosa to form a rich endocrine capillarization.

The corpus luteum represents, structurally and functionally, a temporary endocrine gland. If fertilization does not follow, this formation is called the corpus luteum of menstruation, which exists only for about 14 days. Under hormonal conditions, the corpus luteum undergoes involution after this period. If fertilization succeeds, the corpus luteum persists for 6 months and is called the corpus luteum of pregnancy.

The cells of the corpus luteum of menstruation or pregnancy undergo autolytic degeneration. The cellular debris is phagocytized by macrophages. Residual connective tissue forms a scar, the corpus albicans.

Atresia of the follicles

In humans during the early period of each menstrual cycle, a group of follicles starts to grow, but only one of these is destined to develop according to the concept of the dominant follicle. The others undergo a degenerative process called follicular atresia.

Atresia may begin at any stage of development of the follicle, from the primary or even the preovulatory. The atretic process is evident in the follicular wall as well as in the oocyte (Figure 14). The process of atresia is characterized by a morphological sequence of events as follows:

(1) The cessation of mitotic activity in the granulosa cells;

(2) The degeneration of these cells;

(3) The detachment of these cells from the basal lamina (Figure 14);

(4) The death of the oocyte by pyknosis of the nucleus, followed by changes in the cytoplasm and collapse of the zona pellucida;

(5) The advanced degeneration of the granulosa cells, followed by collapse of the follicular wall;

(6) The filling of the cavity of the atretic follicle with the residue of the zona pellucida and connective tissue; and

(7) The phagocytosis and resorption of the remnants of degenerated granulosa cells.

From puberty to menopause, about 99% of follicles undergo atresia. The postmenopausal ovary has a thin cortex, with a wrinkled surface. Primary and growing follicles are very rare.

ACKNOWLEDGEMENT

The authors express their gratitude to the Department of Histology and Embryology, School of Medicine, University of Zagreb, for the collections of human embryos, fetuses and adult ovaries used for research and documentation.

References

1. Fraser, B. A. and Sato, A. G. (1989). Morphological sex differentiation in the human embryo: a light and scanning electron microscopic study. *J. Anat.*, **165**, 61–74
2. Nicosia, S. V. (1983). Morphological changes of the human ovary throughout life. In Serra, G. B. (ed.) *The Ovary*, pp. 57–81. (New York: Raven Press)

3. Byskov, A. G., Hojer, P: E. and Westergaard, L. (1985). Origin and differentiation of the endocrine cells of the ovary. *J. Reprod. Fertil.*, **75**, 299–306
4. Forabosco, A., Sforza, C. H., De Pol, A., Vizzotto, L., Marzona, L. and Ferrario, V. F. (1991). Morphometric study of the human neonatal ovary. *Anat. Rec.*, **231**, 201–8
5. Byskov, A. G. (1986). Differentiation of mammalian embryonic gonad. *Physiol. Rev.*, **66**, 71–117
6. Fujimoto, T., Miyayama, Y. and Fuyuta, M. (1977). The origin, migration and fine morphology of human primordial germ cells. *Anat. Rec.*, **188**, 315–30
7. Byskov, A. G. and Hoyer, P. E. (1988). Embryology of mammalian gonads and ducts. In Knobil, E. and Neill, J. D. (eds.) *The Physiology of Reproduction*, Vol. I, pp. 265–302. (New York: Raven Press)
8. Ikawa, H., Trelstad, R. L., Hutson, J. M., Manganaro, T. F. and Donahoe, P. K. (1984). Changing patterns of fibronectin, laminin, type IV collagen and a basement membrane proteoglycan during rat Mullerian duct regression. *Dev. Biol.*, **102**, 260–3
9. Wassarman, P. M. (1988). The mammalian ovum. In Knobil, E. and Neill, J. D. (eds.) *The Physiology of Reproduction*, Vol. I, pp. 69–102. (New York: Raven Press)
10. Ozdzénski, W. (1967). Observations on the origin of the primordial germ cells in the mouse. *Zoologica Poloniae*, **17**, 367–79
11. Spiegelman, M. and Bennett, D. (1973). A light- and electron-microscopic study of primordial germ cells in the early mouse embryo. *J. Embryol. Exp. Morphol.*, **30**, 97–118
12. Chiquoine, A. D. (1954). The identification, origin and migration of the primordial germ cells in the mouse embryo. *Anat. Rec.*, **118**, 135–45
13. Witschi, E. (1948). Migration of germ cells of human embryos from yolk sac to primitive gonadal folds. *Contrib. Embryol.*, **32**, 67–80
14. Zamboni, L. and Merchant, H. (1973). The fine morphology of mouse primordial germ cells in extragonadal locations. *Am. J. Anat.*, **137**, 299–336
15. Kuwana, T. and Fujimoto, T. (1983). Active locomotion of human primordial germ cells *in vitro*. *Anat. Rec.*, **205**, 21–6
16. Heath, J. K. (1978). Characterization of a xenogeneic antiserum raised against the fetal germ cells of the mouse: cross-reactivity with embryonal carcinoma cells. *Cell*, **15**, 299–306
17. Hertig, A. T., Rock, J. and Adams, E. C. (1956). Description of 34 human ova within first 17 days of development. *Am. J. Anat.*, **98**, 435–93
18. Satoh, M. (1991). Histogenesis and organogenesis of the gonad in human embryos. *J. Anat.*, **177**, 85–107
19. George, F. W. and Wilson, J. D. (1988). Sex determination and differentiation. In Knobil, E. and Neill, J. D. (eds.) *The Physiology of Reproduction*, Vol. I, pp. 3–26. (New York: Raven Press)
20. Baker, T. G. (1963). A quantitative and cytological study of germ cells in human ovaries. *Proc. R. Soc. (Biol.)*, **158**, 417–33
21. Byskov, A. G. and Saxén, L. (1976). Induction of meiosis in fetal mouse testis *in vitro*. *Dev. Biol.*, **52**, 193–200
22. Grinsted, J. and Aagesen, L. (1984). Mesonephric excretory function related to its influence on differentiation of fetal gonads. *Anat. Rec.*, **210**, 551–6
23. Papadaki, L. and Bleilby, J. O. W. (1971). The fine structure of the surface epithelium of the human ovary. *J. Cell Sci.*, **8**, 445–65
24. Blaustein, A. and Lee, H. (1979). Surface cells of the ovary and pelvic peritoneum: a histochemical and ultrastructure comparison. *Gynecol. Oncol.*, **8**, 34–43
25. Blaustein, A. (1984). Peritoneal mesothelium and ovarian surface cells – shared characteristics. *Int. J. Gynecol. Pathol.*, **3**, 361–75
26. Gillett, W. R. (1990). Two zones of cells of the human ovarian surface epithelium – a new observation. *Proc. Otago Med. Sch.*, **68**, 9–10
27. Gillett, W. R. (1991). Artefactual loss of human ovarian surface epithelium – potential clinical significance. *Reprod. Fertil. Dev.*, **3**, 93–8
28. Gillett, W. R., Mitchell, A. and Hurst, P. R. (1991). A scanning electron microscopic study of the human ovarian surface epithelium: characterization of two cell types. *Hum. Reprod.*, **6**, 645–51
29. Lintern-Moore, S., Peters, H., Moore, G. P. M. and Faber, M. (1974). Follicular development in the infant human ovary. *J. Reprod. Fertil.*, **39**, 53–64
30. Peters, H., Byskow, A. G. and Grinsted, J. (1978). Follicular growth in fetal and prepubertal ovaries in humans and other primates. In Ross, G. T. and Lipset, M. B. (eds.) *Clinics in Endocrinology and Metabolism. Reproductive Endocrinology*, pp. 469–85. (London, Philadelphia, Toronto: W. B. Saunders)
31. Ross, G. T. and Schreiber, J. R. (1986). The ovary. In Yen, S. S. C. and Jaffe, R. B. (eds.) *Reproductive Endocrinology*, 2nd edn., pp. 115–39. (London, Philadelphia, Toronto: W. B. Saunders)
32. Brambell, F. W. R. (1956). Ovarian changes. In Parkes, A. S. (ed.) *Marchall's Physiology of Reproduction*, p. 397. (London: Longmans)
33. Franchi, L. L. and Baker, T. G. (1973). Oogenesis and follicular growth. In Hafez, E. S. E. and Evans, T. N. (eds.) *Human Reproduction*, pp. 53–83. (San Francisco, London: Harper & Row)
34. Wassarman, P. M. (1987). The zona pellucida: a coat of many colors. *Bioessays*, **6**, 161–6
35. Edwards, R. G. and Hollands, P. (1988). New advances in human embryology: implications of the preimplantation diagnosis of genetic disease. *Hum. Reprod.*, **3**, 549–56

36. Bolton, N. (1991). Embryo biopsy. In Chapman, M., Grundzinskas, G. and Chard, T. (eds.) *The Embryo*, pp. 63–81. (Berlin, Heidelberg: Springer-Verlág)
37. Hodgen, G. D., Goodman, A. L., Stouffer, R. L., Williams, R. F., Di-Zerga, G. S., Kreitman, O. L., Marut, E. L. and Schenken, R. S. (1983). Selection and maturation of the dominant follicle and its ovum in the menstrual cycle. In Beier, H. M. and Lindner, H. R. (eds.) *Fertilization of the Human Egg in vitro*, pp. 57–69. (Berlin, Heidelberg, New York, Tokyo: Springer-Verlag)
38. Miller, T. M. and Goodenough, D. A. (1985). Gap junction structures after experimental alteration of junctional channel conductance. *J. Cell Biol.*, **101**, 1741–8
39. Loewenstein, B. R. (1987). The cell-to-cell channel of gap junctions. *Cell*, **48**, 725–6
40. Lipner, H. (1988). Mechanisms of mammalian ovulation. In Knobil, E. and Neill, J. D. (eds.) *The Physiology of Reproduction*, vol. 1, pp. 448–89. (New York: Raven Press)
41. Okamura, H., Takenaka, A. and Yajima, Y. (1980). Ovulatory changes in the wall at the apex of the human Graafian follicle. *J. Reprod. Fertil.*, **58**, 153–5
42. Okamura, H., Virutasamen, P., Wright, K. H. and Wallach, E. E. (1972). Ovarian smooth muscle in the human being, rabbit and cat. *Am. J. Obstet. Gynecol.*, **112**, 183–91
43. Channing, C. P. (1970). Effects of stage of the menstrual cycle and gonadotrophins on luteinization of rhesus monkey granulosa cells in culture. *Endocrinology*, **87**, 49–60
44. Crisp, T. M., Dessouky, D. A. and Denys, F. R. (1970). The fine structure of the human corpus luteum of early pregnancy and during the progestational phase of the menstrual cycle. *Am. J. Anat.*, **127**, 37–70

The physiology and endocrinology of the ovary

2

A. H. Balen and S.-L. Tan

INTRODUCTION

In this chapter we will outline the endocrinological processes that control ovarian function and follicular development – the essential precursors for the release of a healthy oocyte. The gonadotroph is central to reproductive function – its production and secretion of follicle stimulating hormone (FSH) and luteinizing hormone (LH) are directly stimulated by hypothalamic gonadotropin-releasing hormone (GnRH) and are also influenced by integrated feedback mechanisms. FSH provides the initial stimulus for follicular development and also promotes granulosa cell conversion of androgens to estrogens by the aromatase enzymes. LH, previously believed to be important mainly in the luteal phase by promoting progesterone secretion, also has a vital role in the follicular phase, inducing androgen production (the substrate for estrogen synthesis) and initiating oocyte maturation. We shall review these processes and discuss the mechanisms by which complex integrated feedback pathways coordinate the development and release of an appropriately matured oocyte.

HYPOTHALAMIC CONTROL OF THE GONADOTROPH

A single hypothalamic decapeptide, gonadotropin-releasing hormone, stimulates the release of both LH and FSH from the gonadotroph[1]. The action of GnRH is modulated at the level of the pituitary, thereby resulting in differential production and secretion of the two gonadotropins. GnRH both causes release of LH and FSH and has a self-potentiating effect on the gonadotroph[2]. The primary release of gonadotropins and their secondary synthesis and storage have been termed the first and second pools of gonadotropins, respectively[3]. Pituitary responsiveness to GnRH is increased by the self-priming action of GnRH, which is the protein synthesis-dependent increase in GnRH-stimulated gonadotropin release that results from previous exposure of the pituitary gland to GnRH[4].

The sensitivity of the pituitary to stimulation by GnRH varies during the menstrual cycle in apparent synchrony with changes in the circulating estradiol levels[5]. In the early follicular phase, when estradiol levels are low, pituitary sensitivity to GnRH and gonadotropin reserve are at a minimum[3]; as estradiol levels rise, coincident with follicular development, both sensitivity and reserve increase – particularly the latter, as estradiol has a positive effect on pituitary synthesis and storage. At the time of the midcycle LH surge, sensitivity to GnRH greatly exceeds reserve capacity, with the resultant release of large amounts of gonadotropin. Estradiol induces a 'self-priming' effect by GnRH on the pituitary, whereby, during phases of the menstrual cycle when estrogen levels are high, the first pulses of GnRH increase the responsiveness of the pituitary to subsequent GnRH pulses[5]. Estradiol also potentiates GnRH responsiveness in the anterior pituitary by increasing the number of GnRH receptors by directly stimulating the protein synthesis required for receptor formation[6].

The arcuate nucleus of the hypothalamus acts as a transducer of neuronal signals into endocrine signals[7], although the cellular nature of this GnRH 'pulse generator' is still unknown[8]. The GnRH-secreting neurons in the arcuate nucleus act in a pulsatile manner, with varying frequencies throughout the normal ovulatory cycle, resulting in variable frequencies and, possibly, amplitudes of gonadotropin pulses. The control of the rhythmicity of the GnRH pulse generator is not yet fully understood. Although there does not appear to be feedback from within the pituitary itself[8], gonadal steroids and other factors modulate GnRH action at the pituitary level, and possibly also at the level of the hypothalamus.

The precise neuronal mechanisms that underlie GnRH release are presently uncertain. One cannot reliably extrapolate to humans the animal work that has been performed to elucidate the control of the LH surge – in fact there are conflicting data both in different species and between different groups looking at the same species[9]. It is difficult to measure neuronal activity directly as this requires either the precise placement of electrodes in the hypothalamus to measure electrical activity, or catheterization of the hypophyseal portal vessels to measure GnRH concentrations. Clarke and colleagues[10] have examined hypothalamic activity in sheep by measuring GnRH concentrations in hypophyseal portal blood. An increase in the frequency of GnRH pulses was found at the time of an estrogen-induced LH surge, although variable patterns were observed in different individual animals. Rising plasma concentrations of estradiol were also found to have both positive and negative feedback effects at the level of the pituitary and, possibly, hypothalamus[11,12]. Most of these studies were performed on ovariectomized animals to which estradiol had been administered. It has been more difficult to interpret the situation in the normally cycling ewe, in which the data are more ambiguous[13]. Studies of multiunit electrical activity of the hypothalamic GnRH pulse generator in non-human primates further confuse the picture by suggesting that there is, in fact, a cessation of pulse generator activity at the time of the estrogen-induced[14] or spontaneous LH surge[15]. O'Byrne and colleagues[15] hypothesized that high levels of estradiol inhibit pulse generator activity once the LH surge has been initiated.

Studies in women are restricted to the measurement of peripheral circulating LH concentrations as neither hypophyseal portal blood nor pulse generator activity can be directly examined. Most reports agree that LH pulse frequency and amplitude increase during the late follicular phase and remain elevated throughout the LH surge, only falling with the onset of progesterone secretion in the luteal phase[16–21]. The more recent and perhaps somewhat surprising data of O'Byrne and associates[15] may represent a fundamental difference between non-human primates and humans or, alternatively, difficulties in the practical aspects of telemetric recording of neuronal activity.

Some of the factors that have been reported to influence GnRH activity include β-endorphin and opiate peptides, angiotensin II, serotonin, neuropeptide-Y, neurotensin, somatostatin, corticotropin-releasing factor, dopamine, melatonin, norepinephrine, oxytocin and substance P[22]. The precise inter-relationship of these factors is unclear and studies in rodents are more extensive than in non-human primates or humans – and their effects in different species are often different[23].

Melatonin, for example, decreases plasma LH concentrations in humans and serum melatonin levels are at their lowest at the time of ovulation[24], and it has been suggested that low melatonin levels may provide a permissive factor for the preovulatory LH surge. The association between low early morning levels of melatonin and a morning start to the LH surge in many women seemed to support the notion that melatonin was involved in initiating the surge[25,26]. Recent studies using a sensitive radioimmunoassay for melatonin, however, found no changes in plasma melatonin concentrations immediately before or during the LH surge[27] and also found no suppression of serum LH concentrations when melatonin was administered. It is therefore important to distinguish between causal and coincidental hormonal changes in such a dynamic system as the hypothalamo–pituitary–ovarian axis.

Endogenous opioid tone has been extensively studied and has been found to be important in the regulation of both LH and prolactin secretion. Opioids, such as β-endorphin, have been shown to inhibit GnRH release from the human mediobasal hypothalamus[28]. It has been postulated that withdrawal of endogenous opioid tone in the presence of sufficient quantities of estradiol may play a role in mediating the initiation of the LH surge[29]. When endogenous opioid tone decreases, a chain of neurosecretory events is initiated, and Sahu and co-workers[30] hypothesized that, at least in the rat, this activates neuropeptide-Y neurons which then, either alone, or together with adrenergic transmitters, stimulate hypothalamic GnRH secretion. The effects of opioids appear to be dependent upon the steroid hormone environment, in particular estrogen, whose affect is augmented by progesterone[23], as the administration of an opioid antagonist such as naloxone during the early follicular phase has little effect on gonadotropin levels, whilst profound effects are observed mid-cycle[29].

Circulating steroid levels also influence GnRH metabolism, by altering the activity of the proteolytic enzymes that cause its degradation both at the level of the pituitary and also in the peripheral circulation after GnRH administration[31]. Estradiol, for example, has been shown to inhibit GnRH degradation in both rat and monkey pituitaries and may therefore serve to enhance GnRH activity under conditions of high serum estradiol concentrations, such as at midcycle[32]. Perhaps steroids also play such a role in women with the polycystic ovary syndrome.

REGULATION OF THE GONADOTROPH BY GnRH AT THE CELLULAR LEVEL

The effects of GnRH on pituitary secretion and sensitivity have been carefully evaluated over the last decade. GnRH can both sensitize and desensitize the pituitary and it achieves the latter by both receptor down-regulation and inactivation of calcium channels. Calcium serves as the second messenger for the action of GnRH. Intracellular calcium is increased via an alteration of inositol phospholipid metabolism and production of inositol phosphates which promote influx of extracellular calcium. The byproduct of this pathway is diacylglycerol which in turn activates protein kinase C. When GnRH attaches to its receptor it stimulates phospholipase C activity which then generates the inositol phosphates; this effect appears to be mediated by a specific G protein[33]. Calmodulin is a calcium-binding protein which increases calcium levels in the gonadotroph and may have a functional role in LH secretion. While the activation of protein kinase C does not appear to be necessary for GnRH-stimulated LH release, it does appear to be required for the effects of GnRH on LHβ gene expression[33].

THE RESPECTIVE ROLES OF LH AND FSH

LH has several functions in the control of the developing follicle: in the early follicular phase low levels of LH induce a change in function of the theca interstitial cells from production of progesterone to that of androgens[34]. FSH then promotes the conversion of androgens to estradiol by the granulosa cells. Not only does LH initiate theca cell androgen production, it also mediates the change to progesterone secretion at the time of the preovulatory surge.

LH also has a role in the suppression of the 'oocyte maturation inhibitor'. Oocytes are maintained in the first meiotic division from their appearance in the ovary during intrauterine life until just before ovulation, when oocyte maturation is completed, germinal vesicle breakdown occurs and the first polar body is extruded. Since oocytes undergo maturation spontaneously when they are cultured outside the follicle, an intrafollicular oocyte maturation inhibitor has been postulated, itself inhibited at midcycle by the ovulatory stimulus. The precise nature of the oocyte maturation inhibitor is uncertain. It is known, however, that cyclic adenosine monophosphate (cAMP) activates, or is itself, the oocyte maturation inhibitor[35]. The action of this inhibitor is to maintain the meiotic arrest of the oocyte at the diplotene stage of prophase 1. The oocyte does not synthesize cAMP but obtains it from cumulus granulosa cells via processes that traverse the intercellular space. Stimulation by LH leads to disruption of these processes, a fall in intra-oocyte cAMP and then resumption of meiosis[36].

FSH controls major morphological and cellular events during the follicular phase of the cycle, such as acquisition of the antral cavity, activation of the aromatase enzymes, induction of LH receptors and progesterone biosynthesis. Thus FSH facilitates estrogen production, ovulation and luteinization in response to the LH surge[37]. Recruitment and selection of the pre-ovulatory follicle coincides with the intermenstrual rise in serum FSH concentration[38]. Serum FSH concentrations then fall in the latter half of the follicular phase, probably as a result of inhibin secretion by the granulosa cells, which prevents the development of other follicles. It has been shown in non-human primates that once enough FSH has been given for the dominant follicle to be selected, the FSH dose can be decreased and ovulation of the dominant follicle will still occur[39]. Both gonadotropins are required for normal follicular growth and maturation. Fevold in 1941[40] was the first to demonstrate that treatment with highly purified FSH increased ovarian growth and follicle development in immature hypophysectomized rats, without stimulating estrogen secretion. Greep and colleagues[41] then used porcine gonadotropins to show that whole pituitary extract, with presumed LH activity, was required for uterine growth – the biological marker of estrogen production. Many years later it was demonstrated that, whilst both theca and granulosa cells can synthesize steroids *in vitro*, granulosa cell production of estradiol depends upon the close proximity of theca cells, which provide the androgen substrate for estrogen production[42,43]. From this 'two-cell' theory of ovarian steroid synthesis developed the 'two cell, two gonadotropin' theory, when it was demonstrated that the theca cells are driven by LH and the granulosa cells by FSH[44].

As the primordial follicle develops into a primary follicle, FSH receptors appear on the granulosa cells. Steroid receptors then appear in the late secondary and early tertiary stages of development[45]. FSH acts via the granulosa cell receptors to activate adenylate cyclase which synthesizes cAMP, which in turn binds to protein kinase C, resulting in the phosphorylation of regulatory proteins[46]. Estradiol amplifies this action of FSH and stimulates both the proliferation of its own receptors and the mitotic division of granulosa cells. A number of growth factors have been found *in vitro* to augment these processes, yet their precise physiological role has not been determined; they include epidermal, fibroblast and insulin-like growth factors, and insulin[47,48].

FSH is responsible for the development of LH receptors[34] and low levels of LH are usually found in the follicular fluid by about day 7 of the cycle. Estradiol acts synergistically with FSH to increase the number of LH receptors, which are maximal at the time of the preovulatory estradiol peak. The granulosa cells require continual exposure to FSH, albeit at low levels, otherwise they will lose both their FSH and LH receptors as well as their capability for aromatization[49]. The dominant follicle is self-selected by its relative abundance of granulosa cell FSH receptors at a time of diminishing serum FSH concentration. This concentration is insufficient to stimulate the other antral follicles, which then become atretic[50].

The theca interna and externa cells that surround the growing follicle develop their own blood supply[45]. LH receptors develop on the thecal cells, through which LH acts via its second messenger cAMP to achieve androstenedione biosynthesis, which requires the enzymes 3β-hydroxysteroid dehydrogenase, 17α-hydroxylase and 17,20-lyase[34]. Androstenedione diffuses across the follicular basement membrane where it becomes the substrate for granulosa cell aromatase, which metabolizes it to estradiol. An excess of androgen results in follicular atresia, probably because the aromatase system becomes overwhelmed and the enzyme 5α-reductase forms non-aromatizable androgens (dihydrotestosterone and androstenedione)[51].

It is thought that excess androgen production, or deficient androgen aromatization, may be responsible for the increased number of atretic follicles that are found in polycystic ovaries compared with normal ovaries[52,53]. Rosenfield and colleagues[52] postulated that there is dysregulation of cytochrome P_{450}-17α, which is the enzyme that catalyzes the conversion of progesterone to 17α-hydroxyprogesterone and the rate-limiting step in androgen biosynthesis. Alternatively, it was found that granulosa cells from polycystic ovaries cultured *in vitro* were more sensitive to FSH than granulosa cells from normal ovaries[53] and it was postulated that there might be an endogenous inhibitor of FSH action that is increased in women with polycystic ovaries. Franks and Mason[53] demonstrated that epidermal growth factor (EGF) inhibited granulosa cell aromatase and, whilst EGF is not synthesized by the ovary, transforming growth factor-α (TGF-α) is secreted by theca and stromal cells and is homologous to EGF. Insulin-like growth factor-1 (IGF-1) enhances *in vitro* granulosa cell estradiol production[54] and may stimulate aromatase activity in the absence of FSH[53]. The precise inter-relationship of these factors *in vivo* is uncertain, particularly as the role of IGF-1-binding proteins has not been determined. Furthermore, although growth hormone has been found to stimulate estradiol secretion by human granulosa cells, IGF-1 could not be detected in the medium either before or after growth hormone stimulation[55].

Women with the polycystic ovary syndrome often hypersecrete LH and this results in increased theca cell androgen secretion. A number of studies have been performed in which FSH alone has been used to stimulate folliculogenesis and these have provided considerable insight into ovarian physiology. It was initially shown that ovulation induction could be achieved with purified FSH alone in monkeys that had been rendered hypogonadotropic by the administration of GnRH antagonists[56]. It has also been found that women undergoing *in vitro* fertilization after pituitary desensitization with a GnRH agonist, when treated with either human menopausal gonadotropin (hMG) or purified FSH, had similar numbers of mature follicles and serum concentrations of FSH, LH, estradiol and progesterone[57]. It may be, however, that theca cells require very low levels of LH for androgen biosynthesis and neither GnRH antagonists nor agonists achieve complete pituitary suppression[58]. Purified FSH, furthermore, is not completely devoid of LH bioactivity, containing less than one International Unit (IU) of LH for every 75 IU of FSH.

Couzinet and co-workers[59] treated women with hypogonadotropic hypogonadism, due to Kallmann's syndrome or previous hypophysectomy, with either purified FSH or hMG and found that, whilst follicular development could be induced by purified FSH, the estradiol levels were inappropriately low for the number of follicles, the serum androstenedione concentrations were significantly reduced and the rate of ovulation was lower than after treatment with hMG. We performed a similar study in women with isolated hypogonadotropic hypogonadism, using hMG and purified FSH in succeeding cycles in the same patient[60]. The cycles in which purified FSH was used, compared with hMG, required more ampules of the gonadotropin (35.3 vs. 27.6, $p<0.004$) and more days of treatment (22.3 vs. 17.6, $p<0.02$), but resulted in significantly fewer leading follicles (1.2 vs. 2.0, $p<0.05$), lower serum estradiol concentrations (337 vs. 1477 pmol/l, $p<0.002$), a thinner endometrium thickness (6.2 vs. 8.7 mm, $p<0.02$) and lower frequency of ovulation (33% vs. 89%, $p<0.05$).

The inter-relationship between FSH and LH has been studied more closely since the development of recombinantly derived human FSH[61], which is produced by a Chinese hamster ovary cell line and has an intrinsic LH bioactivity of less than 0.025 *milli*-IU per IU of FSH[62]. It was found that when recombinant FSH was administered to hypophysectomized immature rats there was some aromatase activity but this was greatly increased by supplementation with as little as 0.1 IU of human chorionic gonadotropin (hCG), thus confirming the two-cell, two-gonadotropin hypothesis.

An interesting recent discovery has been the finding that LH directly stimulates inhibin production by granulosa cells during preovulatory development[63] and that inhibin also augments androgen production by the theca cells[64]. Thus there appears to be a paracrine amplification of ovarian steroidogenesis which is reciprocally facilitated by androgens and inhibin.

OVARIAN FEEDBACK CONTROL OF LH RELEASE

LH enables the reactivation of meiosis and hence the attainment of oocyte maturity prior to ovulation by reducing cAMP in the oocyte[36]. Inappropriate release of LH may profoundly affect this process so that the released egg is either unable to be fertilized[65] or, if fertilized, miscarries[66]. The precise timing of the preovulatory LH surge is therefore vital for the release of an appropriately mature oocyte. The endocrinological mechanisms that control this process may have evolved with additional safeguards which ensure that the correct physiological sequence is achieved.

STEROIDAL FEEDBACK ON LH SECRETION

In their studies on the functional capacity of the human gonadotroph, with respect to its sensitivity to GnRH and its reserve storage of gonadotropins, Lasley and associates[67] examined the effects of estradiol and progesterone administration on GnRH-stimulated gonadotropin secretion in normal women in the follicular phase of the cycle. They found that estradiol increased pituitary gonadotropin secretion and this was augmented by the addition of progesterone – the effects being similar on FSH and LH secretion. The physiological significance of the amplification effect of progesterone on the estrogen-primed pituitary is uncertain and there have been conflicting views about the onset of progesterone secretion. Some studies have indicated that progesterone levels do not significantly rise until after the onset of the surge[68], whilst, more recently, other studies have suggested that progesterone levels are elevated 12 h before the onset of the surge[69]. It has been suggested, in fact, that progesterone may function as a secondary signal in the maintenance of the mid-cycle surge[67] and a small increment of progesterone secretion from the preovulatory follicle is required to establish the normal dimension of the LH surge[70].

Hoff and colleagues[69] carefully evaluated the changing levels of hormones by sampling blood at 2 h intervals from five normal women over 5 consecutive days. During the 50 h preceding the onset of the surge, there were similar incremental rates of secretion of estradiol, progesterone and LH, with doubling times of approximately 60 h. Both LH and FSH surges started abruptly, with LH doubling within 2 h. The onset of the surge correlated with the attainment of peak serum estradiol concentrations and occurred 12 h after the initiation of a rapid rise in progesterone. The mean duration of the surge was 48 h, with a rapidly ascending limb, which had a doubling time of 5.2 h and lasted 14 h. Estradiol levels declined rapidly whilst progesterone concentrations continued to rise. Both gonadotropins and progesterone plateaued for 14 h and then the gonadotropins declined over 20 h, with a halving time of 9.6 h, whilst the levels of progesterone began a second rapid increase 12 h before the end of the surge. Thus there is a lapse of about 36 h between the onset of the surge and early luteal activity. The LH surge lasts about 48 h and by performing frequent blood sampling a precise picture of the endocrine events surrounding the surge has been developed. It was interesting that Hoff and associates[69] reported that serum testosterone and androstenedione concentrations increased significantly at the time of the decline in estradiol concentrations, suggesting, perhaps, that progesterone inhibits aromatase activity when granulosa cell function switches from estradiol to progesterone production.

Both estradiol and progesterone can also exert inhibitory influences on pituitary gonadotropin secretion and the differential effects may be dose- and time-dependent[71]. *In vitro* studies, using pituicyte cultures, demonstrated that estradiol, estrone and 2-hydroxyestradiol sensitized gonadotrophs to GnRH, but not estriol or 2-hydroxyestrone. Progesterone antagonized this estradiol-induced sensitization[71] and this antagonist effect is now more widely accepted than the amplificatory effect that had previously been shown by Lasley and colleagues[67] and Karsch[72]. The main feedback effect of progesterone has been proposed as being mediated at the level of the hypothalamus[72], although the finding of progesterone receptors on monkey gonadotrophs suggests a direct effect at the level of the pituitary also[73].

The precise role of estrone in gonadotropin secretion is not known. Plasma concentrations of estrone are elevated in postmenopausal women and women with the polycystic ovary syndrome[74] and it has been postulated that estrone may play a role in the hypersecretion of LH that is seen in these women[74,75]. The hydroxyestrogens are estrogen metobolites which may compete for pituitary estrogen receptors and it is possible that 2-hydroxyestradiol prolongs the effect of estradiol on the pituitary whilst 2-hydroxyestrone terminates it[71].

Estrogens have also been shown to be inhibitory to GnRH-mediated gonadotropin secretion, usually in a biphasic pattern, with a subsequent stimulatory effect[76] which may be secondary to a direct effect on the number of available GnRH receptors[6,77]. It appears that a 4-h exposure to estradiol decreases the rat pituitary response to GnRH, whilst a longer exposure of 24–48 h is required before the GnRH response is augmented[6,77]. The cellular mechanisms that result in this inhibitory effect are still to be elucidated. The concentration of estradiol is critical, as high concentrations decrease the response, creating a bell-shaped dose–response curve[78].

Different studies have reported both stimulation and inhibition of transcription of the α-subunit and LHβ messenger RNAs by estradiol[79–81] as well as regulation of GnRH receptor levels[82]. It has also been suggested that the actions of estradiol could be mediated indirectly by either a modulation of GnRH secretion[83] or gonadotropin gene transcription[84–86]. Furthermore, estradiol may produce a combination of both direct and indirect effects on the gonadotroph[73]. The time-course of pituitary exposure to estrogen regulates whether there is short-term negative, short-term positive or long-term negative feedback[86].

Androgens have been shown to inhibit gonadotropin secretion by decreasing the number of GnRH receptors in a pituicyte culture[87] and post-receptor events also appear to be affected by androgens[88]. Androgens, however, are thought not to play a part in the LH surge as suggested by their inability to induce an LH surge in estradiol-treated men in whom a surge could be induced after castration[89]. Studies in female-to-male transsexuals, however, demonstrated that large doses of testosterone failed to block an estradiol-induced LH surge[90]. It therefore appears that androgens do not play a significant role in the genesis of the LH surge, or, for that matter, in normal secretion of LH.

NON-STEROIDAL FEEDBACK ON LH SECRETION

In recent years a number of groups have proposed the existence of an inhibitory factor, different from inhibin, that is produced by ovarian follicles and which suppresses GnRH-stimulated LH, and possibly also FSH, secretion. This factor has been named gonadotropin surge inhibiting[91] or attenuating[92] factor (GnSIF/GnSAF). The postulated theory is that GnSAF antagonizes the priming of the pituitary gland by GnRH and raises its threshold to the action of GnRH, preventing a premature LH surge. The surge may then occur when elevated estradiol levels increase the sensitivity of the pituitary to GnRH, thus overriding the inhibitory factor. As the action of GnSAF appears to be at the level of the pituitary, it is reasonable to expect an effect on both types of GnRH-induced LH release. If GnSAF also influences tonic LH secretion, a deficiency of GnSAF may result in LH hypersecretion.

THE EFFECT OF INHIBIN ON FSH AND LH SECRETION

Inhibin is a glycoprotein hormone, produced by the granulosa cells, which inhibits pituitary gonadotropin production and/or secretion, preferentially FSH[93], and thus preserves the dominance of the leading follicle in natural cycles[50]. At high concentrations it may also inhibit GnRH-stimulated LH release, by reducing pituitary GnRH receptors[94]. Serum inhibin concentrations increase significantly during superovulation induction[95] and then decrease during the LH surge[96].

There are several isoforms of human inhibin and there are so far no immunoassays that satisfactorily differentiate between them. Furthermore, inhibin has been shown to have effects, at different concentrations and in differing conditions, on both basal secretion of FSH and GnRH-stimulated FSH and LH. Until reliable assays are available, it will not be possible to determine which are the physiologically active forms of inhibin in the circulation. Paracrine roles have been postulated for inhibin and its related peptide hormones, both in the gonad and in the pituitary, where messenger RNA for activin and inhibin has been found. Thus, in order to say with certainty that GnSAF is different from inhibin, it will have to be isolated and characterized. It should then be possible to assess the action of the hormone once antibodies are available to construct a reliable assay that provides a parallel measurement of immuno- and bioactivity.

CONCLUSION

We have reviewed the current thinking behind the complex subject of the endocrinological control of ovulation. Whilst many issues have yet to be fully clarified, it is important to have a basic understanding of the inter-relationship between the ovary, pituitary and hypothalamus when considering abnormalities of ovulation and ovarian ultrasonography.

References

1. Schally, A. V., Arimura, A., Kastin, A. J., Matsuo, H., Baba, Y., Redding, T. W., Nair, R. M. G., Debeljuk, L. and White, W. F. (1971). Gonadotropin-releasing hormone: one polypeptide regulates secretion of luteinizing and follicle stimulating hormones. *Science*, **173**, 1036–7
2. Pickering, A. J. M.C. and Fink, G. (1976). Priming effect of luteinising hormone-releasing factor: *in-vitro* and *in-vivo* evidence consistent with its dependence upon protein and RNA synthesis. *J. Endocrinol. Metab.*, **69**, 373–9
3. Yen, S. S. C. and Lein, A. (1976). The apparent paradox of the negative and positive feedback control system on gonadotropin secretion. *Am. J. Obstet. Gynecol.*, **126**, 942–54
4. Aiyer, M. S., Chiappa, S. A. and Fink, G. (1974). A priming effect of luteinizing releasing factor on the pituitary gland in the female rat. *J. Endocrinol.*, **62**, 573–88
5. Wang, C. F., Lasley, B. L., Lein, A. and Yen, S. S. C. (1976). The functional changes of the pituitary gonadotrophs during the menstrual cycle. *J. Clin. Endocrinol. Metab.*, **42**, 718–28
6. Menon, M., Peegel, H. and Katta, V. (1985). Estradiol potentiation of gonadotrophin-releasing hormone responsiveness in the anterior pituitary is mediated by an increase in gonadotrophin-releasing hormone receptors. *Am. J. Obstet. Gynaecol.*, **151**, 534–40
7. Knobil, E. (1980). The neuroendocrine control of the menstrual cycle. *Recent Prog. Horm. Res.*, **36**, 53–88
8. Knobil, E. (1990). Electrophysiological approaches to the hypothalamic GnRH pulse generator. In Yen, S. S. C. and Vale, W. W. (eds.) *Neuroendocrine Regulation of Reproduction*, pp. 3–8. (Norwell, USA: Serono Symposia)
9. Clarke, I. J., Phillips, D. J., Mercer, J. E. and Robertson, D. M. (1990). Mechanisms involved in the LH surge. In Yen, S. S. C. and Vale, W. W. (eds.) *Neuroendocrine Regulation of Reproduction*, pp. 29–38. (Norwell, USA: Serono Symposia)
10. Clarke, I. J. and Cummins, J. T. (1985). Increased GnRH pulse frequency associated with estrogen-induced surges in ovariectomized ewes. *Endocrinology*, **116**, 2376–83
11. Clarke, I. J. and Cummins, J. T. (1984). Direct pituitary effects of estrogen and progesterone on gonadotropin secretion in the ovariectomized ewe. *Neuroendocrinology*, **39**, 267–74
12. Caraty, A., Locatelli, A. and Martin, G. B. (1989). Biphasic response in the secretion of gonadotrophin-releasing hormone in ovariectomized ewes injected with estradiol. *J. Endocrinol.*, **123**, 375–9
13. Clarke, I. J., Thomas, G. B., Yao, B. and Cummins, J. T. (1987). GnRH secretion throughout the ovine estrous cycle. *Neuroendocrinology*, **46**, 82–8
14. Kesner, I. S., Wilson, R. G., Kaufman, J. M., Hotchkiss, J., Chen, Y., Yamamoto, H., Pardo, R. R. and Knobil, E. (1987). Unexpected response of the hypothalamic gonadotropin-releasing hormone 'pulse-generator' to physiological estradiol inputs in the absence of the ovary. *Proc. Natl. Acad. Sci. USA*, **84**, 8745–9
15. O'Byrne, K. T., Thalabard, J.-C., Grosser, P. M., Wilson, R. C., Williams, C. L., Chen, M.-D., Ladendorf, D., Hotchkiss, J. and Knobil, E. (1991). Radiotelemetric monitoring of hypothalamic gonadotropin-releasing hormone pulse generator activity throughout the menstrual cycle of the rhesus monkey. *Endocrinology*, **129**, 1207–14
16. Yen, S. S. C., Tsai, C. C., Naftolin, F., Vandenberg, G. and Ajabor, L. (1972). Pulsatile patterns of gonadotropin release in subjects with and without ovarian function. *J. Clin. Endocrinol. Metab.*, **34**, 671–5
17. Djahanbakhch, O., Warner, P., McNeilly, A. S. and Baird, D. T. (1984). Pulsatile release of LH and oestradiol during the preovulatory period in women. *Clin. Endocrinol. (Oxf.)*, **20**, 579–89
18. Soules, M. R., Steiner, R. A., Clifton, D. K., Cohen, N. L., Aksel, S. and Bremner, W. J. (1984). Progesterone modulation of pulsatile luteinizing hormone secretion in normal women. *J. Clin. Endocrinol. Metab.*, **58**, 378–83
19. Filicori, M., Santoro, N., Merriam, G. R. and Crowley, W. F. (1986). Characterisation of the physiological pattern of episodic gonadotropin secretion throughout the human menstrual cycle. *J. Clin. Endocrinol. Metab.*, **62**, 1136–44
20. Clayton, R. N., Royston, J. P., Chapman, J., Wilson, M., Obhrai, M., Sawers, R. S. and Lynch, S. S. (1987). Is changing hypothalamic activity important for control of ovulation? *Br. Med. J.*, **295**, 7–12
21. Rossmanith, W. G., Liu, C. H., Laughlin, G. A.,

Mortola, J. F., Suh, B. Y. and Yen, S. S. C. (1990). Relative changes in LH pulsatility during the menstrual cycle: using data from hypogonadal women as a reference point. *Clin. Endocrinol. (Oxf.)*, **32**, 647–60
22. Kordon, C. and Drouva, S. V. (1990). Interplay between hypothalamic hormones and sex steroids in the control of neuroendocrine reproductive functions. In Yen, S. S. C. and Vale, W. W. (eds.) *Neuroendocrine Regulation of Reproduction*, pp. 259–68. (Norwell, USA: Serono Symposia)
23. Plosker, S. M., Marshall, L. A., Martin, M. C. and Jaffe, R. B. (1990). Opioid, catecholamine and steroid interaction in prolactin and gonadotropin regulation. *Obstet. Gynecol.*, **45**, 441–53
24. Wetterberg, L., Arendt, J., Paunier, L., Sizonenko, P. C., Van Donselaar, W. and Heyden, T. (1976). Human serum melatonin changes during the menstrual cycle. *J. Clin Endocrinol. Metab.*, **42**, 185
25. Seibel, M. M., Shine, W., Smith, D. M. and Taymor, M. L. (1982). Biological rhythm of the luteinising hormone surge in women. *Fertil. Steril.*, **37**, 709–12
26. Testart, J., Frydman, R. and Roger, M. (1982). Seasonal influence of diurnal rhythms in the onset of the plasma luteinising hormone surge in women. *J. Clin. Endocrinol. Metab.*, **55**, 374
27. Zimmermann, R. C., Schroder, S., Baars, S., Schumacher, M. and Weise, H.-C. (1990). Melatonin and the ovulatory LH surge. *Fertil. Steril.*, **54**, 612–18
28. Rasmussen, D. D., Liu, J. H., Wolf, P. L. and Yen, S. S. (1983). Endogenous opioid regulation of gonadotrophin-releasing hormone release from the human fetal hypothalamus *in-vitro*. *J. Clin. Endocrinol. Metab.*, **57**, 881–4
29. Rossmanith, W., Mortola, J. and Yen, S. S. C. (1988). Role of endogenous peptides in the initiation of the mid-cycle luteinising surge in normal cycling women. *J. Clin. Endocrinol. Metab.*, **67**, 695
30. Sahu, A., Crowley, W. R. and Kalra, S. P. (1990). An opioid–neuropeptide-Y transmission line to LHRH neurons: a role in the induction of the LH surge. *Endocrinology*, **126**, 876–83
31. Griffiths, E. C., Hooper, K. C., Jeffcoate, S. L. and Holland, D. T. (1975). The effects of gonadectomy and gonadal steroids on the activity of hypothalamic peptidases inactivating luteinizing hormone-releasing hormone (LHRH). *Brain Res.*, **88**, 384
32. Danforth, D. R., Elkind-Hirsch, K. and Hodgen, G. (1990). *In-vivo* and *in-vitro* modulation of GnRH metabolism by estradiol and progesterone. *Endocrinology*, **127**, 319–24
33. Waters, S. B. and Conn, P. M. (1991). Regulation of the pituitary gonadotrope by GnRH: multiple intracellular effectors. *Chinese J. Physiol.*, **34**, 1–26
34. Erickson, G. F., Magoffin, D. A., Dyer, C. A. and Hofeditz, C. (1985). The ovarian androgen producing cells: a review of structure/function relationships. *Endocrinol. Rev.*, **6**, 371–99
35. Downs, S. M. (1990). Maintenance of meiotic arrest in mammalian oocytes. In Bavister, B. D., Cummins, J. and Roldan, E. R. S. (eds.) *Fertilisation in Mammals*, pp. 5–16. (Norwell, USA: Serono Symposia)
36. Dekel, N., Galiani, D. and Aberdam, E. (1990). Regulation of rat oocyte maturation: involvement of protein kinases. In Bavister, B. D., Cummins, J. and Roldan, E. R. S. (eds.) *Fertilisation in Mammals*, pp. 17–24. (Norwell, USA: Serono Symposia)
37. Zeleznik, A. J. and Hillier, S. G. (1984). The role of gonadotrophins in the selection of the preovulatory follicle. *Clin. Obstet. Gynecol.*, **27**, 927–40
38. diZerega, G. S. and Hodgen, G. D. (1981). Folliculogenesis in the primate ovarian cycle. *Endo. Rev.*, **2**, 27–34
39. Zeleznik, A. J. and Kubik, C. J. (1986). Ovarian responses in macaques to pulsatile infusion of FSH and LH: increased sensitivity of the maturing follicle to FSH. *Endocrinology*, **119**, 2025–30
40. Fevold, H. L. (1941). Synergism of follicle stimulating hormone in producing estrogen secretion. *Endocrinology*, **28**, 33–6
41. Greep, R. O., VanDyke, H. B. and Chow, B. F. (1942). Gonadotropins of the swine pituitary. I. Various biological effects of purified thylakentrin (FSH) and pure metakentrin (ICSH). *Endocrinology*, **30**, 635–49
42. Short, R. V. (1962). Further observations of the defective synthesis of ovarian steroids in the Stein–Leventhal syndrome. *J. Endocrinol.*, **24**, 359–63
43. Ryan, K. J., Petro, Z. and Kaiser, J. (1968). Steroid formation by isolated and combined ovarian granulosa and theca cells. *J. Clin. Endocrinol. Metab.*, **28**, 355–9
44. Erickson, G. F. (1978). Normal ovarian function. *Clin. Obstet. Gynecol.*, **21**, 31–41
45. Erickson, G. F. (1986). An analysis of follicle development and ovum maturation. *Semin. Reprod. Endocrinol.*, **4**, 233–52
46. Seibel, M. M. (1990). Oocyte maturation and follicle development. In Seibel, M. M. (ed.) *Infertility, A Comprehensive Text*, pp. 37–49. (Norwalk, Connecticut: Appleton & Lange)
47. Poretsky, L., Grigorescu, F., Seibel, M., Moses, A. and Flier, J. S. (1985). Distribution and characterisation of insulin and insulin-like growth factor-1 receptors in normal human ovary. *J. Clin. Endocrinol. Metab.*, **61**, 728–35
48. Hammond, J. M. and English, H. F. (1987). Regulation of DNA synthesis in cultured porcine granulosa cells by growth factors and hormones. *Endocrinology*, **120**, 1039–46
49. Uilenbroek, J. T. H., Woutersen, P. J. A. and Van der Shoot, P. (1980). Atresia of preovulatory follicles: gonadotropin binding and steroidogenic activity. *Biol. Reprod.*, **23**, 219–26

50. Hodgen, G. D. (1982). The dominant ovarian follicle. *Fertil. Steril.*, **38**, 281–300
51. Hillier, S. G., Van den Boogaard, A. M. J., Reichert, L. E. and Van Hall, E. V. (1980). Intraovarian sex steroid interactions and the regulation of follicular maturation: aromatization of androgens by human granulosa cells *in vitro*. *J. Clin. Endocrinol. Metab.*, **50**, 640–9
52. Rosenfield, R. L., Barnes, R. B., Cara, J. F. and Lucky, A. W. (1990). Dysregulation of cytochrome P450c17-alpha as the cause of polycystic ovarian syndrome. *Fertil. Steril.*, **53**, 785–91
53. Franks, S. and Mason, H. D. (1991). Polycystic ovary syndrome: interaction of follicle stimulating hormone and polypeptide growth factors in oestradiol production by human granulosa cells. *J. Steroid Biochem. Mol. Biol.*, **40**, 405–9
54. Erickson, G. F., Garzo, V. G. and Magoffin, D. A. (1989). Insulin-like growth factor-1 regulates aromatase activity in human granulosa and granulosa luteal cells. *J. Clin. Endocrinol. Metab.*, **69**, 716–24
55. Mason, H. D., Martikainen, H., Beard, R. W., Anyaoku, V. and Franks, S. (1990). Direct gonadotrophic effect of growth hormone on oestradiol production by human granulosa cells *in vitro*. *J. Endocrinol.*, **126**, R1–R4
56. Kenigsberg, D., Littman, B. A., Williams, R. F. and Hodgen, G. D. (1984). Medical hypophysectomy: II. Variability of ovarian response to gonadotrophin therapy. *Fertil. Steril.*, **42**, 116–26
57. Bentick, B., Shaw, R. W., Iffland, C. A., Burford, G. and Bernard, A. (1988). A randomised comparative study of purified follicle stimulating hormone and human menopausal gonadotrophin after pituitary desensitisation with buserelin for superovulation and IVF. *Fertil. Steril*, **50**, 79–84
58. Loumaye, E. (1990). The control of endogenous secretion of LH by gonadotrophin-releasing hormone agonist during ovarian hyperstimulation for *in-vitro* fertilisation and embryo transfer. *Hum. Reprod.*, **5**, 357–76
59. Couzinet, B., Lestrat, N., Brailly, S., Forest, M. and Schaison, G. (1988). Stimulation of ovarian follicular maturation with pure FSH in women with gonadotrophin deficiency. *J. Clin. Endocrinol. Metab.*, **66**, 552–6
60. Shoham, Z., Balen, A. H., Patel, A. and Jacobs, H. S. (1991). Results of ovulation induction using human menopausal gonadotrophins or purified follicle stimulating hormone in hypogonadotrophic hypogonadism patients. *Fertil. Steril.*, **56**, 1048–53
61. Van Wezenbeek, P., Draaier, J., Van Meel, F. and Olijve, W. (1990). Recombinant follicle stimulating hormone I. Construction, selection and characterization of a cell line. In Crommelin, D. J. A. and Schellekens, H. (eds.) *From Clone to Clinic, Developments in Biotherapy*, vol. 1, pp. 245–51. (Amsterdam: Kluwer Academic Publishers)
62. Mannaerts, B., de Leeuw, R., Geelen, J., Van Ravestein, A., Van Wezenbeek, P., Schuurs, A. and Kloosterboer, H. (1991). Comparative *in vitro* and *in vivo* studies on the biological characteristics of recombinant human follicle stimulating hormone. *Endocrinology*, **129**, 2623–30
63. Hillier, S. G., Wickings, E. J., Illingworth, P. I., Yong, E. L., Reichart, L. E., Baird, D. T. and McNeilly, A. S. (1991). Control of immunoreactive inhibin production by human granulosa cells. *Clin. Endocrinol.*, **35**, 71–8
64. Hillier, S. G., Yong, E. L., Illingworth, P. I., Baird, D. T., Schwall, R. H. and Mason, A. J. (1991). Effect of recombinant inhibin on androgen synthesis in cultured human thecal cells. *Mol. Cell Endocrinol.*, **75**, R1–R6
65. Homburg, R., Armar, N. A., Eshel, A., Adams, J. and Jacobs, H. S. (1988). Influence of serum luteinising hormone concentrations on ovulation, conception and early pregnancy loss in polycystic ovary syndrome. *Br. Med. J.*, **297**, 1024–6
66. Regan, L., Owen, E. J. and Jacobs, H. S. (1990). Hypersecretion of luteinising hormone, infertility and miscarriage. *Lancet*, **336**, 1141–4
67. Lasley, B. L., Wang, C. F. and Yen, S. S. C. (1975). The effects of estrogen and progesterone on the functional capacity of the gonadotrophs. *J. Clin. Endocrinol. Metab.*, **41**, 820–6
68. Abraham, G. E., Odell, W. D., Swerdloff, R. S. and Hopper, K. (1972). Simultaneous radioimmunoassay of plasma FSH, LH, progesterone, 17-hydroxyprogesterone and estradiol-17 beta during the menstrual cycle. *J. Clin. Endocrinol. Metab.*, **34**, 312–18
69. Hoff, J. D., Quigley, M. E. and Yen, S. S. C. (1983). Hormonal dynamics at midcycle: a reevaluation. *Clin. Endocrinol. Metab.*, **57**, 792–6
70. Liu, J. H. and Yen, S. S. C. (1983). Induction of midcycle gonadotropin surge by ovarian steroids: a critical evaluation. *J. Clin. Endocrinol. Metab.*, **57**, 792–802
71. Hsueh, A. J. W., Erickson, G. F. and Yen, S. S. C. (1979). The sensitizing effect of estrogens and catechol estrogen on cultured pituitary cells to LHRH: its antagonism by progestins. *Endocrinology*, **104**, 807–13
72. Karsch, F. J. (1987). Central actions of ovarian steroids in the feedback regulation of pulsatile secretion of luteinising hormone. *Annu. Rev. Physiol.*, **49**, 365–82
73. Sprangers, S. A., Brenner, R. M. and Bethea, C. L. (1989). Estrogen and progesterone receptor immunocytochemistry in lactotropes versus gonadotropes of monkey pituitary cell cultures. *Endocrinology*, **124**, 1462–70
74. DeVane, G. M., Czekala, N. M., Judd, H. L. and Yen, S. S. C. (1974). Circulating gonadotropins, estrogens and androgens in polycystic ovarian disease. *Am. J. Obstet. Gynecol.*, **38**, 476–81

75. Rebar, R., Judd, H. L., Yen, S. S. C., Rakoff, J., Vandenberg, G. and Naftolin, F. (1976). Characterization of the inappropriate gonadotropin secretion in polycystic ovary syndrome. *J. Clin. Invest.*, **57**, 1320–9
76. Frawley, L. S. and Neill, J. D. (1984). Biphasic effects of estrogen on GnRH-induced LH release in monolayer cultures of rat and monkey pituitary cells. *Endocrinology*, **114**, 659–63
77. Emons, G., Hoffmann, H. G., Brack, C., Ortmann, O., Sturm, R., Ball, P. and Knuppen, R. (1988). Modulation of GnRH receptor concentration in cultured female pituitary cells by estradiol treatment. *J. Steroid Biochem.*, **31**, 751–6
78. Emons, G., Knuppen, R., Ball, P. and Catt, K. J. (1984). Biphasic modulation of pituitary sensitivity to GnRH by oestrogens: the effect of A- and D-ring substitution on LH release in cultured pituitary cells. *Acta Endocrinol. Copenh.*, **107**, 317–27
79. Landefeld, T. D., Kepa, J. and Karsch, F. J. (1983). Regulation of alpha-subunit synthesis by gonadal steroid feedback in the sheep anterior pituitary. *J. Biol. Chem.*, **258**, 2390–3
80. Landefeld, T. and Kepa, J. (1984). Regulation of LH beta subunit mRNA in the sheep pituitary gland during different feedback states of estradiol. *Biochem. Biophys. Res. Comm.*, **122**, 1307–13
81. Nilson, J. H., Nejedlik, M. T., Virgin, J. B., Crowder, M. and Nett, T. M. (1983). Expression of alpha subunit and luteinizing hormone beta genes in the ovine anterior pituitary. *J. Biol. Chem.*, **258**, 12087–90
82. Adams, T. E., Norman, R. L. and Spies, H. G. (1983). Gonadotrophin-releasing hormone receptor binding and pituitary responsiveness in estradiol-primed monkeys. *Science*, **213**, 1388–90
83. Plant, T. M. (1986). Gonadal regulation of hypothalamic GnRH release in primates. *Endocrinol. Rev.*, **7**, 75–88
84. Lalloz, M. R. A., Detta, A. and Clayton, R. N. (1988). Gonadotropin-releasing hormone is required for enhanced LH subunit gene expression *in-vivo*. *Endocrinology*, **122**, 1681–8
85. Lalloz, M. R. A., Detta, A. and Clayton, R. N. (1988). Gonadotropin-releasing hormone desensitization preferentially inhibits expression of the LH beta-subunit gene expression *in-vivo*. *Endocrinology*, **122**, 1689–94
86. Mercer, J. E., Clements, J. A., Funder, J. W. and Clarke, I. J. (1988). Luteinizing hormone-beta mRNA levels are regulated primarily by GnRH and not by negative estrogen feedback on the pituitary. *Neuroendocrinology*, **47**, 563–6
87. Giguere, V., Lefebvre, F. A. and Labrie, F. (1981). Androgens decrease LHRH binding sites in rat anterior pituitary cells in culture. *Endrocrinology*, **108**, 350–2
88. Drouin, J., Lavoie, M. and Labrie, F. (1978). Effect of gonadal steroids on the luteinising hormone follicle stimulating hormone response to 8-bromo-adenosine-3′,5′-monophosphate in anterior pituitary cells in culture. *Endocrinology*, **102**, 358–64
89. Barbarino, A. and De Marinis, L. (1980). Estrogen induction of luteinising hormone release in castrated adult human males. *J. Clin. Endocrinol. Metab.*, **51**, 280–6
90. Goh, H. H. and Ratnam, S. S. (1990). The gonadotrophin surge in humans: its mechanism and role in ovulatory function – a review. *Ann. Acad. Med.*, **19**, 524–9
91. Sopelak, V. M. and Hodgen, G. D. (1984). Blockade of the estrogen-induced luteinising hormone surge in monkeys: a nonsteroidal, antigenic factor in porcine follicular fluid. *Fertil. Steril.*, **41**, 108–13
92. Messinis, I. E. and Templeton, A. (1989). Pituitary response to exogenous LHRH in superovulated women. *J. Reprod. Fertil.*, **87**, 633–9
93. Burger, H. G. and Igarashi, M. (1988). Inhibin – definition and nomenclature. *J. Clin. Endocrinol. Metab.*, **66**, 885–6
94. Wang, Q. F., Farnworth, P. G., Findlay, J. K. and Burger, H. G. (1988). Effect of purified 31k bovine inhibin on the specific binding of gonadotrophin-releasing hormone to rat anterior pituitary cells in culture. *Endocrinology*, **123**, 2161–6
95. McLachlan, R. I., Robertson, D. M., de Kretser, D. M. and Burger, H. G. (1988). Advances in the physiology of inhibin and inhibin-related peptides. *Clin. Endocrinol.*, **29**, 77–114
96. Tsonis, C. G., Messinis, I. E., Templeton, A. A., McNeilly, A. S. and Baird, D. T. (1988). Gonadotropic stimulation of inhibin secretion by the human ovary during the follicular and early luteal phase of the cycle. *J. Clin. Endocrinol. Metab.*, **66**, 915–21

Diagnosis and management of fetal ovarian cysts

3

G. Volpe, V. D'Addario and A. Kurjak

FOLLICULAR GROWTH IN THE DEVELOPING FETUS

Most fetal ovarian cysts are of follicular origin. It is therefore reasonable to start this chapter with a discussion of follicular growth in the developing fetus.

In a broad sense two major classes of follicles have proved most useful for analyzing follicular development: non-growing follicles and growing follicles. The non-growing or primordial follicles account for the majority (90–95%) of the ovarian follicles at any given time in the life of a female. Once a primordial follicle has been recruited to initiate growth, its size and relative position in the ovary change in a progressive manner forming a primary, secondary or preantral, antral, large antral (or Graafian) follicle and atretic follicle[1] (Figure 1).

A *primordial follicle* consists of a small primary oocyte arrested in the dictyate stage of the first prophase of the first meiotic division (a resting stage between prophase and metaphase), derived from a primordial germ cell, surrounded by a single layer of squamous epithelial cells, termed pregranulosa or follicle cells, and a thin extracellular matrix, the basal lamina[2]. Every preovulatory follicle that develops during the reproductive life of a female comes from the pool of these non-growing follicles. In the human and the monkey, follicular growth starts during fetal life. The first small primordial follicles appear during the fourth month of gestation and all the primordial follicles present in the woman's ovaries are formed before the ninth month of gestation. Because the entire stock of oocytes in primordial follicles is in meiotic prophase, all the oocytes capable of participating in reproduction during a woman's life are present at birth[3]. The process of recruitment begins soon after the formation of the primordial follicles in the fetus and then continues at a relatively constant rate thereafter[4,5]. As a result of continued recruitment of primordial follicles into the pool of growing follicles, the total number of primordial follicles is reduced progressively. The maximal number of primordial follicles is reached at approximately 20 weeks of gestation, at which time 6–7 million are present. Subsequently, their number is gradually decreased by a process termed atresia, so that by the time of birth, only 1–2 million primordial follicles have survived. This process, which appears to be independent of hormonal changes, continues throughout childhood and, at the time of puberty, 300 000–400 000 primordial follicles are present within the ovaries. Of these, approximately 300–400 will be ovulated during the woman's reproductive life from menarche to menopause, while the remainder undergo atresia[6].

A *primary follicle* contains a growing oocyte surrounded by a single layer of cuboidal granulosa cells. The first indication that a primordial follicle has been recruited to progress into the primary stage is that pregranulosa cells begin to round up and appear cuboidal rather than squamous in shape[7]. The oocyte increases in size and an extracellular matrix begins to develop around the oocyte, termed the zona pellucida. At the end of the primary stage the oocyte is almost fully grown (100 μm in diameter); it is completely surrounded by a thin zona pellucida, a single layer of cuboidal granulosa cells and a basal lamina[8].

A *preantral follicle* (called a secondary, medium follicle) enters the growing phase. By the end of the secondary stage, the follicle is organized into a multilayer structure that is strikingly symmetri-

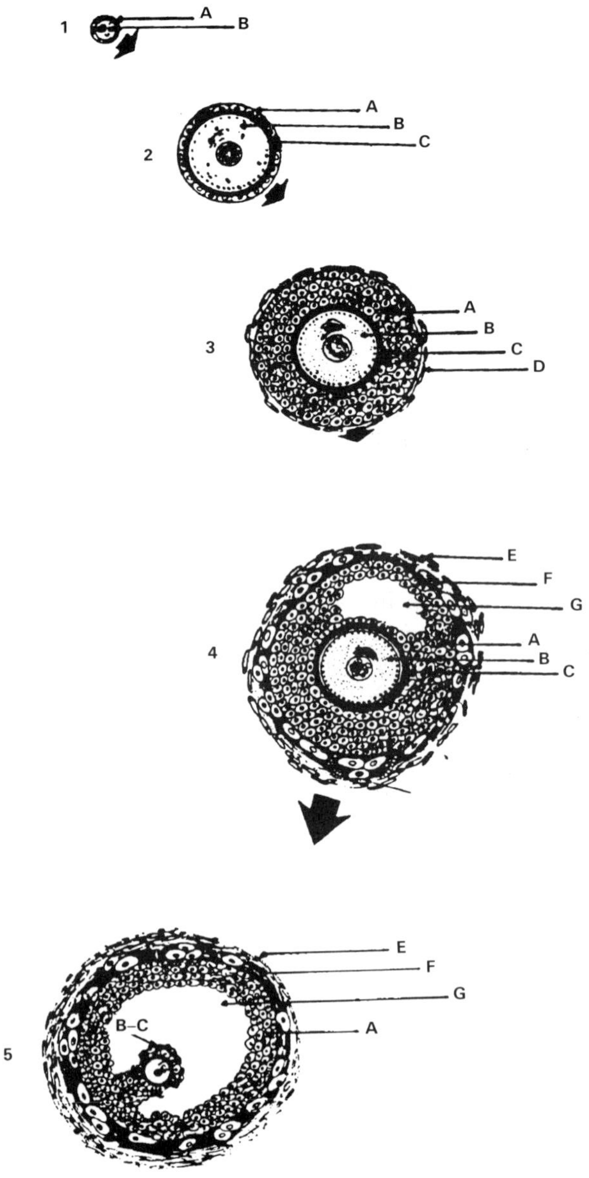

Figure 1 Classification of follicles in human ovary: (1) primordial follicle; (2) primary follicle; (3) preantral follicle; (4) small antral follicle; (5) Graafian follicle. (A) Basal lamina and granulosa; (B) oocyte; (C) zona pellucida; (D) presumptive theca; (E) theca externa; (F) theca interna; (G) antrum

cal. In the center is a full-grown oocyte (about 120 μm in diameter) covered by a thick zona pellucida and four to eight layers of granulosa cells. One of the major structural changes occurring during the preantral follicle development is the acquisition of the prospective theca from the cells of the ovarian stroma[8].

An *antral follicle* contains a fully grown oocyte, several layers of granulosa cells, an antrum filled with fluid and, outside the basement membrane, well differentiated theca layers. In all mammals this basic event occurs when follicles reach about 400 μm in diameter[9]. Antrum formation is termed 'cavitation'. It begins with the accumulation of follicular fluid between a specific set of granulosa cells, resulting in the formation of a small internal cavity at one pole of the oocyte. This event does not depend on pituitary hormones, but rather seems to result from an autocrine/paracrine activity found within the follicle itself[10]. As a consequence of cavitation, the follicle takes on a characteristic polarity and internal organization that remains throughout Graafian follicle development. Following this change, the theca interstitial cells acquire the ultrastructure typical of active steroid-synthesizing cells[11]. As cavitation progresses, a relatively large number of gap junctions are present between the granulosa cells that fill the follicle. Thus ions, amino acids and regulatory molecules like cyclic adenosine monophosphate (cAMP) can pass freely from cell to cell[8].

During the primary, preantral and antral stages an oocyte undergoes a striking growth, increasing from 20 μm to about 120 μm in diameter. A principle in ovarian physiology is that the growth of the follicle relative to that of the oocyte can be divided into two distinct phases. Initially, the oocyte and follicular diameters are positively and linearly correlated until the follicle reaches the cavitation stage. Then the oocyte ceases to grow while follicular growth continues. The conclusion is that a human oocyte completes its growth very early in follicular development at cavitation, when the early follicle reaches about 400 μm in diameter[8].

While primordial follicles do not have an independent blood supply, this comes with the acquisition of theca tissue.

The *large antral follicle* (referred to as a Graafian follicle) which reaches its maximum diameter, is fully responsive to a preovulatory surge of gonadotropins.

Small antral follicles are found as early as 5 months of fetal life and become larger and more numerous during the last two months of pregnancy. The ovary of the newborn is often crowded with large antral follicles[12]. However, these follicles do not ovulate but rather show signs of degeneration or atresia and irregular growth[13].

Anencephalic human fetuses have a greatly reduced pituitary gland which contains only about 2% of the normal gonadotropin content[14]. Ovaries of such fetuses at term weigh less than those of normal fetuses and contain few preantral and no antral follicles[15]. Also, hypophysectomy *in utero* of rhesus monkeys resulted in impaired growth of follicles. These studies suggest that the failure of fetal pituitary led to inadequate support for follicles in fetal ovaries and that maturation beyond the primary follicle stage requires ongoing gonadotropic support.

STEROID HORMONE FUNCTION IN THE DEVELOPING FETUS

During the first half of gestation the only ovarian cells that show ultrastructural features suggestive of steroidogenic potential are interstitial cells, which appear at about 12 weeks of age[16]. After 24 weeks, multiplication of granulosa cells leads to the formation of multilayered primary follicles and a few antral follicles. These, in turn, become encapsulated by epithelioid theca interna cells which, on the basis of electron-microscopic criteria, are thought to be capable of steroidogenesis[12].

Increases in blood steroid levels following gonadotropin-releasing hormone (GnRH) administration to fetal rhesus monkeys imply that fetal gonadotropin levels also rise. The synthesizing capacity of the fetal ovary during gestation has been demonstrated as early as 12–18 weeks' gestation for androgens and as early as 20–22 weeks for progesterone[17,18]. Winter, Faiman and Reyes detected a low concentration of estradiol (0.5 pg/mg) in human fetal ovaries at 10–22 weeks' gestation[19].

In vitro studies of fetal ovarian homogenates have suggested that some biosynthesis of dehydroepiandrosterone (DHEA) and androstenedione from acetate or steroid precursors is possible by mid-gestation[20].

Payne and Jaffe, using pregnenolone sulfate as a precursor, identified 17-OH pregnenolone, DHEA, and androstenedione in incubations of fetal ovarian tissue but did not find progesterone, testosterone, estrone or estradiol[17]. George and colleagues, using testosterone and androstenedione as precursors, found that the fetal ovary was capable of aromatization *in vitro*[21]. Wilson and Jawad concluded that, whereas the steroidogenic enzymes may be present in the midterm fetal ovary, functional tropic hormone receptors are deficient.[22].

Total circulating estrogen concentrations in the fetus resemble those of the maternal peripheral circulation, although the distribution of estrone, estradiol and estriol may be different. In addition, fetal and maternal serum estrogen levels rise in parallel throughout gestation. This finding, plus the observation that umbilical venous estrogen levels consistently exceed those in the umbilical artery, support the notion that all fetal estrogens are of placental origin[23,24].

These results suggest that the fetal ovary is biochemically competent to produce sex steroids *in utero*, but a deficiency of gonadotropin receptors and/or an intrinsic enzyme in receptor-coupled adenylate cyclase may compromise steroidogenesis and prohibit testosterone production prior to 22 weeks[12].

Many of the biological effects of human chorionic gonadotropin (hCG) are similar but not identical to those of luteinizing hormone (LH)[25]. It has been shown that hCG is capable of inducing ovulation of follicles previously primed by follicle-stimulating hormone (FSH) and LH. Follicular cells are luteinized under the influence of hCG, and the corpus luteum formed during the menstrual cycle or in pregnancy is stimulated to produce more progesterone when hCG is added *in vitro* or *in vivo*. Some effects of hCG are negated by inhibitors of RNA and protein synthesis, suggesting a locus of action involving protein (enzyme) synthesis. Cyclic AMP, LH and hCG raise luteal progesterone production, and this increase is associated with expanded synthesis of RNA and protein. Thus cAMP may be an intracellular messenger for LH and hCG. Certainly a major consequence of the effect of hCG on gonads is increased steroid production. Like LH and adrenocorticotropic hormone (ACTH), hCG appears to stimulate steroidogenesis by increasing the rate of one of the steps in the conversion of cholesterol to pregnenolone.

Thus the placental hormone hCG, perhaps via adenylate cyclase, enhances the synthesis of steroids in the gonads as well as in its own cells. The possibility that the placenta controls its own steroid synthesis is intriguing, but evidence is not yet available to allow us to accept or reject it. By means of its gonadal effects, hCG prolongs the life span of the corpus luteum and regulates the developing fetal gonads[25].

HYPOTHALAMIC AND PITUITARY FUNCTION IN THE DEVELOPING FETUS

Although the functioning of the fetal pituitary–hypothalamic axis may become operational as soon as the respective structures are anatomically discernible, target organs elsewhere in the body are more sluggish.

Considerable indirect evidence has accumulated in both the monkey and the human that implicates the fetal pituitary in ongoing gonadotropin secretion; secretory granules similar to those found in adult pituitaries have been identified in human fetal pituitaries; and immunoreactive and bioreactive gonadotropins have been extracted from both human and monkey fetal pituitaries.

Evidence for early function has been well demonstrated by *in vitro* and *in vivo* studies that show the human fetal pituitary gland to be producing all tropic hormones by 20 weeks' gestation[26–31].

The pituitary portal system connects the primitive hypothalamus with the anterior hypophysis. It begins to form as early as 7–8 weeks' gestation, from mesenchymal cells adjoining Rathke's pouch. However, a complete system capable of transport of blood and endocrine substances is probably not present before 18–20 weeks[32,33]. Hormones have been identified by 6–8 weeks' gestation[26,32,34,35]. Functional development of the hypothalamus begins with formation of its nuclei by 8 weeks. As early as 10 weeks, the presence of biogenic amines in the human fetus has been confirmed by fluorescence techniques. Dopamine seems to be present in higher concentrations than the other monoamines[36]. Immunochemical techniques have been used to identify hypothalamic releasing factors as early as 8 weeks[37].

Steroid hormones are furnished to the fetal nervous system (CNS) and pituitary by maternal adrenal glands and ovaries, the placenta and the fetal gonads and adrenals. Many experimental observations, such as those to be described, indicate the importance of steroid hormones in the development of the fetus, especially its nervous system.

The fetal pituitary and hypothalamus are affected by stimulatory and inhibitory substances *in vitro* by 10–13 weeks. By midgestation in humans, the hypothalamic–pituitary axis can be shown to be a functional unit[38]. There is a regulatory hierarchy in the neuroendocrine system. The hypothalamus responds to messages from many brain centers and is modulated by target organ and peripheral organ products and functions.

There is a critical period during which the steroid-sensitive centers of the brain that control reproductive behavior and gonadotropin release are not fully differentiated. In the rhesus monkey and probably in the human, maturation occurs in the late prenatal period. There are receptors for both estrogens and androgens in many parts of the brain, but especially in the medial preoptic area of the hypothalamus, the basal medial hypothalamus and the amygdalae. The brain and the anterior pituitary can convert testosterone to dihydrotestosterone (catalyzed by 5 α-reductase). The hypothalamus and the limbic system have aromatizing enzymes that convert testosterone to estradiol[25]. Estrogens are metabolized in the central nervous system and anterior pituitary of both adult and fetus[25].

FSH is present in the fetal pituitary by 9 weeks. It rises slowly until 12–20 weeks and levels are higher in female fetuses than in males. Perhaps that is a reflection of the later developmental characteristic of the ovary, since the surrounding hormonal environment will influence later FSH levels to decrease. From 20–29 weeks, LH and FSH levels are higher in the female fetus than in the males[29,31].

Immunochemically identifiable luteinizing hormone-releasing factor (LRF) is present in the hypothalamus at 10 weeks and is found in fetal blood by 14 weeks[37]. It is assumed that the LRF effect is dependent upon the development of the portal system. Takagi and associates[31] have studied LRF effect *in vivo* in fetuses and draw the following conclusions:

(1) Infusion of LRF will increase fetal release of LH and FSH;

(2) Levels of FSH are higher in the female fetus in the second but not in the third trimester; and

(3) The increases in FSH and LH are greater in the second, as compared to the third trimester.

In the mid- and late portions of pregnancy the hypothalamic–pituitary axis is operational in the human fetus and under the influence of feedback mechanisms by way of circulating steroid hormones[38]. In the late portion of pregnancy, especially in the last weeks of gestation, in the fetal hypothalamic–pituitary–ovarian axis, there is an increasing negative feed-back sensitivity with ovarian hyperstimulation by steroid hormones (gonadal and placental steroids). In the premature newborn, the increase in the hypothalamic–pituitary–ovarian axis was found to be greater when compared to normal controls[39].

FROM THE OVARIAN FOLLICLE TO THE OVARIAN CYST

Occasionally, single follicles may contain more than the usual amount of fluid and may measure several centimeters in diameter. Estrogenic hormone was demonstrated in the fluid of a 2 cm follicle, and in another that was 12 cm in greatest diameter, the lining resembled granulosa cells[40].

It is possible for the cells of the theca interna to become luteinized. Enlarged ovaries with prominent cystic follicles have been reported, as well as remarkable numbers of follicles with luteinized theca interna detected during the third trimester and immediately post-partum[41,42]. Luteinized follicles are also found at other ages, and it is apparent that such luteinization may occur in the absence of ovulation[43].

The reported cases of corpus luteum cysts in the first year of life bear scrutiny since ovulation must be a most rare event at this period of life. Marshall[43] reported 45 cases of enlarged ovaries in children, with 23 having the diagnosis established in the first 37 days of life (7 follicular cysts, 9 serous or simple cysts, 2 theca lutein cysts, 4 corpus luteum cysts, and 1 granulosa cell cyst). Autopsy data of female stillbirths and neonatal deaths have shown a higher frequency (32–34%) of small follicular ovarian cysts. De Sa[44] found 113 in 332 stillborns or infants (34%) who died within 28 days of birth and Doshi and associates[45] found such cysts in 32% of 40 neonates at autopsy. Most of these small cysts involute within the first few months of life and have no clinical significance.

Discrepancy between prenatally diagnosed fetal ovarian cysts and ovarian cysts found in stillbirths and neonates is probably due to the fact that only large cysts causing complications are detected clinically or by sonography. Benign cysts, including follicle cysts and theca lutein cysts, constitute the most common types of fetal ovarian cyst[46].

A follicle cyst is a follicle which does not rupture at the time of ovulation. Subsequently, the liquor accumulates within the follicle and the structure becomes cystic, the so-called hydrops folliculi. Pathologically, follicle cysts are thin-walled structures lined, in the early stages of development, by both granulosa and theca cells. Later, as the cyst enlarges and intracystic pressure increases, the normal cellular morphology is destroyed; eventually only luteinized connective tissue remains, making it almost impossible to distinguish the origin of the cyst.

Although the etiology of follicular cysts is unclear, it is probable that they result from disordered folliculogenesis[47]. Maternal hypothyroidism has also been postulated as a possible cause of fetal follicular cysts. In one patient, non-specific pituitary glycoprotein hormone synthesis secondary to hypothyroidism was considered the explanation for accelerated sexual development and consequent cyst formation[48].

Whereas ovulation precedes development of a corpus luteum cyst, the theca-lutein cyst develops in the absence of ovulation. It is a result of a disturbance in the normal hypothalamic–pituitary–gonadal axis, in which an elevated gonadotropin level is observed. Its lining consists of large luteinized cells (granulosa and theca) surrounded by a connective-tissue stroma which, in turn, is surrounded by a well developed theca interna[49]. There are three mechanisms or clinical situations involved in the pathogenesis of theca-lutein cysts[46]:

(1) The transplacental diffusion of maternal hCG may result in theca-lutein cysts in the newborn;

(2) Owing to the faulty utilization and metabolism of maternal hCG by the fetoplacental unit in cases of Rh incompatibility, pre-eclampsia, eclampsia and diabetes mellitus, multiple theca-lutein cysts may develop in infants[49,50]; and

(3) Increased hCG production that often accompanies multiple pregnancy, hydatiform mole, chorioadenoma destruens, and choriocarcinoma may result in multiple bilateral theca-lutein cysts[51].

SONOGRAPHIC EVALUATION OF COMPLICATED AND UNCOMPLICATED FETAL OVARIAN CYSTS

Although the sonographic features of a pelvic mass frequently do not permit a specific histopathological diagnosis, sonography usually provides clinically important parameters for the management of the mass. Sonographic criteria in the diagnosis of fetal ovarian cysts include[52–61] (Figure 2):

(1) Presence of a cystic structure that is regular in shape and usually located on one side of the fetal abdomen;

(2) Presence of normally structured and functioning organs of the urinary and gastrointestinal tracts; and

(3) Female sex of the fetus.

Once the diagnosis of fetal ovarian cyst has been made, the following parameters should be evaluated:

(1) Establishment of the mono- or bilateral site of the ovarian mass;

(2) Detailed evaluation of the size, internal echo patterns and contour of the mass;

(3) Establishment of the anatomic relationship of the mass to other pelvic structures; and

(4) Evaluation of intraperitoneal fluid.

Masses arising in the fetal ovary are usually cystic, non-neoplastic and of follicular origin[62]. In the

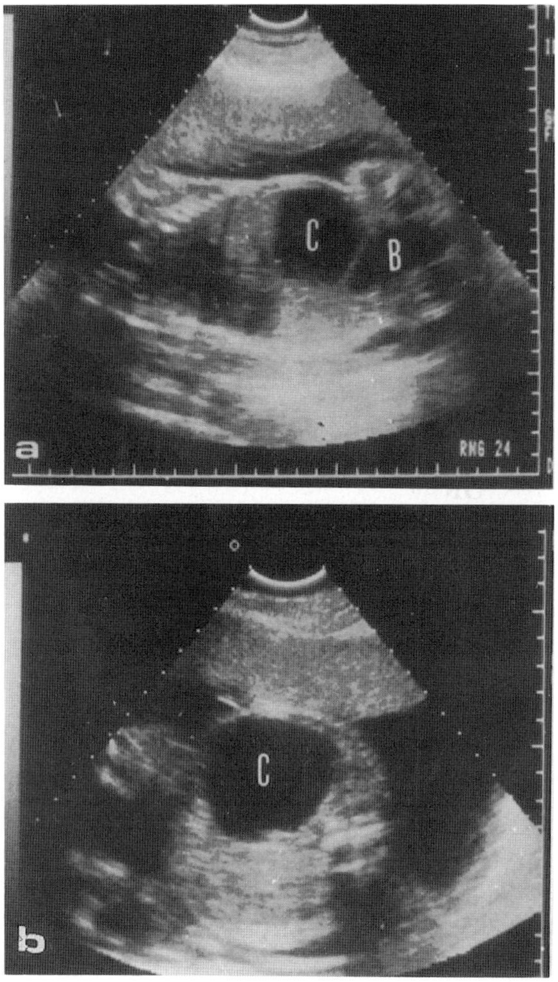

Figure 2 Fetal ovarian cyst appearing as an anechoic structure in the fetal abdomen. The longitudinal section (a) shows the close correlation of the cyst (C) to the fetal bladder (B); the transverse section (b) shows the location of the cyst on one side of the fetal abdomen

literature, as well as in our own data, most follicular and theca-lutein cysts do not appear earlier than 27 weeks of pregnancy at ultrasound (165 out of 173) despite the widespread use of sonography as a screening test for fetal malformations at 20–24 weeks of gestation (Table 1).

This late development of the fetal ovarian cyst is probably due to the fact that the majority of the cysts have a functional origin as confirmed by the high levels of estradiol, progesterone and testosterone found in ovarian cysts[47–82]. The fetal ovary is biochemically competent to produce sex steroids *in utero*, but the deficiency of gonadotropin receptors and/or intrinsic enzyme deficiency in receptor-coupled adenylate cyclase may compromise steroidogenesis and prohibit testosterone production prior to 22 weeks[12]. Meizner and colleagues[90] are the only authors reporting cases diagnosed earlier in pregnancy (19 weeks) but they do not offer any explanation of the phenomenon.

Sometimes the cysts decrease in size throughout the remainder of gestation, reflecting the drop in gonadotropins occurring at term, and presumably resulting from maturation of the hypothalamus due to the negative feedback of estrogens[35].

Table 1 Fetal age at diagnosis and site of fetal ovarian cysts in 173 cases reported in the literature

Authors	*Fetal age at diagnosis* (weeks)	*Site*	*Cases* (*n*)
Valenti *et al.*[63]	36	Mo	1
Montag *et al.*[47]	30	Mo	1
Jafri *et al.*[48]	32–39	Mo–Bi	3
Kirkinen and Jouppila[54]	32–41	Mo–Bi	8
Borin *et al.*[64]	37	Bi	1
Sandler *et al.*[65]	31	Bi	1
Suita *et al.*[66]	35–41	Mo	2
Preziosi *et al.*[67]	32–34	Mo	2
Landrum *et al.*[68]	27	Mo	1
Calì *et al.*[69]	27	Mo	1
Bruno *et al.*[70]	28	Mo	1
Suma *et al.*[71]	28–35	Mo–Bi	5
De Rosi *et al.*[72]	36	Mo	1
Gesmundo *et al.*[73]	37	Mo	1
Centini *et al.*[74]	31–36	Mo–Bi	4
Ikeda *et al*:[75]	32–40	Mo	9
Nussbaum *et al.*[76]	30–40	Mo	11
La Prova *et al.*[77]	33–36	Mo	4
D'Addario *et al.*[78]	30–41	Mo–Bi	25
Gonzales *et al*[79]	27–40	Mo	3
Valenti *et al.*[80]	31	Mo	1
Giorlandino *et al.*[81]	30	Mo	1
Holzgreve *et al.*[53]	37	Mo	1
Shozu *et al.*[82]	29	Mo	1
Lee and Blake[83]	41	Mo	1
Crade *et al.*[84]	40	Mo	1
Mitsutake *et al.*[85]	36	Mo	1
Tabsh Khalil[86]	33	Mo	1
Rizzo *et al.*[87]	28–36	Mo	13
Bagolan *et al.*[88]	28–39	Mo–Bi	25
Garel *et al.*[89]	28–38	Mo–Bi	27
Meizner *et al.*[90]	19–35	Mo–Bi	15

Mo = monolateral, Bi = bilateral

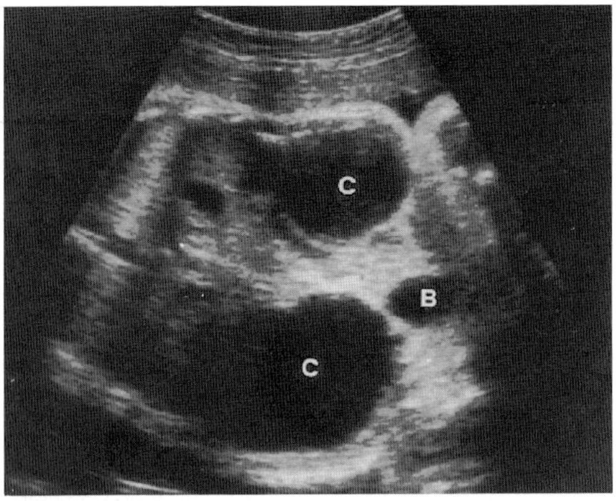

Figure 3 Bilateral fetal ovarian cysts (C) located above the bladder (B)

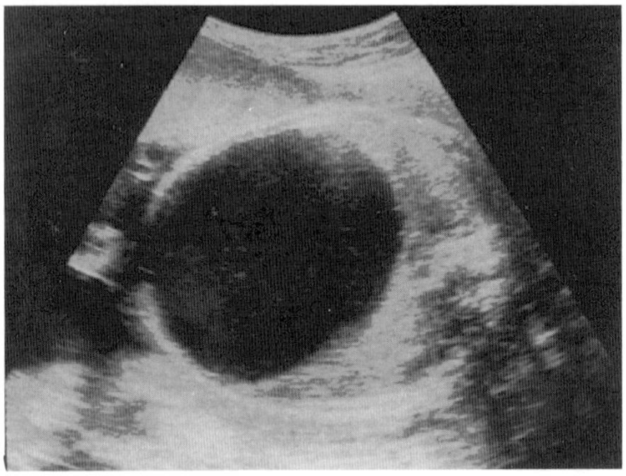

Figure 4 Huge ovarian cyst entirely occupying the fetal abdomen

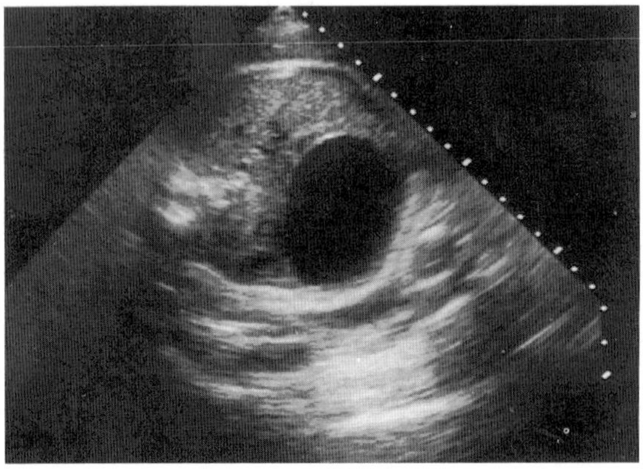

Figure 5 Type A fetal ovarian cyst; the mass is unilocular, homogeneously anechoic with smooth borders

Table 2 Prenatal sonographic data of fetal ovarian cysts

Authors	*Site*	*Maximum size* (cm)	*Type* *A*	*B*	*C*	*Cases* (*n*)
Valenti *et al.*[63]	Mo	9.0 × 9.0	1			1
Montag *et al.*[47]	Mo	7.0 × 7.0	1			1
Jafri *et al.*[48]	Mo–Bi	9.0 × 5.0	3			3
Kirkinen and Jouppila[54]	Mo–Bi	8.0 × 10.0	8			8
Preziosi *et al.*[67]	Mo	5.4 × 4.4	1		1	2
Landrum *et al.*[68]	Mo	11.0 × 11.0	1			1
Calì *et al.*[69]	Mo	5.0 × 5.0	1			1
Bruno *et al.*[70]	Mo	3.1 × 2.5	1			1
Suma *et al.*[71]	Mo–Bi	5.1 × 5.0	5			5
De Rosi *et al.*[72]	Mo	5.7 × 7.5	1			1
Gesmundo *et al.*[73]	Mo	5.1 × 4.8	1			1
Nussbaum *et al.*[76]	Mo	8.8 × 8.8	3		8	11
D'Addario *et al.*[78]	Mo–Bi	8.0 × 6.0	17	5	3	25
Gonzales *et al.*[79]	Mo	6.0 × 6.2	3			3
Valenti *et al.*[80]	Mo	4.0 × 3.5		1		1
Giorlandino *et al.*[81]	Mo	8.0 × 8.0	1			1
Holzgreve *et al.*[53]	Mo	10.0 × 9.0	1			1
Rizzo *et al.*[87]	Mo		11		2	13
Shozu *et al.*[82]	Mo	6.5 × 6.1	1		1	
Muller-Leisse *et al.*[91]			39		5	44

Mo = monolateral, Bi = bilateral

The unilateral fetal ovarian cyst is more common than the bilateral cyst (Figure 3). The size varies and ranges from small cysts to structures filling the entire abdomen (Figure 4, Table 2). The widest cyst (11.0 × 11.0 cm) was reported by Landrum and colleagues[68] who successfully aspirated the cyst *in utero* to avoid pulmonary hypoplasia. The sonographic patterns of fetal ovarian cysts may be put into the following groups[78]:

Type A Unilocular homogeneous anechoic mass with smooth borders;

Type B Cystic mass containing internal echoes and/or septa; and

Type C Cystic mass containing echogenic debris.

Uncomplicated ovarian cysts appear ultrasonically as a homogeneous anechoic mass with thin and regular walls (type A) (Figure 5). This is the most common type of ultrasonically diagnosed

Table 3 Characteristics of fetal ovarian cysts

	Uncomplicated	*Complicated*
Ultrasonic patterns	type A	types B, C
Histological findings	follicular, luteinic, serous ovarian cysts	hemorrhagic cysts (resulting from torsion and associated infarction)
Clinical course	(a) spontaneous resolution (decreasing size) during fetal life and first few months after birth; (b) increasing size; (c) solid components inside the cyst (types B, C) resulting from torsion and hemorrhage	(a) surgical treatment; (b) rarely, spontaneous resolution

fetal ovarian cyst in the literature as well as in our own series, accounting for 81% of the reported cases (Table 3). Histologically they may be identified as follicular, luteinic and serous. The most common course of this type of ovarian mass is spontaneous resolution during fetal life or during the first few months after birth. At times they may increase in size and show solid components during intrauterine life. If solid components appear inside the cyst, as in types B and C, a complication (hemorrhage or torsion) is suspected.

A complicated fetal ovarian cyst contains septa (type B) and/or fluid and debris (type C) and often has a thick wall (Figures 6, 7 and 8). Histologically it is represented as a hemorrhagic cyst almost uniformly resulting from torsion and associated infarction. A fluid–debris level is formed by cyst fluid and liquid hematoma. A cyst

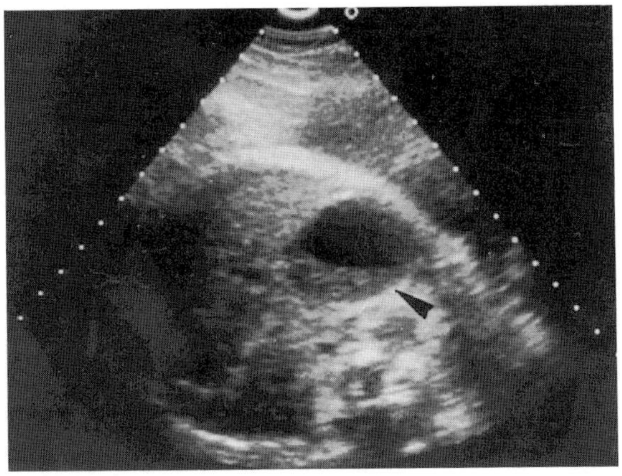

Figure 7 Type C fetal ovarian cyst; echogenic debris can be seen in the lower pole of the cyst (arrow)

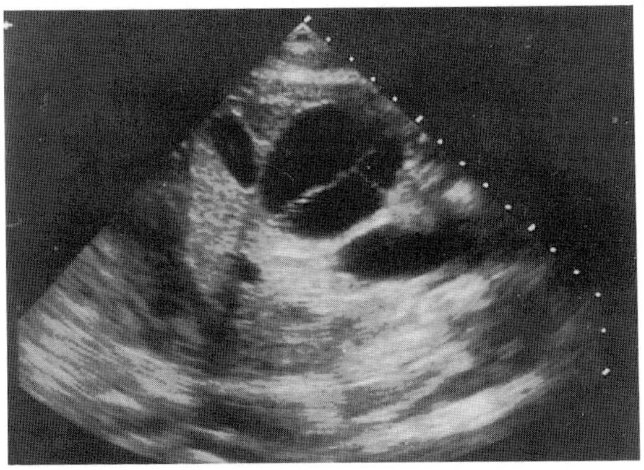

Figure 6 Type B fetal ovarian cyst; multiple septa can be seen inside the cyst

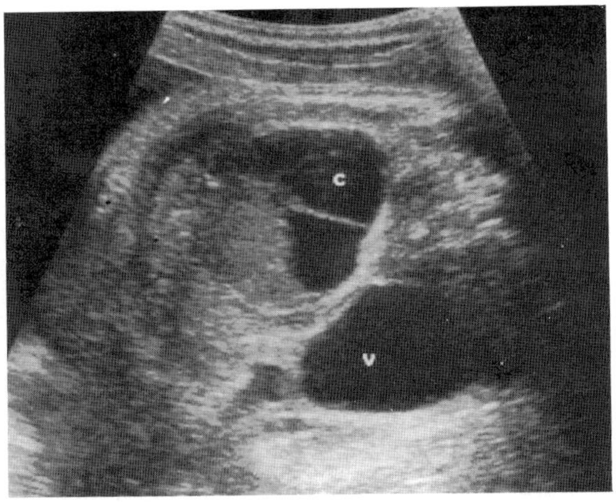

Figure 8 Complicated fetal ovarian cyst showing both septum and debris

that contains liquid and organized hematoma will show internal echo patterns generated by retracting clot. The septa are presumably formed by strands of organized hemorrhage. Blood is known to have a variable sonographic appearance, mostly related to the temporal sequence of clot formation and lysis[76].

The appearance of solid components in the cyst, after a previous finding of homogeneous cystic mass, suggests the possibility of a twisted cyst and/or endocystic bleeding during fetal life, but as yet no sonographic criteria aid the sonographer to the conclusive diagnosis.

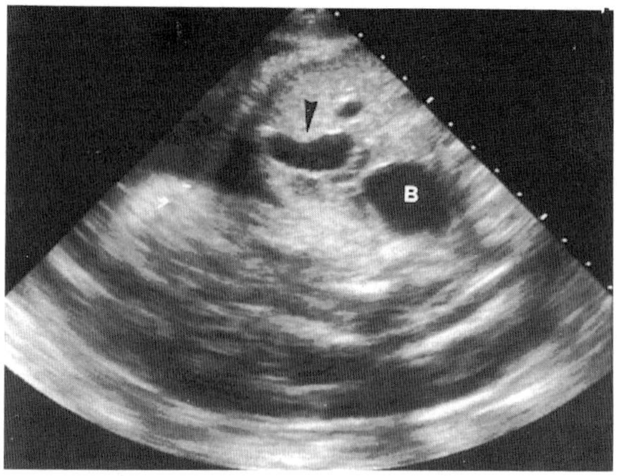

Figure 9 Urachal cyst mimicking ovarian cyst. The cystic structure, however, (arrow) is close to the fetal abdominal wall and extends from the bladder (B) to the umbilicus

SONOGRAPHIC DIFFERENTIAL DIAGNOSIS OF FETAL OVARIAN CYSTS

The sonographic differential diagnosis of fetal ovarian cysts includes:

(1) Mesenteric and enteric cysts, whose sonographic appearance is indistinguishable from fetal ovarian cysts[52,92–95];

(2) Enteric bowel duplication, whose shape tends to be more tubular than round or ovoid, but this is not enough for differential diagnosis[52];

(3) Urachal cyst – single, tubular in shape and extending from the bladder to the umbilicus (Figure 9);

(4) Duodenal atresia with a typical double bubble appearance; polyhydramnios is the rule;

(5) Bowel obstruction showing multiple dilated bowel loops and increased peristalsis;

(6) Hydrometrocolpos, appearing as a cystic mass with low level echoes posterior to the bladder and extending into the fetal abdomen[96–101] (Figure 10);

(7) A cyst of renal origin tending to be located more dorsally and in close proximity to the spine (Figure 11). If the cystic mass is a large pelvic abdominal mass, the diagnosis is quite difficult;

(8) Anterior meningocele.

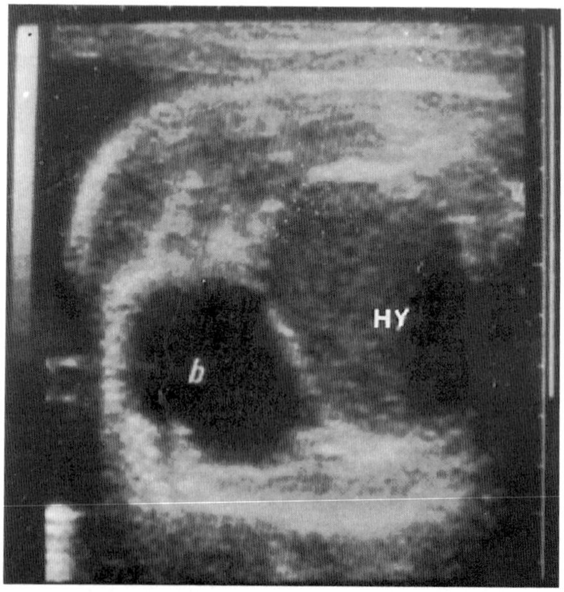

Figure 10 Hydrometrocolpos (HY) appearing as a cystic mass with low-level echoes, posterior to the fetal bladder (b)

COMPLICATIONS OF FETAL OVARIAN CYSTS

The course of fetal ovarian cysts most often seems to be postnatal involution even though prenatal disappearance is not unusual.

If we take into account the fact that antenatal

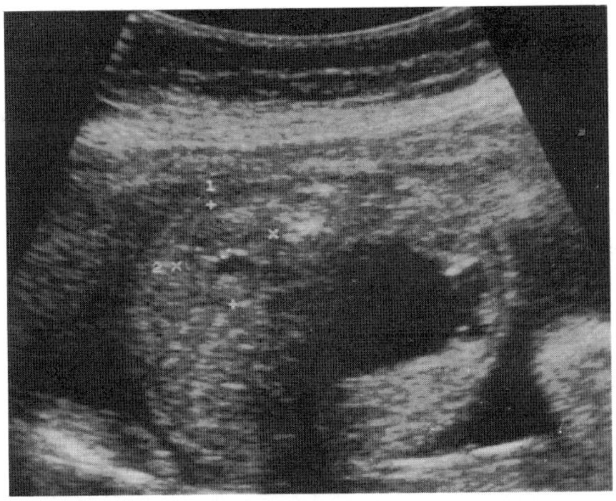

Figure 11 Renal cyst mimicking ovarian cyst. The cystic structure, however, is located dorsally and close to the spine

diagnosis of pelvic cysts is made incidentally by sonographic examination, it suggests that a large number of fetal ovarian cysts may remain undiagnosed if routine screening during late pregnancy is not done. This also strongly suggests that the true incidence of fetal ovarian cysts may be somewhat greater than supposed.

The complications of fetal ovarian cysts, to the fetus (or to the newborn) and to the mother, are shown in Table 4. The main fetal complications may be primarily related to the cyst (torsion, rupture and infarction or hemorrhage) or can affect other organs (bowel obstructions, compression of fetal thorax with pulmonary hypoplasia, or incarceration within an inguinal hernia). All these complications may have great postnatal clinical importance[102–106].

Table 4 Complications of fetal ovarian cysts

Fetal complications		*Maternal complications*
Primary	*Secondary*	
Torsion	bowel obstruction	polyhydramnios
Rupture	thorax compression (with pulmonary hypoplasia)	vaginal dystocia at delivery
Hemorrhage	urinary tract obstruction	

The presence of ascites in association with fetal ovarian cysts raises the possibility of a potentially lethal cyst rupture, or peritonitis from cyst torsion with infarction or bowel obstruction[76].

Maternal implications related to fetal ovarian cysts are dystocia and cyst rupture during vaginal delivery and the polyhydramnios related to the small bowel obstruction or compression of the umbilical cord[80,86,106]. The frequency with which these accidents occur *in utero* is unknown. At present, it is not possible to predict if some fetuses will have disturbances in ovarian–pituitary function during intrauterine development. Associated congenital anomalies such as hypertrophic pyloric stenosis, congenital hypothyroidism, hydrocephalus and absence of corpus callosum and of the pyramidal system have been reported[107].

MANAGEMENT OF FETAL OVARIAN CYSTS

The management of a fetus affected by an ovarian cyst mainly depends on the antenatal sonographic appearance of the cyst and on its evolution throughout pregnancy.

Homogeneously anechoic cysts of small to moderate size (less than 6 cm) are usually uncomplicated, and can undergo spontaneous resolution either in prenatal life or in the first few months after birth.

Larger cysts can cause mechanical complications such as abdominal distension and consequent dystocia, partial gastrointestinal obstruction with consequent polyhydramnios, and renal and lung compression with consequent respiratory distress. Further complications of the larger cysts are torsion and intracystic bleeding[78,79] (Figures 12–14).

However, even small simple cysts can undergo this last type of complication. Due to this variable evolution of the disease, once the prenatal diagnosis of fetal ovarian cyst has been made, it is most important to plan serial ultrasound examinations on a weekly basis to detect any structural change in the mass.

The prenatal follow-up can demonstrate the disappearance of the cyst or its persistence. Persistent simple cysts smaller than 6 cm should be monitored after birth, since their spontaneous

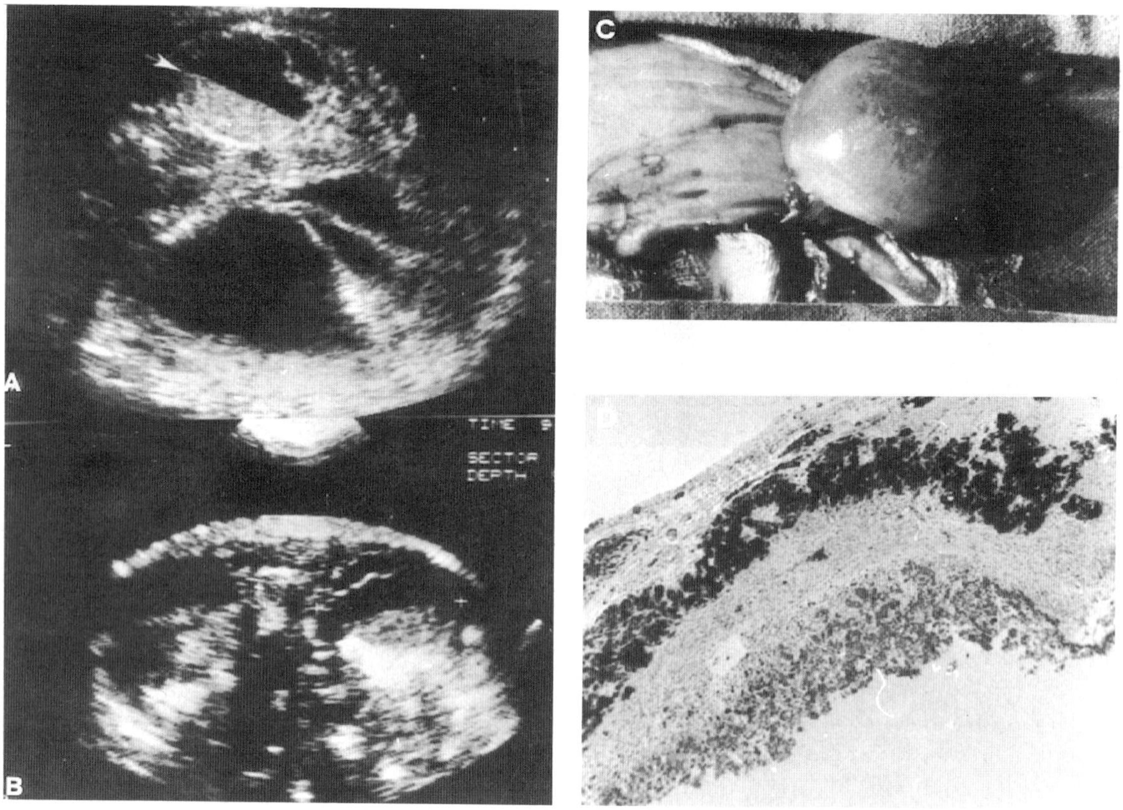

Figure 12 Complicated bilateral fetal ovarian cysts. A, B: ultrasonic prenatal appearance; C, D: macro- and microscopic findings

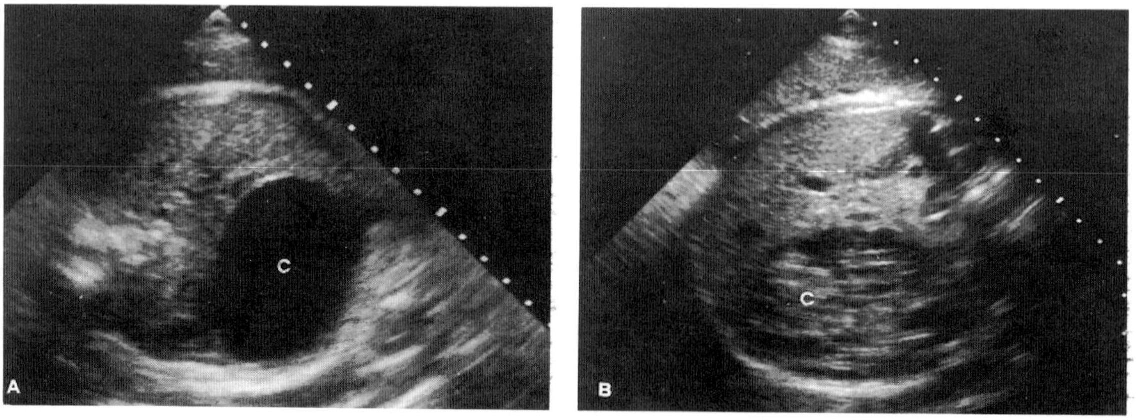

Figure 13 Intrauterine torsion of a large fetal ovarian cyst (c). After the torsion, the simple unilocular cyst (A) modifies into a complex mass (B)

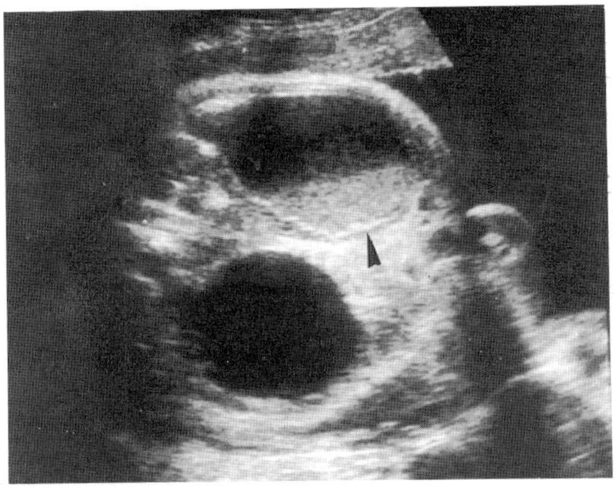

Figure 14 Intracystic hemorrhage in one of the bilateral ovarian cysts (arrow)

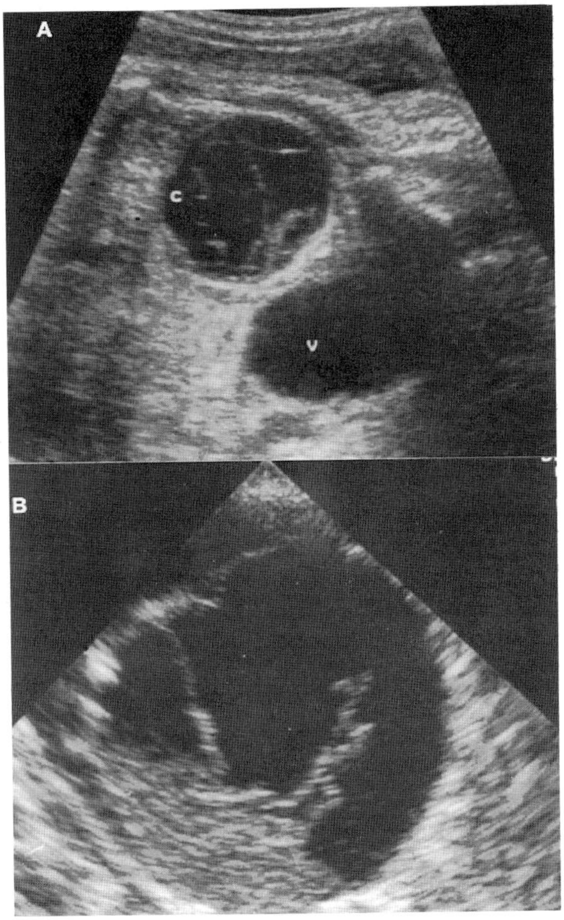

Figure 15 Complicated fetal ovarian cyst (A) confirmed by neonatal sonography (B) and requiring surgery. C, cyst; v, bladder

resolution is possible in the first 6 months of life. Cysts larger than 6 cm or rapidly increasing in size during the prenatal follow-up must be treated with particular attention, due to their higher risk of complications. If the cyst is so large as to be suspected as a cause of dystocia, a Caesarean delivery should be contemplated.

An alternative approach is the ultrasound-guided needle aspiration of the cyst[81]. The benefit of this procedure, however, is controversial. The aspiration may avoid the need for a Caesarean section and theoretically diminish the risk of intrauterine torsion, but puncture of the cyst may carry some risks to the fetus, such as rupture of the cyst with intraperitoneal bleeding or, for instance, the inadvertant puncture of a choledochal cyst, erroneously diagnosed as an ovarian one, which can be a catastrophic event[53].

When the cyst shows signs of torsion or hemorrhage, the pediatric surgeon should be alerted for a prompt neonatal intervention in order to avoid further complication, such as adhesions or ovarian necrosis[53] (Figure 15).

If a simple cyst begins to show signs of recent torsion during follow-up and if the fetus is viable, induction of labor may be considered to permit early surgical intervention in an effort to save an ovary[90].

However, even small complicated fetal ovarian cysts may undergo rare spontaneous resolution. This may be the case in intracystic bleeding which resolves spontaneously as in the hemorrhagic corpus luteum of the adult or hemorrhagic neonatal ovarian cyst[78,108]. For this reason, the follow-up is the most important step in the decision-making process regarding fetal ovarian cysts.

References

1. Erickson, G. F. and Schreiber, J. R. (1990). Morphology and physiology of the normal ovary. In Becker, K. L. (ed.) *Principles and Practice of Endocrinology and Metabolism*, pp. 776–87. (Philadelphia: J. B. Lippincott)
2. Tsafriri, A., Reich, R. and Obisogun, A. O. (1987). Ovarian regulation of oocyte maturation. In Genazzani, A. R., Volpe, A. and Facchinetti, F. (eds.) *Gynecological Endocrinology*, p. 109. (Carnforth, UK: Parthenon Publishing)
3. Ohno, S., Klinger, H. P. and Atkin, N. B. (1962). Human oogenesis. *Cytogenetics*, **1**, 42
4. Pryse-Davis, J. and Dewhurst, C. J. (1971). The development of the ovary and uterus in the foetus, newborn and infant: a morphological and enzyme histochemical study. *J. Pathol.*, **103**, 5
5. Peters, H., Himelstein-Braw, R. and Faber, M. (1976). The normal development of the ovary in childhood. *Acta Endocrinol.*, **82**, 617
6. Baker, T. G. and Sum, O. W. (1976). Development of ovary and oogenesis. *Clin. Obstet. Gynecol.*, **3**, 3
7. Gougeon, A. and Chainy, G. B. N. (1987). Morphometric studies of small follicles in ovaries of women at different ages. *Reprod. Fertil.*, **81**, 433
8. Erickson, G. F. (1991). Follicular growth and development. In Sciarra, J. J. (ed.) *Gynecology and Obstetrics*, Vol. 5, Chap. 77, Revised Edition. (Philadelphia: J. B. Lippincott)
9. Gougeon, A. (1979). Qualitative changes in medium and large antral follicles in the human ovary during the menstrual cycle. *Ann. Biol. Anim. Biochem. Biophys.*, **19**, 1461
10. Eshkol, A., Lunenfeld, B. and Peters, H. (1972). Gonadotropic regulation of ovarian development in mice during infancy. In Saxena, B. B., Belina, C. G. and Gandy, H. M. (eds.) *Gonadotropins*, pp. 335–46. (New York: John Wiley and Sons)
11. Erickson, G. F., Magoffin, D. A. and Dyer, C. A. (1985). The ovarian androgen producing cells: a review of structure/function relationships. *Endocr. Rev.*, **6**, 371
12. Di Zerega, G. S. and Ross, G. Y. (1980). Clinical relevance of fetal gonadal structure and function. *Clin. Obstet. Gynecol.*, **23** (3), 849
13. Tsafriri, A., Braw, R. H. and Reich, R. (1986). Follicular development and mechanism of ovulation. In Insler, V. and Lunenfeld, B. (eds.) *Infertility*, p. 75. (Edinburgh: Churchill Livingstone)
14. Grumbach, M. M. and Kaplan, S. L. (1973). Ontogenesis of growth hormone, insulin, prolactin and gonadotropin secretion in the human foetus. In *Fetal and Neonatal Physiology*, p. 362. (Cambridge: Cambridge University Press)
15. Baker, T. G. and Scrimegeour, J. B. (1980). Development of the gonad in normal and ancephalic human fetuses. *J. Reprod. Fertil.*, **60**, 193
16. Gondos, B. (1979). Classification of tumors of the ovary: developmental and ultrastructural considerations. *Ann. Clin. Lab. Sci.*, **9**, 179
17. Payne, A. H. and Jaffe, R. B. (1974). Androgen formation from pregnenolone sulfate by the human fetal ovary. *J. Clin. Endocrinol. Metab.*, **39**, 300
18. Jungman, R. A. and Schweppe, J. S. (1968). Biosynthesis of sterols and steroids from acetate 14 C by human fetal ovaries. *J. Clin. Endocrinol. Metab.*, **28**, 1599
19. Winter, J. S. D., Faiman, C. and Reyes, F. I. (1977). Sex steroid production by the human fetus: its role in morphogenesis and control by gonadotropins. *Birth Defects*, **13**, 41
20. Jost, A. (1960). The role of fetal hormones in prenatal development. *Harvey Lect.*, **55**, 201
21. George, F. W., Catt, K. J. and Wilson, J. D. (1979). Regulation of the onset of steroid hormone synthesis in fetal gonads. In Hamilton, T. H., Clark, J. H. and Sadler, W. A. (eds.) *Ontogeny of Receptors and Reproductive Hormone Action*. (New York: Raven Press)
22. Wilson, E. A. and Jawad, M. J. (1979). The effects of trophic agents on fetal ovarian steroidogenesis in organ culture. *Fertil. Steril.*, **32**, 73
23. Kaplan, S. L. and Grumbach, M. M. (1978). Pituitary and placental gonadotropin and sex steroids in the human and sub-human primate fetus. *Clin. Endocrinol. Metab.*, **7**, 487
24. Bloch, E. (1979). Fetal gonadal endocrine activity and reproductive tract differentiation. *Contrib. Gynecol. Obstet.*, **5**, 21
25. Page, E. W., Villee, C. A. and Villee, D. B. (1981). *Human Reproduction*, 3rd. edn., p. 18. (Philadelphia: W. B. Saunders)
26. Fisher, D., Dussault, J. H., Sack, J. and Chopra, I. J. (1977). Ontogenesis of hypothalamic, pituitary, and thyroid function and metabolism in man, sheep, and rat. *Rec. Prog. Horm. Res.*, **33**, 59
27. Hagen, C. and McNeilly, A. J. (1975). Identification of hormones LH, FSH, LH β-subunit and gonadotropin α-subunit in fetal and adult pituitary glands. *J. Endocrinol.*, **67**, 49
28. Levina, S. E. (1978). Hypothalamic control of the development of endocrine functions in the human fetus. In Borgman, W., Oksche, A., Polenov, A. and Scharrer, B. (eds.) *Neurosecretion and Neuroendocrine Activity Evolution, Structure and Function*, pp. 76–90. (Berlin: Springer-Verlag)
29. Reyes, F. I., Winter, J. S. D. and Faiman, D. (1976). *Gonadotropins in Gonadal Interrelationships in*

the Fetus in Diabetes and Other Endocrine Disorders During Pregnancy and in the Newborn, pp. 83–106. (New York: Alan R. Liss)

30. Siler-Khodr, T. M., Morgenstern, L. L. and Greenwood, F. C. (1974). Hormone synthesis and release from human fetal adenohypophyses *in vitro*. *J. Clin. Endocrinol. Metab.*, **39**, 891
31. Takagi, S., Yoshida, J., Tsubata, K., Ozaki, H., Fujii, T. R., Nomura, Y. and Swada, M. (1977). Sexual differentiation in fetal gonads and androgens. *J. Steroid Biochem.*, **8**, 609
32. Goodyer, G. C., Guyda, H. and Giroud, C. J. P. (1979). Development of hypothalamus–pituitary axis in the human fetus. In Tolis, G., Labrie, G., Martin, J. B. and Naftolin, F. (eds.) *Clinical Neuroendocrinology: A Pathophysiological Approach*, pp. 199–214. (New York: Raven Press)
33. Marchetti, B., Cioni, M. and Scapagnini, U. (1987). Neuropsico endocrinologia della riproduzione: basi molecolari e implicazioni cliniche. In De Cecco, L. and Venturini, P. L. (eds.) *Neuropsicoendocrinologia Ostetrica e Ginecologica* (Padova: Liviana).
34. Gorski, R. A., Harlan, R. R. and Christensen, L. H. (1977). Perinatal hormonal exposure and development of the neuroendocrine regulatory process. *J. Toxicol. Environ. Health.*, **33**, 97
35. Kaplan, S. L., Grumbach, M. M. and Aubert, M. L. (1976). The ontogenesis of pituitary hormones and hypothalamic factors in the human fetus: maturation of central nervous regulation of anterior pituitary function. *Rec. Prog. Horm. Res.*, **32**, 161
36. Hyppa, M. (1992). Hypothalamic monoamines in the human fetus. *Neuroendocrinology*, **9**, 257
37. Curtis, A., Lyous, V. and Fink, G. (1984). In Labriel, F. and Raulx, L. (eds.) *Endocrinology*, p. 361. (Amsterdam: Elsevier Science Publishers)
38. DeCherney, A. and Naftolin, F. (1980). Hypothalamic and pituitary development in the fetus. *Clin. Obstet. Gynecol.*, **23** (3), 749–62
39. Tapaninen, J., Koivisto, M., Vihko, R. and Huhtaniemi, I. (1981). Enhanced activity of the pituitary-gonadal axis in premature human infants. *J. Clin. Endocrinol. Metab.*, **52**, 235
40. Potter, E. L. and Craig, J. M. (1975). *Pathology of the Fetus and the Infant*, 3rd edn., pp. 476–99. (Chicago: Year Book Medical Publishers)
41. Dehner, L. P. (1975). Female reproductive systems. In Kissane, J. M. (ed.) *Pathology of Infancy and Childhood*, 2nd edn., pp. 719–45. (St Louis: Mosby)
42. Ober, W. B. and Bernstein, J. (1996). Observations on the endometrium and ovary in the newborn. *Pediatrics*, **16**, 445
43. Marshall, J. R. (1965). Ovarian enlargements in the first year of life: review of 45 cases. *Am. Surg.*, **161**, 375
44. De Sa, D. J. (1975). Follicular ovarian cysts in stillbirth and neonates. *Arch. Dis. Child.*, **50**, 45–50
45. Doshi, N., Fujikura, T. and Kaubaur, A. (1977). Vaginal adenosis and polycystic ovaries during infancy and childhood. *Am. J. Obstet. Gynecol.*, **129**, 374–8
46. Bird, C. C., McElin, T. W. and Victor, T. A. (1985). Benign neoplasms of the ovary. In Sciarra, J. J. (ed.) *Gynecology and Obstetrics*, Vol. 1, Chap. 18. (Philadelphia: Harper Row)
47. Montag, T. W., Auletta, F. J. and Gibson, M. (1983). Neonatal ovarian cyst: prenatal diagnosis and analysis of the cyst fluid. *Obstet. Gynecol.*, **61**, 385
48. Jafri, S. Z. H., Bree, R. L., Silver, T. M. and Ouimette, M. (1984). Fetal ovarian cysts: sonographic detection and association with hypothyroidism. *Radiology*, **150**, 809–12
49. Ahlvin, R. C. and Bauer, W. C. (1957). Luteinized cysts in ovaries of infants born of diabetic mothers. *Am. J. Dis. Child.*, **93**, 107
50. Nguyen, K. T., Reid, R. L. and Sauerbrei, E. (1986). Antenatal sonographic detection of a fetal theca lutein cyst: a clue to maternal diabetes mellitus. *J. Ultrasound Med.*, **5**, 665
51. Miles, P. S. and Penney, L. L. (1983). Corpus luteum formation in the fetus. *Obstet. Gynecol.*, **61**, 523
52. Romero, R., Pilu, G., Jeanty, P., Ghidini, A. and Hobbins, J. C. (1988). *Prenatal Diagnosis of Congenital Anomalies*. (Norwalk: Appleton-Lange)
53. Holzgreve, W., Winde, B., Willital, G. H. and Beller, F. K. (1985). Prenatal diagnosis and perinatal management of a fetal ovarian cyst. *Prenat. Diagn.*, **5**, 155–9
54. Kirkinen, P. and Jouppila, P. (1985). Perinatal aspects of pregnancy complicated by fetal ovarian cyst. *J. Perinat. Med.*, **13**, 245–51
55. Kurjak, A., Latin, V. and D'Addario, V. (1982). Abnormalities of the fetus, placenta and umbilical cord. *Prog. Med. Ultrasound*, **3**, 87
56. Jurkovic, D. and Kurjak, A. (1989). Prenatal diagnosis and management of fetal tumors. In Cagnazzo, G. and D'Addario, V. (eds.) *The Fetus as a Patient*, p. 49–68. (Amsterdam: Excerpta Medica)
57. Fariello, G., Perale, R., Perri, G. and Tomà, P. (1991). *Ecografia Pediatrica*, p. 498. (Milan: Ambrosiana)
58. Fleischer, A. C., Romero, R., Manning, G. F. A., Jeanty, P. and James, A. E. Jr. (1991). *Ultrasonography in Obstetrics and Gynecology*, 4th edn., p. 270. (Norwalk: Appleton-Lange)
59. Eggermont, E., Lecoutere, D. and Bevlieger, H. (1988). Ovarian cysts in newborn infants. *Am. J. Dis. Child.*, **142**, 702
60. Volpe, G., D'Addario, V. and Lituania, M. (1988). The diagnosis and management of the fetal ovarian cysts: a collaborative study. *New Trends Obstet. Gynecol.*, **4**, 115

61. Wu, A. and Soegel, M. J. (1987). Sonography of pelvic masses in children: diagnostic predictability. *Am. J. Roentgenol.*, **148**, 1199
62. Babcock, D. S. and Han, B. K. (1984). The pediatric pelvis. In Steel, W. B. and Cochrane, W. J. (eds.) *Gynecologic Ultrasound*, Clinic in Diagnostic Ultrasound, Vol. 15. (Edinburgh: Churchill Livingstone)
63. Valenti, C., Kassner, E. G., Yermakov, V. and Cromb, E. (1975). Antenatal diagnosis of a fetal ovarian cyst. *Am. J. Obstet. Gynecol.*, **123**, 216
64. Borin B., Fabris, C. and Monari, G. (1985). Diagnosi ecografica di cisti ovariche bilaterali fetali. Presentazione di un caso clinico. *Ultr. Ost. Gin.*, **3**, 171–4
65. Sandler, R. M. A., Smith, S. J., Pope, S. G. and Madrazo, B. L. (1985). Prenatal diagnosis of septated ovarian cysts. *J. Clin. Ultrasound*, **13**, 55–7
66. Suita, S., Ikeda, K., Koyanagi, T. and Nakano, H. (1984). Neonatal ovarian cyst diagnosed antenatally: report of two patients. *J. Clin. Ultrasound*, **12**, 517–18
67. Preziosi, P., Fariello, G., Maiorana, A., Malena, S. and Ferro, F. (1986). Antenatal sonographic diagnosis of complicated ovarian cysts. *J. Clin. Ultrasound*, **14**, 196–8
68. Landrum, B., Ogburn, P. Jr, Feinberg, S., Bendel, R., Ferrara, B., Johnson, D. E. and Thompson, T. R. (1986). Intrauterine aspiration of a large ovarian cyst. *Obstet. Gynecol.*, **68**, 118
69. Calì, G., Li Calsi, L., Re, F. M., Orlando, G. and Lo Cascio, S. (1986). Diagnosi prenatale e trattamento di cisti ovarica. *Ultr. Ost. Gin.*, **4**, 319–21
70. Bruno, P., Mastrantonio, P., Lampariello, C., Muzi, H., Palazzo, A. and Guida, M. (1986). Diagnosi prenatale di cisti ovarica funzionante. *Ultr. Ost. Gin.*, **4**, 354–6
71. Suma, V., Marini, A. and Ciccolallo, G. (1988). Gli ultrasuoni nella diagnosi prenatale di cisti ovariche fetali. *Ultrasonica*, **3**(3), 179–83
72. De Rosi, A., Benedetti, T. and Pontoriero, G. (1988). Un caso di diagnosi intrauterina di cisti ovarica fetale e suo riscontro ecografico in epoca post natale. *Atti VII Congr. n. 2 SIEOG*, Siena, CIC edn., p. 489
73. Gesmundo, G., Russo, P., Carucci, A. and Milito, M. G. (1988). Diagnosi ecografica pre-natale della patologia ovarica. *Atti VII Congr. in 2 SIEOG*, Siena CIC edn., p. 597
74. Centini, G., Colosi, E., Vinciarelli, E., Scisca, C., Miceli, M. G. and Severi, F. M. (1988). Diagnosi ecografica prenatale e management delle cisti ovariche fetali. *Atti VII Congr. n. 2 SIEOG*, Siena CIC edn., p. 473
75. Ikeda, K., Suita, S. and Nakano, H. (1988). Management of ovarian cyst detected antenatally. *J. Pediatr. Surg.*, **23**(5), 432–5
76. Nussbaum, A. R., Sanders, R. C., Hartman, D. S., Dudgeon D. L. and Parmley, T. H. (1988). Neonatal ovarian cysts: sonographic–pathologic correlation. *Pediatr. Radiol.*, **168**, 817–21
77. La Prova, A., Viora, E. and Campogrande, M. (1985). Diagnosi e prognosi di cisti ovariche fetali. *Ultr. Ost. Gin.*, **4**, 241
78. D'Addario, V., Volpe, G., Kurjak, A., Lituania, M. and Zmijanac, J. (1990). Ultrasonic diagnosis and perinatal management of complicated and uncomplicated fetal ovarian cysts: a collaborative study. *J. Perinat. Med.*, **18**, 375–81
79. Gonzales, G., Lo Cascio, S. and Graziano, R. (1992). Le cisti ovariche fetali: problemi diagnostici e di trattamento. *Giorn. It. Ost. Gin.*, **5**, 307–9
80. Valenti, V., Amenta, A., Grifo, S., Adile, B., Ansaldi, R. and Cataliotti, F. (1989). Su un caso di cisti ovarica fetale torta sul peduncolo: diagnosi ecografica prenatale e trattamento. *Riv. Ost. Gin. Perin.*, **2**, 208–13
81. Giorlandino, C., Rivosecchi, M., Bilancioni, E., Bagolan, P., Zaccara, A., Taramann, C. and Vizzone, A. (1990). Successful intrauterine therapy of a large fetal ovarian cyst. *Prenat. Diagn.*, **10**, 473–4
82. Shozu, M., Akasofu, K., Iida, K. and Harada, T. (1991). Treatment of an antenatally diagnosed fetal ovarian cyst by needle aspiration during the neonatal period. *Arch. Gynecol. Obstet.*, **249**(2), 103–6
83. Lee, T. G. and Blake, S. (1977). Prenatal fetal abdominal ultrasonography and diagnosis. *Radiology*, **124**, 475
84. Crade, M., Gillooly, L. and Taylor, K. J. W. (1980). *In utero* demonstration of an ovarian cystic mass by ultrasound. *J. Clin. Ultrasound*, **8**, 251
85. Mitsutake, K., Abe, T. and Masumoto, R. (1981). Prenatal diagnosis of fetal abdominal masses by real-time ultrasound. *Kurume Med. J.*, **28**, 329
86. Tabsh Khalil, M. A. (1982). Antenatal sonographic appearance of a fetal ovarian cyst. *J. Ultrasound Med.*, **1**, 329
87. Rizzo, N., Gabrielli, S., Perolo, A., Pilu, G., Cacciari, A., Domini, R. and Bovicelli, L. (1989). Prenatal diagnosis and management of fetal ovarian cysts. *Prenat. Diagn.*, **9**, 97
88. Bagolan, P., Rivosecchi, M., Giorlandino, C., Bilancioni, E., Nahon, A., Zaccara, A., Trucchi, A. and Ferro, E. (1992): Prenatal diagnosis and clinical course of ovarian cysts. *J. Pediatr. Surg.*, **27**(7), 879–81
89. Garel, L., Filia Trault, D., Brandt, M., Grignon, A., Baisvert, J., Perreault, G. and Patriquin, H. (1991). Antenatal diagnosis of ovarian cysts: natural history and therapeutic implications. *Pediatr. Radiol.*, **21**, 182–4
90. Meizner, I., Levy, A., Katz, M., Maresh, A. J. and Glezerman, K. (1991). Fetal ovarian cysts: prenatal ultrasonographic detection and postnatal evaluation and treatment. *Am. J. Obstet.*

Gynecol., **164**, 874–8
91. Muller-Leisse, C., Bick, U., Paulussen, K., Troger, L., Zachariou, Z., Holzgreve, W., Schuhmacher, R. and Horvitz, A. (1992). Ovarian cysts in the fetus and neonate: changes in sonographic pattern in the follow-up and their management. *Pediatr. Radiol.*, **22**, 395–400
92. Haller, J. O., Schneider, M. and Kassner, E. G. (1978). Sonographic evaluation of mesenteric and omental masses in children. *Am. J. Radiol.*, **130**, 269
93. Girdany, B. R. (1985). The abdomen and gastrointestinal tract. In Silverman, F. N. (ed.) *Caffey's Pediatric X-Ray Diagnosis*, Vol. II, 8th edn., pp. 1398–9. (Chicago: Year Book Medical Publishers)
94. Takiff, H. Calabria, R. and Yin, L. (1985). Mesenteric cysts and intraabdominal cystic lymphangiomas. *Arch. Surg.*, **120**, 1266
95. Kurtz, R. J., Heimann, T. M. and Beck, A. R. (1986). Mesenteric and retroperitoneal cysts. *Ann. Surg.*, **203**, 109
96. Janus, C. and Godine, L. (1986). Newborn with hydrometrocolpos and ambiguous genitalia: clinical significance. *J. Clin. Ultrasound*, **14**, 739
97. Behrman, R. E. and Vaughan, V. C. (1987). *Nelson Textbook of Pediatrics*, 13th edn. (London: W. B. Saunders)
98. Davis, G. H., Wapner, J. R. and Kurtz, A. B. (1984). Antenatal diagnosis of hydrometrocolpos by ultrasound examination. *J. Ultrasound Med.*, **3**, 271–4
99. Hill, S. J. and Hirsch, J. H. (1985). Sonographic detection of fetal hydrometrocolpos. *J. Ultrasound Med.*, **4**, 323–5
100. Muckle, C. W. (1985). Developmental abnormalities of the female reproductive organs. In Sciarra, J. J. (ed.) *Gynecology and Obstetrics*, Vol. 1, Chap. 4. (Philadelphia: Harper-Row Publishers)
101. Volpe, G., D'Addario, V. and Volpe, P. (1988). L'uso dell'ecografia nella diagnosi prenatale di idrometrocolpo. *Ultrasonica*, **2**, 108–10
102. Dieter, R. A. Jr, Kindrachuk, W. and Muller, E. P. (1980). Neonatal intestinal obstruction due to torsion of an ovarian cyst. *J. Fam. Pract.*, **10**, 533–4
103. Mainolfi, F., Standiford, W. and Hubbard, T. (1968). Ruptured ovarian cyst in the newborn. *J. Pediatr. Surg.*, **3**, 612
104. Monson, R., Rodgers, B. M. and Nelson, R. M. (1978). Ruptured ovarian cysts in newborn infants. *J. Pediatr.*, **93**, 324–5
105. Ahmed, S. (1971). Neonatal and childhood ovarian cysts *J. Pediatr. Surg.*, **6**, 702–8
106. Carson, D. H. and Griscom, N. T. (1972). Ovarian cysts in the new born. *Am. J. Radiol.*, **116**, 664–72
107. Evers, J. L. and Roland, R. (1981). Primary hypothyroidism and ovarian activity: evidence for an overlap in the synthesis of pituitary glycoproteins. Case report. *Br. J. Obstet. Gynaecol.*, **88**, 195
108. Zamora, M. and Gonzales, N. (1992). Spontaneous resolution of a sonographically complicated fetal ovarian cyst. *J. Ultrasound Med*, **11**, 567–9

The ovary in pediatric and adolescent ages: place of sonography

4

V. Dramusic, Y. C. Wong and B. Funduk

INTRODUCTION

In the recent few decades it has become evident that gynecological disorders of children and adolescents warrant more attention than had been formerly devoted to them. Children and adolescents have their own particular gynecological problems[1–5]. These disorders are often more difficult to diagnose and treat than those of adults. Furthermore, as they are less common, even well experienced gynecologists are not adequately familiar with them. Examination and investigation of the child and the adolescent pose special problems. Manual pelvic examination of a child or an adolescent may be difficult and is frequently unrewarding. Ultrasonography is a simple alternative method to examination under anesthesia or laparoscopy, with no risk of irradiation to these young age groups.

Pediatric gynecology is concerned with the period from birth to about 10 years. This is a relatively quiet period, when the influence of hormones on the pelvic organs is minimal. Although they are not common, malformations can be detected in childhood. They are often multiple and associated with anomalies of the urinary or intestinal tracts. Unquestionably, the most disturbing of all gynecological conditions of childhood is intersexuality or ambiguous genitalia[6,7]. Uncertainty about a child's sex, if not investigated and appropriately managed at the earliest possible time, may lead to life-long frustration. Precocious puberty as well as any of its manifestations must likewise be immediately assessed in order not to overlook some organic cause. Though fortunately rare, tumors in childhood, the majority of which are of ovarian origin, are highly malignant; hence early diagnosis of these is of paramount importance.

High-resolution pelvic sonography has been extremely useful in the diagnosis and management of these problems. Not only does it have a high degree of accuracy in delineating many of these abnormalities, but it is both non-invasive and painless, making it an extremely suitable diagnostic technique in the evaluation of these patients[8].

The period of puberty and adolescence involves the complex transition from childhood to maturity and is associated with multiple somatic and psychic changes influencing the health, reproductive potential and sexuality of the future woman[9,10]. Adolescence is a long, dynamic period, difficult to define precisely but generally accepted to be between the 10th and 20th years of life. Puberty should be singled out as a biological phase of growth and maturation during which the body attains sexual maturity and the differentiation between the sexes becomes complete. Puberty coincides with the last effort of the human body towards generalized growth; it occurs between the 10th and 16th years. Usually two years before overt puberty, there is period of so-called 'biochemical puberty', with no physical signs of puberty visible but hormonal changes suggesting its onset. There is an increase in the adrenal production of dehydroepiandrosterone (DHEA) and its sulfate (DHEA-S), triggering the pubertal program. Androgens themselves will cause attainment of critical body weight inducing the pubertal growth spurt. Some adrenal androgens will convert into estrogens, causing a cascade of metabolic processes ending with increased release of gonadotropin-releasing hormone (GnRH), maturation of the hypothalamic center and increased response of the pituitary.

Table 1 Major events of female human puberty and adolescence

Event	*Age* (years)	*Characteristics*
Adrenarche	8–10	onset of prepubertal increase of adrenal function (biochemical puberty)
Pubertal growth spurt	10–13	starts around 10 years and reaches peak velocity at 12–13 years
Telarche	10–12	onset of breast development divided into 5 stages by Tanner[12]
Pubarche	10–13	onset of pubic hair growth, divided into 5 stages by Tanner[12]
Menarche	10–16	first menstrual period (nowadays most common at 12–14 years)
Growth of axillary hair	> 12	divided into 3 stages

Puberty is associated with two kinds of alterations in the reproductive system: changes in the gonads, and changes wrought by the secretions of the gonads. In 1965 it was thought that changes of the first kind can only be discovered by direct observation of the gonads[11]. The second group of effects is seen as the development of distinctive structural modifications denoted as secondary sexual characteristics. Today, fortunately, direct observation of the gonads is possible easily and reliably by ultrasonography. The events of normal puberty are judged by certain parameters which are not applicable in adults (Table 1). Specific parameters to be considered in adolescence are:

(1) *Chronological age* – age counted from birth;

(2) *Bone/skeletal age* – measure of general somatic maturity (radiography of wrists[13]);

(3) *Gynecological age* – years counted from menarche.

SONOGRAPHIC TECHNIQUES

The great majority of obstetric and gynecological sonography done today is with real-time gray-scale B-mode scanning. This technique allows a very precise characterization of tissues and allows visualization of motion such as fetal heart action. Sector scanning is particularly good for visualization of pelvic structures through a small acoustic window.

Transabdominal sonography is most commonly used during childhood and puberty[14–17]. For infants and young children, it could be said to be the only technique used. Accuracy of findings depends significantly on the 'acoustic window' for pelvic structures obtained by a full urinary bladder which allows adequate visualization of the pelvis. Distension of the bladder will also displace gas-filled bowel loops that may interpose between the transducer and pelvic organs. An additional benefit of a distended bladder is a more satisfactory position of the uterus, which becomes less anteflexed and rather more elongated. Simple oral intake of fluids is sufficient to meet the necessary conditions and children and adolescents generally have no problems in keeping good bladder volume. Their abdominal walls are thin and unscarred in the majority of cases, making them ideal subjects for pelvic ultrasonography.

In general, a 3.5-MHz transducer is used for older children and a 5-MHz transducer for infants, because more resolution is desirable and less penetration required in the small patient. An electronic sector transducer is preferred over a mechanical, because of the better resolution and image quality obtained[18–20].

Although the ovaries may be difficult to evaluate sonographically in the child under 2 years, an accurate assessment of their presence, size, and acoustic character usually can be made in the older child. Distortion of the normal pelvic anatomy by pelvic masses (including pregnancy) may make it impossible to visualize the ovaries.

Transvaginal sonography has improved resolution and visualization of pelvic organs due to closer proximity of the transducer to pelvic structures and allows the use of a higher frequency of transducer (5–7 MHz). However, this method is not used in childhood due to anatomical, technical and psychological reasons. Similarly, it has very low applicability even during puberty and adolescence and is reserved for special cases, often combined with transabdominal scanning[21].

The assessment of the female pelvis can be improved by the use of color flow and duplex Doppler, mainly in conditions where vascularity plays a major role in obtaining diagnoses as in cases of ovarian torsion, tumor, ectopic pregnancy and deep venous thrombosis[21]. However, its use is very limited during childhood and adolescence, and it may have its place only in evaluating ovarian tumors and their response to treatment by observing changes in vascularity.

In general, during childhood and adolescence, transabdominal sonography is the method of choice and only in exceptional cases can other modes be thought of in specialized institutions.

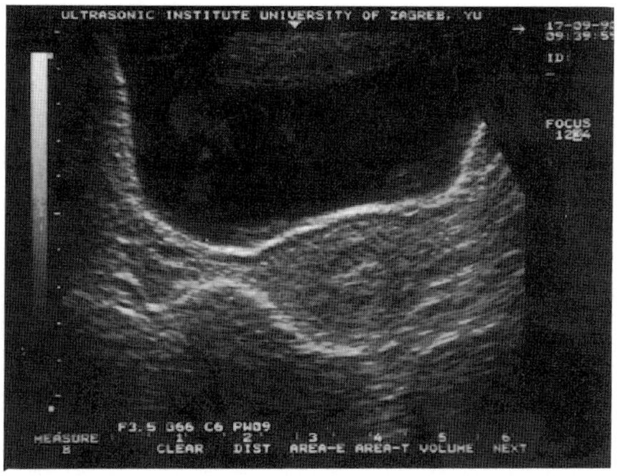

Figure 1 Transverse scan of the uterus and both ovaries lateral to it in a pubertal girl

NORMAL ANATOMY – SONOGRAPHY OF OVARIES DURING CHILDHOOD AND ADOLESCENCE

Ovaries can be identified in the majority of children. They lie within the broad ligament. Their relationship to the uterus varies because of the mobility of the ligamentous attachments. They may be located cephalad, lateral, or posterior to the uterus. There is great variability in the shape of the ovaries, although they characteristically have an ovoid appearance. Because of the variability in the shape of the ovaries, their size is typically expressed in terms of volume rather than planar measurements. Ovarian volumes are determined by the formula for a prolate ellipsoid (volume = 0.523 × longitudinal × anteroposterior × transverse diameter) and expressed in cubic centimeters (cm^3).

The most important part of ovaries is the germ cells. There are around 5 000 000 in fetal life; at term 1–2 000 000; by puberty, the average number of follicles is 300 000–500 000; by the early forties, less than 10 000; and they are totally depleted by menopause. On the basis of anatomical studies, it has been suggested that the ovaries are not resting and that follicular growth and atresia occur continuously during childhood resulting in a progressive increase in ovarian size[22]. Using high resolution sonography this follicular development can also be successfully assessed *in vivo* and it confirms that ovarian maturation continues during childhood and that remarkable morphological changes occur before the visible onset of puberty[23]. Ovarian size is relatively stable before puberty, after which there is a rapid increase in volume. A broad range of ovarian volume measurements has been noted in postpubertal women, reflecting the dynamic nature of the organ[24–26]. The mean ovarian volume in various studies has been reported as 0.7–4.0 cm^3 in prepubertal girls, 1.8–5.7 cm^3 during puberty and 4–9.8 cm^3 in postpubertal women[27–31]. Throughout life, follicles are developing to a certain degree and then undergoing atresia. Reproductive function is affected, as well as levels of estradiol (E_2), the principal female estrogen, being very low in childhood, increasing in puberty, reaching a peak during reproductive age (average 150–200 pg/ml) and dropping to 10–15 pg/ml postmenopausally.

In childhood ovarian morphology can be studied reliably and fairly easily by a real-time mechanical sector scanner. On a transverse scan it is fairly easy to identify the uterus and both ovaries in the same plane due to the small dimensions of the organs. The uterus is always in the medial line, with the ovaries lateral to it in a slightly curved line upwards (under ideal anatomic conditions) (Figure 1).

With increased use of pelvic sonography in children and adolescent girls, physicians are likely to observe physiologic events, such as ovarian follicular development. Because many sonograms are performed when a patient presents with symptoms, there is a tendency to associate sonographic findings with the symptoms that necessitated medical care. Sometimes, physiological

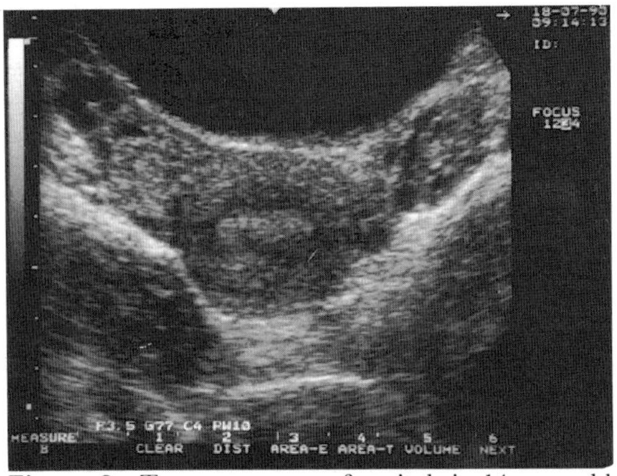

Figure 2 Transverse scan of genitals in 14-year-old girl with late onset of puberty, showing typical microcystic ovary of premenarchal phase of puberty

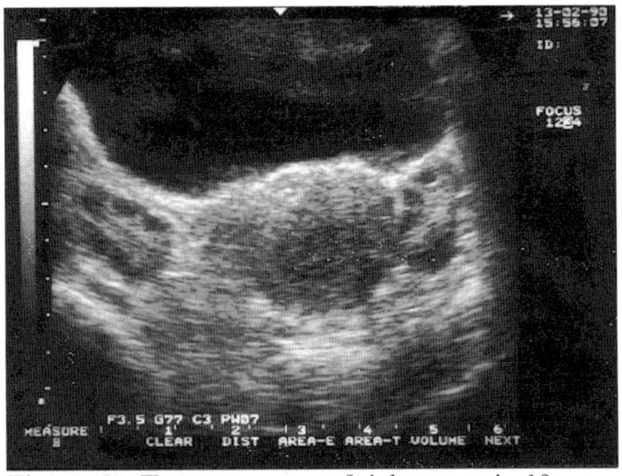

Figure 3 Transverse scan of right ovary in 13-year-old premenarchal girl. Typical multicystic appearance; cysts of varying size, one exceeding 9 mm

events are considered to represent disease processes[32]. Such misinterpretation may lead to unnecessary interventions with their inherent potential for complications. For that reason it is important to understand the physiological changes of ovarian growth.

A solid, homogeneous ovarian morphology is very common in younger girls and is observed in virtually all normal girls aged under 6–7 years. From this age, microcystic aspects become more and more frequent, but microcysts do not exceed 9 mm up to the age of 12. There is also a steady increase in the size of ovaries, as well as the uterus, in particular the corpus. Most researchers agree that ovarian morphology can be classified according to the presence or absence of functional cystic structures[33–35]:

(1) Homogeneous ovarian morphology, with no cystic structures detectable in ovaries, reflects the very low sex-hormone stimulation of childhood;

(2) Microcystic ovarian morphology with several clearly outlined cysts, not exceeding 9 mm, present from the stage of biochemical puberty till the age of 10–12 years, mainly in premenarchal girls (Figure 2); and

(3) Macrocystic ovarian morphology where some cysts may exceed 9 mm (Figure 3). The number of cysts in this group is important to distinguish physiological conditions due to acceleration of sex hormone production, and the site of the cysts within the ovary is important to indicate pathological hormonal influences such as polycystic ovarian syndrome. Symmetrical bilateral ovarian growth has been noted with increasing age, correlating well with the increase in uterine length.

During the period between 10 and 12.5 years, ovaries are multifollicular or multicystic in the majority of girls and there is good correlation between ovarian volume and levels of follicle-stimulating hormone (FSH), luteinizing hormone (LH) and estradiol. For those below 10 years, the increment in follicular growth detected by ultrasound is related only to the level of FSH. Apter and colleagues[23,36] in recent studies have shown that sequences of maturation related to increase of ovarian volume begin just around the time of FSH increase, but before any signs of puberty appear, and correlate well with breast development stage 1. Breast development into stage 2 (telarche) is accompanied by a significant increase in FSH, LH and estradiol and on ultrasound presents with multifollicular or microcystic ovaries, when cysts reach 5–9 mm in size, marking the early pubertal but usually premenarchal phase. Our own results on maturational processes in the peripubertal period are very much in the same line, both for hormonal[4] and sonographic findings which fit well with the major happenings during female puberty (Figure 4c). We have performed endocrine assessment of 75 peripubertal girls, divided according to breast development stages (each group containing 15 girls), who were premenarchal in the first three stages. We first noted a marked increase in FSH, followed by further increases in FSH, LH and estradiol. Towards the end of puberty (breast stage 5), FSH reached a plateau and progesterone started to be present, all indicating maturation of both negative and positive feedback mechanisms (Figure 4a). Sonographic assessment was made of 105 healthy girls aged between 7 and 17 years (unpublished data – ongoing research project, National Singapore University). Premenarchal girls were judged by bone age and postmenarchal girls by gynecological age. A gradual increase in ovarian volume was noted throughout these years, but was more marked after 10 years (Figure 4b). Morphological changes may be even more marked, with homogeneous ovaries in all 7-year-old girls, gradually changing towards multicystic ovaries in all girls from the age of 11 years. By the age of 13 years, all the girls were postmenarchal and their ovarian texture started to change towards the normal adult morphology, particularly after the 3rd gynecological year. By the age of 16 or 17 years, only one out of all in each group still had multicystic ovaries. This suggests that by the 5th gynecologic year, ovaries reach their normal adult features. Sonographic changes, which closely correlate with the onset of puberty, may be useful in assessment of gonadal development during puberty and at times avoid the need for repeated hormonal investigations in follow up of pubertal development.

The mean number of five follicles exceeding 5 mm in diameter per ovary was found in most girls over 10 years. These ovaries differed sonographically from polycystic ovaries in which the stromal component is increased, and small cysts are located just under the capsule, which is thickened. In normal pubertal multicystic ovaries, the stromal component appears scanty. When the right and left ovaries were compared in size, they were similar, suggesting bilateral, even growth. Unilateral ovarian enlargement may indicate adnexal pathology and the need for further evaluation. There is a close correlation

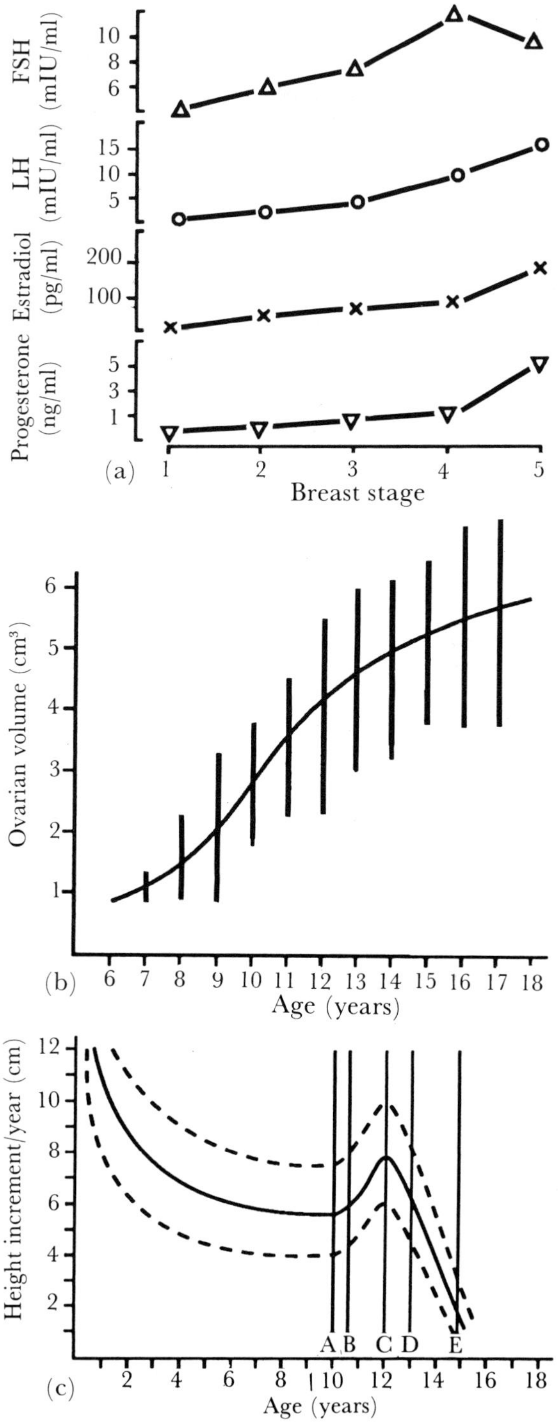

Figure 4(a) Patterns of increase of hormones in puberty; (b) increase in ovarian volume during puberty (mean ± 2SD); (c) pubertal growth. A, thelarche; B, pubarche; C, peak height velocity; D, menarche; E, ovulation

between uterine length and ovarian volume. Ovarian enlargement without a corresponding increase in uterine length may represent neoplastic ovarian growth indicating the need for further evaluation[37,38].

PRECOCIOUS PUBERTY

Sexual maturation of girls involves increase in growth, development of breast tissue, pubic and axillary hair, enlargement of the uterus and ovaries and onset of menstruation. However, development of secondary sexual characteristics or any other signs of maturation before the age of 8 years is considered precocious. This may occur in true precocious puberty or pseudo-precocious puberty. True precocious puberty involves early activation of the hypothalamic–pituitary–ovarian axis resulting in the increase in size and activity of the gonads and consequently leading to ovulation. In approximately 80% of girls, no etiology of precocious puberty is found. The sex difference in the response to GnRH suggests that the pituitary gonadotropes of prepubertal females are more sensitive to GnRH than those of prepubertal males. Further, prepubertal girls have a larger readily-releasable pool of pituitary FSH than have prepubertal or pubertal males[2,9]. This sex difference in sensitivity to GnRH and releasable FSH may be a factor in the higher frequency of idiopathic precocious puberty in girls and the higher prevalence of constitutional delayed adolescence in boys. Girls with precocious puberty have more advanced biological age when compared with children of the same chronological age. Clinical presentation in these girls shows typical sequences as in normal puberty, but at an earlier age. Bone age is much more advanced compared to chronological age. Nowadays, sonography gives very reliable findings supporting the diagnosis of true precocious puberty. The uterus increases as in normal puberty and has a pear-shaped appearance, but most typical are the findings of ovaries which are multifollicular–microcystic, or even macrocystic[39] (Figure 5). However, a variety of lesions may cause pseudo-precocious puberty, such as intracranial neoplasms, hydrocephalus, postencephalitis or post-

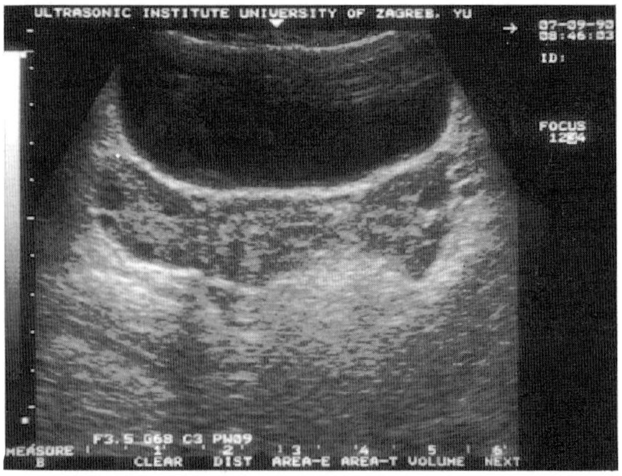

Figure 5 Longitudinal scan in 8-year-old girl with true precocious puberty showing uterus and ovaries reaching adult size with the texture of microcystic ovaries

traumatic scars, ovarian and adrenal hormone-secreting tumors, or exogenous estrogens. As some of these conditions are life-threatening, a clear-cut diagnosis of the etiology of precocious puberty must be obtained. The advent of sonography, showing the prepubertal appearance of the uterus and ovaries, has made differential diagnosis in such cases much easier.

True precocious puberty will not affect health and life, but will result in short stature due to osseous growth acceleration and bone closure. In the beginning, the sexually precocious person may be the tallest and heaviest among her peers, but due to fast epiphyseal closure, more than 50% will not reach a height of 150 cm. Interruption of fast and premature maturation and early treatment may help in achieving reasonably normal height (Figure 4c). The suppression of gonadotropin secretion by exposure to high doses of superactive GnRH analogs (GnRH-A) is now well established as a highly effective therapy for central precocious puberty due to down-regulation of the pituitary gonadotropin-secreting cells. Subsequently, the output of gonadal sex steroids decreases until it is again in the prepubertal range, followed by an arrest and even regression of the gonadotropin-dependent signs (gonadarche). Growth velocity and bone maturation are also reduced to prepubertal rates, thus improving the final height prognosis, which is the main goal of treatment.

The girls who may need treatment are not only those with true precocious puberty but also those with early and fast puberty, i.e. those in whom puberty has started close to the early physiological age limit but has progressed at an accelerated rate.

Numerous authors[40–42] have shown that pelvic ultrasonography before and during treatment is of great value. Before therapy, all girls had an enlarged uterus and ovaries which decreased to prepubertal dimensions during therapy. Ovarian cysts, present in all prior to therapy, disappeared within 6 months. Some workers have advocated the use of ultrasonography as an alternative means for follow-up of girls with precocious puberty undergoing treatment with GnRH-A, with the aim of avoiding numerous laboratory examinations[43].

MONITORING OF OVARIAN GROWTH AFTER ONCOTHERAPY

Sonographic monitoring of pelvic organs during pubertal maturation in girls undergoing oncotherapy for leukemia or other malignancies is important for long-term survivors and their future reproductive capacities. Several studies[44–46] have shown that the uterus and ovaries in the prepubertal stage (8–10 years) of these patients are smaller than those of controls. Ovarian ultrasonography has shown during puberty that subsequent growth is slower than in healthy females, leading to reduced ovarian volume in the most mature long-term survivors, though pubertal maturation of the hypothalamo–pituitary–ovarian axis is normal. That could be related to the decrease in the follicle numbers due to cytotoxic gonadal damage during childhood. Therefore, the slower pubertal growth of the ovaries may suggest the presence of long-term ovarian sequelae related to the previous oncotherapy.

DELAYED DEVELOPMENT OF PUBERTY

Delayed puberty, or primary amenorrhea (as we used to call it before), is defined as the absence of secondary sexual characteristics by age 14 years, or some secondary sexual characteristics and no menstruation by the age of 16 years. Causes are numerous and may be summarized as follows:

(1) *Chromosomal* (chromosomally incompetent gonadal failure) gonadal dysgenesis;

(2) *Gonadal* (chromosomally competent gonadal failure) true gonadal agenesis;

(3) *Hypothalamo–pituitary* panhypopituitarism, partial pituitarism, Kallman's syndrome, prepubertal polycystic ovarian syndrome;

(4) *End-organ insensitivity* testicular feminization, resistant ovary syndrome;

(5) *Adrenal* congenital adrenal hyperplasia;

(6) *Gynatresia* congenital absence of uterus and vagina, vaginal septi, imperforated hymen; and

(7) *Delayed puberty* late maturers.

Primary amenorrhea is not a benign entity because:

(1) There is a high incidence of infertility. Our experience has found this in 36.7% of cases (genetic disorders, ovarian dysgenesis, Müllerian duct aplasia, etc.);

(2) Patients may need long-standing hormone replacement treatment, surgical procedures or, later, some form of ovulation stimulation and assisted reproduction when possible.

Ultrasonography has become an important diagnostic method in the majority of cases of delayed puberty, but especially in evaluating anomalies[47–49].

EVALUATION OF CONGENITAL ANOMALIES OF THE GENITAL TRACT

Utero-vaginal agenesis or Mayer–Rokitansky–Kistner–Hauser syndrome can be clearly demonstrated. A severely atretic uterus is identified as streak tissue with non-visualization of the endometrial echo. Total or partial vaginal agenesis may be differentiated similarly, by a thin uncanalized vaginal plate with the absence of the

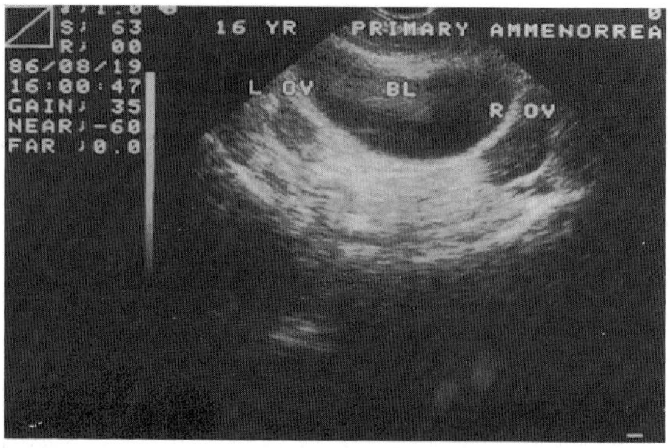

Figure 6 Transverse scan in 16-year-old girl with primary amenorrhea showing two seemingly normal, adult ovaries and absence of central uterine echo

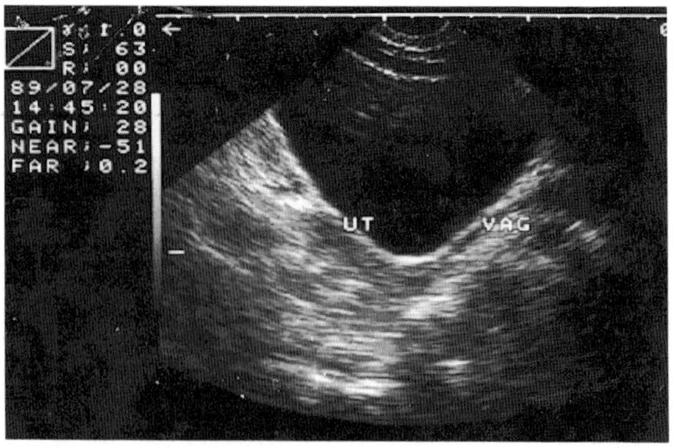

Figure 7 Longitudinal scan showing very small, infantile uterus (UT) and vagina (VAG) and no ovaries in a 13-year-old girl with ovarian dysgenesis

characteristic midline vaginal echo. Ovaries are visualized (Figure 6).

We had 17 cases with classical presentation of absent menstruation in otherwise normally developed pubertal girls. On rectal examination, the uterus was not palpable, and the hymen had a blind ending. Sonographic examination confirmed a clear diagnosis of uterovaginal dysgenesis. However, five of our cases had a small, rudimentary, non-functional uterus; no uterine cavity and endometrium were present. In our experience, from the psychological point of view, it may be better not to tell girls about the existence of rudimentary uteruses, as too much hope may be given regarding reproductive possibilities. In all girls ovaries were well visualized, and they were of normal adult morphology in 15 girls; two had classical findings of polycystic ovarian syndrome.

When streak gonads are suspected clinically, the absence or streaks of ovaries can be demonstrated by the non-visualization of ovarian tissue over both adnexae[50,51], but the uterus and vagina are visualized (Figure 7). Ovaries develop from primitive gonads in the presence of two X chromosomes and absence of a Y chromosome. If there are XY chromosomes, testes form. If testes form normally and function normally, the genitalia become male. If there is no Y chromosome, testes do not form and genitalia become female. However, sometimes in early fetal life, damage to testes may occur or they do not develop. Genitalia will then develop as 'XY gonadal dysgenesis', phenotypically female.

INTERSEX

There are other circumstancs where 46,XY individuals may have a female phenotype as in so-called 'androgen insensitivity' (previously used to be called 'testicular feminization')[1,2,6]. In this case, there is a failure of the tissue to respond to androgens but anatomically and functionally normal testes are present. Non-responsiveness of body androgen receptors will result in a female phenotype. However, during fetal life, Müllerian inhibitor will cause disappearance of the uterus, tubes and upper portion of the vagina. Similar findings will be found in rare cases of enzymatic failure of androgen synthesis. Such cases are clinically fairly easy to recognize, but final diagnosis can be confirmed by sonography, by identifying testicular tissue, as well as the extent of upper genital tract anomalies. In rare cases these conditions may present as partial androgen or enzymatic insensitivity, causing variations of ambiguous genitals where sonography is of great diagnostic help.

An extremely rare condition of unexplained genetic origin is true hermaphroditism with the presence of the tissue of both ovary and testis, in separate gonads or combined, causing again ambiguous genitals. Secondary sexual development may be heterosexual.

Excess of androgens as in congenital adrenal hyperplasia and adrenal tumor, masculinizing ovarian tumor or Cushing's syndrome, need prompt investigations which may be eased by sonographic assessment of the gonads and the presence or absence of parts of the genital tract, avoiding all surgical or more aggressive investigations. In particular, ambiguity of genitals in the neonate[52,53] requires urgent medical attention to settle the sex of rearing as early as possible. While the results of hormonal and genetic screening are awaited, ultrasound may have a particularly useful role, because the presence of a uterus and ovaries will point to a virilized female, whereas their absence suggests male pseudohermaphroditism.

Presence of testes or Y chromosome (streak gonads) in a phenotypic female has potential for malignant transformation and it is generally accepted that the testes need to be removed after pubertal development is completed even if gonads are just mere streaks of tissue.

The ability of ultrasound to detect fusion anomalies of the uterus depends on deformity of the external uterine contour, the recognition of two endometrial cavities, and the observation of the number of cervices and vaginal canals (Figure 8).

In all cases of genital tract anomalies, a thorough evaluation of the urinary tract must be done, as associated urinary tract anomalies are present in about 20% of these patients.

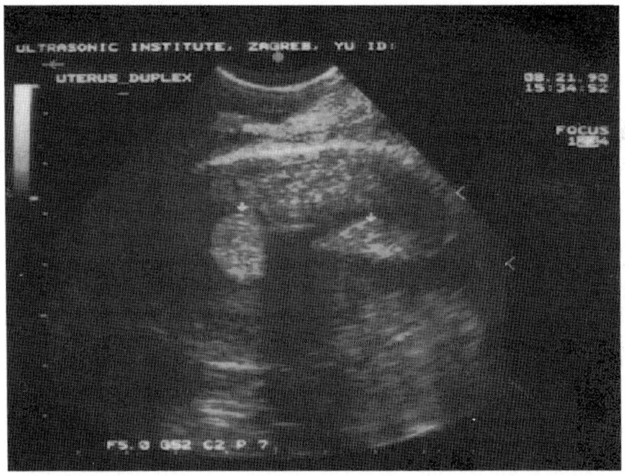

Figure 8 Transvaginal scan in a 17-year-old girl demonstrating two uteruses with endometrial cavities (and two cervices and two vaginas)

MENSTRUAL DYSFUNCTIONS IN ADOLESCENCE

Maturation of the hypothalamo–pituitary–ovarian axis, which is responsible for cyclical activity occurring during the menstrual cycle, is a gradual and relatively slow process[1,3,54]. It has been reported that up to 80% of menstrual cycles during the first year after menarche are anovulatory in nature. In most instances, menstrual dysfunctions in adolescence are short-lived or can be managed with simple medical treatment, but in some cases, the early manifestations of reproductive disorders may persist longer. In the Adolescent Clinic at the National University Hospital and School Health Clinic in Singapore, between mid-1984 and the end of 1991, a total of 1200 adolescents were seen with the following menstrual disorders:

(1) Secondary amenorrhea (41.1%);

(2) Primary amenorrhea (18.3%);

(3) Dysfunctional uterine bleeding (23.9%); and

(4) Oligomenorrhea (16.7%).

Adolescent girls with polycystic ovary syndrome (PCOS) were found in all the four major groups with menstrual disorders (24.3%), indicating that this syndrome occurs more often and earlier than once thought. Analysis of our 179 cases of adolescents with PCOS revealed the following:

(1) Most patients, except those with primary amenorrhea, were seen in their 3rd gynecological year;

(2) Acne and hirsutism were found in a very high proportion, 55% and 43% of girls, respectively;

(3) The ages of these patients ranged from 12–20, with 77.2% between 15 and 17 years, suggestive that symptoms of PCOS develop fairly early in adolescents;

(4) A large proportion of girls, 57.6%, were early maturers, having their menarche between 9 and 12 years old – not forgetting that 14% had primary amenorrhea;

(5) All the girls had menstrual disorders; and

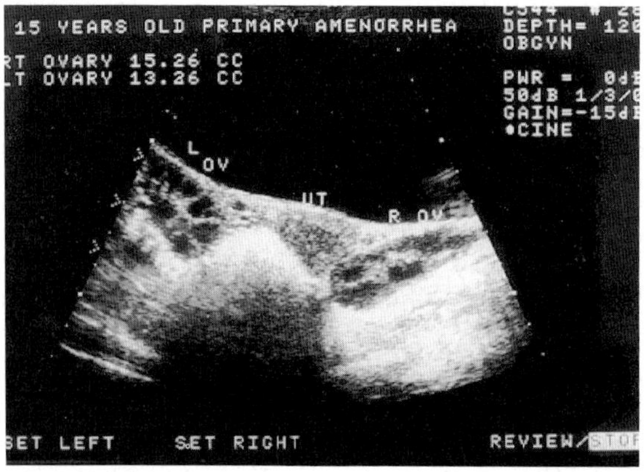

Figure 9 Transverse scan in a 15-year-old girl with primary amenorrhea showing typical features of polycystic ovarian syndrome: bilaterally enlarged ovaries, thickened capsule, dense stroma and multiple subcapsular cysts

(6) Raised testosterone levels and a reversed LH/FSH ratio were two common endocrine features in this group of girls.

Ultrasound scanning was of major importance for confirming a diagnosis of PCOS. Sonographic diagnostic criteria of PCOS are bilateral ovarian enlargement, thickened capsules, multiple subcapsular cysts of 8 mm or less, with a central ovarian matrix (Figure 9). The uterine–ovarian ratio may reach 0.8 to 1.0. These ultrasound features correlate well with biochemical parameters like the LH/FSH ratio and increased testosterone level. Among our cases ovarian enlargement varied depending on advancement of untreated PCOS. The majority of our adolescents (34.1%) had ovarian volumes of 10–15 cm^3. Further enlargement of 15–20 cm^3 was seen in 13.5% and in very advanced cases of PCOS ovarian volumes of 20–28 cm^3 were found (in 4.8%), interestingly more often in the right ovary.

The majority of patients (140) were treated with antiandrogen (cyproterone acetate) for 6 to 18 months. Following the treatment, acne was completely resolved in 44.5% of cases, improved in 47.8%, and remained the same in 5.5%. Varying degrees of improvement in hirsutism were noted in 21.4% of girls only following higher doses of cyproterone acetate. Cyclic function either was normalized or improved in 56.7% of girls.

Analysis of ultrasound scans, following treatment, showed a certain reduction of ovarian size, interestingly, more pronounced on the left compared to the right ovary. The mean volume of the right ovary before and after treatment was 13.1 cm^3 and 11.7 cm^3, respectively. For the left ovary, the mean volume before and after treatment was respectively 9.7 and 8.9 cm^3. Reduction of ovarian size was noted in 44.4% of cases and morphology reversed from PCOS features to multicystic in 31.1%.

Until recently PCOS was considered to be a problem confined to adult women; however, recent studies suggest that its onset may take place in adolescence[55–57].

It has been suggested that PCOS may be caused by early or exaggerated adrenarche leading to increased anabolism (obesity), increased androgen stimulation (acne and hirsutism) and inadequate feedback (chronic anovulation) presenting with various menstrual disorders.

Ultrasound plays an important diagnostic role not only in establishing diagnosis but for follow-up of response to treatment. Ultrasound is also a very valuable parameter for diagnosis, as well as follow-up of other menstrual dysfunctions where progression to PCOS may occur, impairing future fertility of adult women, bringing them into a higher cancer risk group and possibly giving rise to onset of hirsutism. Hormonal investigations may sometimes be omitted and diagnosis based on the clinical picture and ultrasound findings. For follow-up of such cases, similar guidelines can be adopted. These groups of menstrual dysfunctions are:

(1) *PCOS-like syndrome* – where not all features of PCOS are present. This endocrine entity is significantly influenced by early or fast maturational processes and often combined with excessive obesity (Figure 10);

(2) *Oligomenorrhea* – a very common menstrual dysfunction that seldom requires treatment. Ultrasound monitoring of cases with obesity or signs of androgenization can easily and reliably point to a group of patients in need of treatment;

(3) *Acne* – common during pubertal maturational processes, may suggest hyperandrogenism

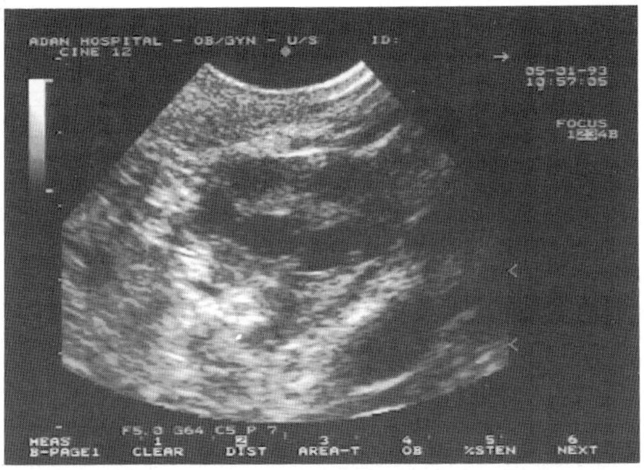

Figure 10 Transvaginal scan of enlarged right ovary (volume 16 cm^3) with thickened wall, minimal proliferation of central stroma and multicystic appearance in an 18-year-old girl with secondary amenorrhea, obesity and hirsutism

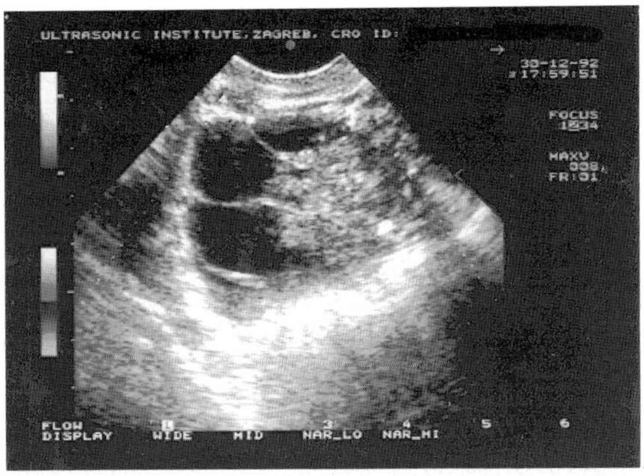

Figure 11 Transvaginal scan of an 18-year-old adolescent with subacute pelvic inflammatory disease showing cystic left ovary with extraovarian mass, irregularly outlined; typical appearance for tubo-ovarian complex

and PCOS, where ultrasound may be the only parameter needed to decide if hormonal treatment is needed; and

(4) *Hirsutism* – a very complex entity that has its onset in adolescence and may reliably be supported in diagnosis and management by ultrasonography.

OVARIAN TORSION

Ovarian torsion results from rotation of the ovarian pedicle on its axis, causing compromise of the arterial supply and venous drainage. The adnexae demonstrate increased mobility in young girls. Therefore, torsion of the ovary is usually noted before the onset of menarche[21,58].

Clinical symptoms are usually very distinct: acute abdomen or nausea, vomiting, diarrhea, abdominal and pelvic pain. Sonography may help in assessment of cases, particularly color flow Doppler, but diagnosis cannot be based on ultrasound only.

PELVIC INFLAMMATORY DISEASE

Pelvic inflammatory disease (PID) refers to the infection of the upper genital tract involving Fallopian tubes and/or adjacent structures. The earlier onset of puberty, changed moral norms, earlier onset of sexual activity often combined with promiscuity, and poor knowledge of contraception and protection from sexually transmitted diseases (STD), has led to epidemic proportions of the spread of both STD and PID among adolescents. Most infections occur in young persons of 15–24 years of age, but in the parts of the world where very young, early teenagers become sexually active, PID is hitting that age group as well. Most common causes are *Neisseria gonorrhoeae* and *Chlamydia trachomatis*. Possible sequelae are ectopic pregnancy, chronic pain and infertility. If not treated in time, tubes will become thickened and filled with purulent exudate, but if pressure increases, this may lead to pyosalpinx, and at a much later stage, hydrosalpinx. If inflammation progresses, a tubo-ovarian complex may develop (Figure 11) as periovarian adhesions fuse the inflamed tube and ovary into what eventually may lead to formation of a tubo-ovarian abscess. During the acute stage, clinical findings may be sufficient for diagnosis and fast treatment which is most important. However, if the condition goes into the subacute and chronic stages, ultrasonography may be very helpful in distinguishing clearly the pathological occurrences in the tubes and ovaries[59,60].

Ectopic pregnancy, a complication of PID, must be kept in mind where ultrasound may be useful in excluding the diagnosis[61,62]. As ectopic pregnancy mainly occurs in the Fallopian tube,

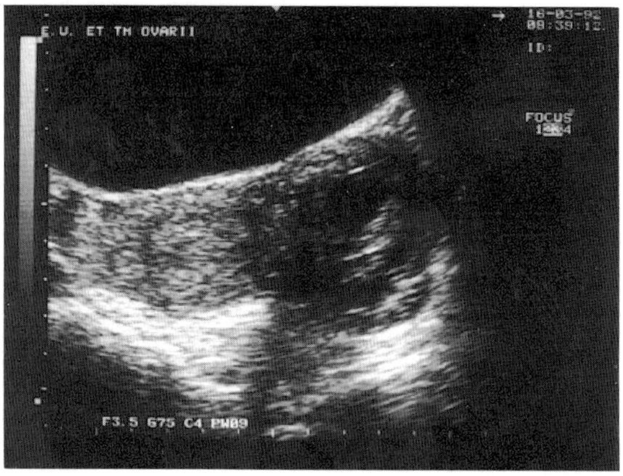

Figure 12 Transvaginal scan showing the typical echogenic rims of trophoblastic tissue surrounding ectopic gestation; normal ovary is visualized laterally

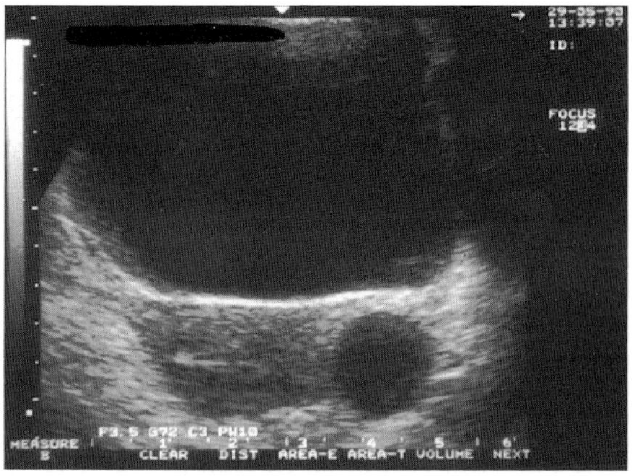

Figure 14 Corpus luteum with typical internal echoes and well defined borders in a 19-year-old girl with pelvic pain

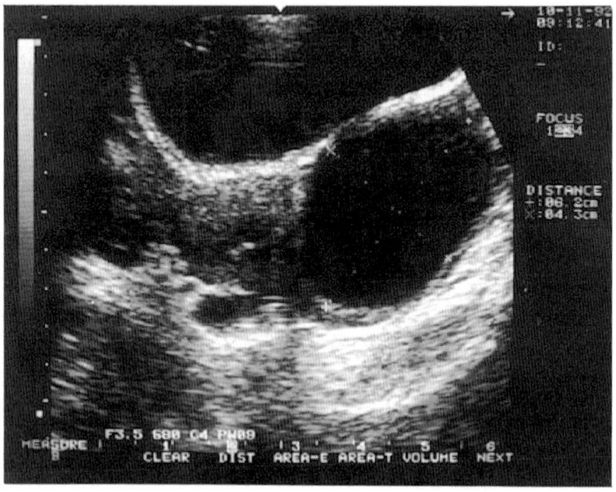

Figure 13 Transverse scan of clear, very anechoic follicular cyst on the left in a 20-year-old girl; uterus and right ovary normal

there is only the need here for a reminder that any mass near the ovary in a sexually active adolescent should be considered as a possible ectopic pregnancy (Figure 12).

OVARIAN CYSTS

The majority of ovarian cysts are either follicular or corpus luteal cysts. Follicular cysts result when the mature follicle does not ovulate. Functional cysts are frequent incidental findings on pelvic sonograms[23,63] (Figure 13). If they achieve a large size, they may be palpated as an abdominal or pelvic mass. Pelvic pain from hemorrhage, rupture, or torsion is another presentation. Follicular cysts are anechoic, whereas corpus luteal cysts frequently contain internal echoes due to intracystic hemorrhage. Septations or fluid–debris levels may be present or the cyst may look primarily hyperechoic (Figure 14). Distinction between a hemorrhagic cyst and other adnexal masses may not be possible on the initial sonogram. Color flow Doppler sonography can be useful in assessing such cases.

Small ovarian cysts are seen in many peripubertal girls, but larger cysts may be present in some postmenarchal girls. Ovarian follicular cysts demonstrate typical characteristics of a simple cyst (thin, smooth walls, completely anechoic, unilocular, increased through transmission of sound), and are usually no larger than 2.5 cm in diameter[64]. Simple cysts that are larger than 2.5 cm in diameter may still represent follicular cysts, but may also suggest other causes of ovarian enlargement, including neoplasms. Sonography is non-specific and cannot provide definitive diagnoses. Therefore, follow-up sonographic evaluations are performed to confirm resolution of the cyst, as functional cysts usually resolve after the next menstrual period. If the cyst resolves spontaneously, no further intervention is required.

Neonatal ovarian cysts have previously been considered uncommon. With the increased use of

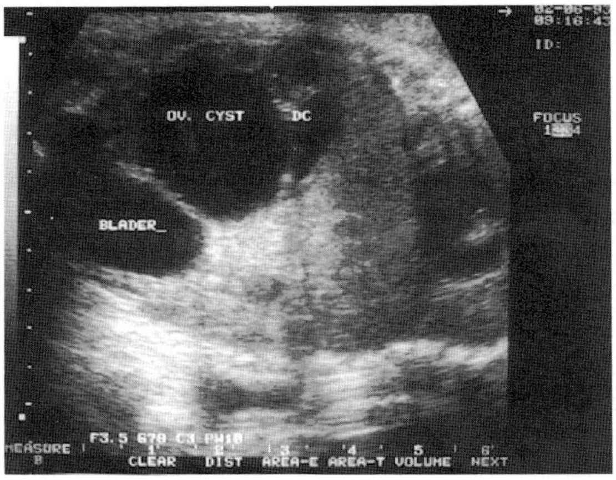

Figure 15 Antenatal scan at 35 weeks showing fetal ovarian cyst; anechoic cystic structure above the bladder in a female fetus

sonography, prenatal and postnatal detection of both small and large cysts has increased. Obstetric ultrasound enables those concerned with the pregnant patient to observe fetal growth and development. With the increase in sophistication of imaging techniques over the last 10 years, fetal organs can be carefully scrutinized. The abnormal fetal ovary can be seen early in the third trimester and fetal ovarian cysts can be diagnosed and followed in the late fetal, neonatal, and postnatal period[21,65,66]. The ultrasonographic diagnosis of a perinatal ovarian cyst has resulted in referrals to pediatric gynecologists and pediatric surgeons for management decisions. A dilemma for appropriate treatment results from the lack of experience with the clinical features and evolution of ovarian cysts developing in the perinatal period.

A cyst may be discovered incidentally on a prenatal sonogram (Figure 15) or postnatally in an infant with symptoms or a palpable abdominal mass. Discoveries of an ovarian cyst *in utero* have increased in frequency[67]. In many cases, recognition of the sonographic features of an ovarian cyst aids in establishing a preoperative diagnosis and in the obstetric management of the mother and postnatal treatment of the infant.

Ovarian cysts in fetuses and neonates are thought to be due to excessive maternal hormonal stimulation. These infants usually present with an asymptomatic abdominal mass unless the cyst undergoes torsion. Neonatal ovarian cysts are of variable size. The larger cysts may fill the entire abdomen. Neonatal cysts occasionally undergo spontaneous resolution[68]. Perinatal ovarian cysts may result from disturbed folliculogenesis. When the gonadotropins fall physiologically, the cyst can be expected to regress. The presence of small follicular cysts is a common and normal finding in neonatal ovaries. This has been demonstrated by autopsy studies, one of which showed small follicular cysts in 34% of stillbirths and neonates within the first 28 days of life[65]. Neonatal ovaries are functionally and anatomically similar to pubertal and adult ovaries. These small cysts, which measure 1–7 mm in diameter, regress spontaneously and are thought to result from excessive stimulation from maternal placental chorionic gonadotropin. Maternal hormones probably cause larger ovarian cysts in infants of mothers with diabetes, toxemia, or rhesus isoimmunization, all of which result in a greater release of placental chorionic gonadotropins.

GYNECOLOGICAL TUMORS

Pediatric gynecological tumors are rare. Although sonography plays an important role in the initial evaluation of these masses, computed tomography or magnetic resonance imaging is usually required for further characterization and staging of malignant neoplasms. The majority of ovarian tumors found in children or adolescents are benign. In fact, many series have found the overall malignancy rate to be only 15–32%. Only 2–5% of malignant pediatric tumors occur in the female reproductive organs. Of these, ovarian cancers are most frequent (65–70%). Ovarian malignancies are most likely to occur at puberty, and are mainly of germ cell origin[69]. As a special chapter in this book is devoted to ovarian tumors, we will mention here only a few benign ovarian tumors.

The mature teratoma or dermoid cyst is the most common ovarian tumor in the pediatric and adolescent age groups. It is a benign lesion that arises from pluripotential primitive germ cells and is composed of tissues derived from all three germ layers. Ectoderm is the predominant element. Adipose tissue, teeth and fragments of bone may also be found[70–72]. They are usually unilateral, although bilateral tumors can occur. Clinical presentation may result from a palpable mass, but is often an accidental finding in adolescence when ultrasound scanning is required for other reasons. We had five cases where PCOS was suspected and ultrasound revealed unilateral dermoids smaller than 5 cm in diameter (Figures 16 and 17). In all cases, laparoscopic cystectomy was performed, decreasing hospitalization to 1–2 days. One of the girls had recurrence of a dermoid cyst in the contralateral ovary 2 years later. It is important to repeat ultrasound examinations every year in adolescents with dermoid cysts. The sonographic appearance of mature teratoma is variable due to the heterogeneous internal architecture, predominantly solid complex mass, and at times complex mass with cystic portions or echogenic areas representing calcifications, teeth or fat.

Serous cystadenoma is a benign tumor rather uncommon in younger age groups. It is a large, cystic and epithelial tumor. One patient, otherwise symptomless, has seen us because of secondary amenorrhea and the tumor was found accidentally (Figure 18).

Ovarian fibromas have a variable appearance on sonography; they may be primarily cystic, solid or have a mixed echotexture. These tumors are rarely seen.

ACKNOWLEDGEMENTS

We would like to thank the staff of Adolescent Clinic in National University Hospital as well as School Health Clinic in Singapore for their assistance in our study of adolescent menstrual disorders. Equally we are thankful to the staff of the ultrasound section of Antenatal Diagnostic Centre in National University Hospital for their expert technical assistance. Without financial support from the National University of Singapore our study would not have been possible.

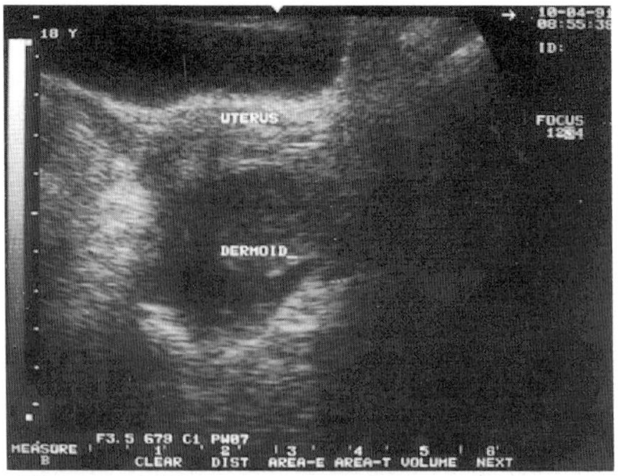

Figure 16 Transverse sectional scan showing complex predominantly cystic tumor on the left; a case of dermoid cyst

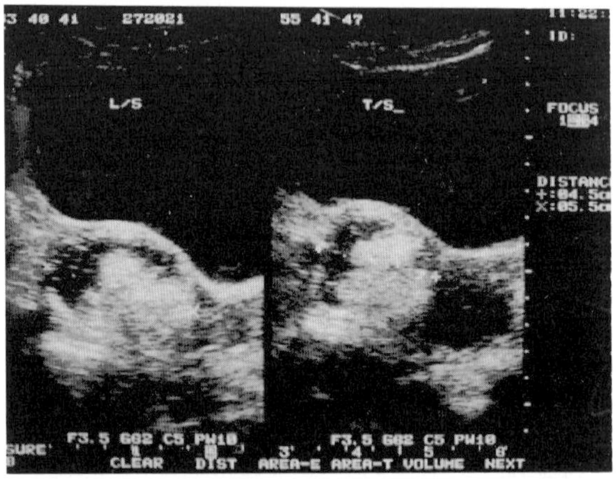

Figure 17 Transverse scan showing dermoid cyst. Note cystic and markedly echogenic components

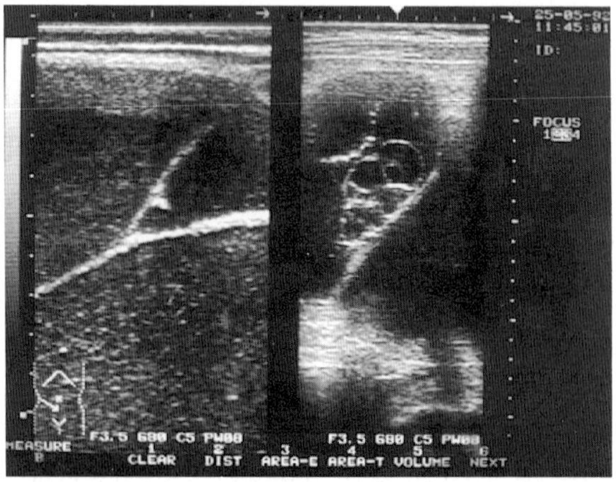

Figure 18 Transverse scan of ovary showing multilocular large cystadenoma with well defined septa in a 19-year-old asymptomatic girl seen for menstrual dysfunction

References

1. Huffman, J., Dewhurst, Y. and Caproaro, V. (1981). *The Gynecology of Childhood and Adolescence*, 2nd edn. (Philadelphia: W. B. Saunders Co.)
2. Dewhurst, J. (1982). *Integrated Obstetrics and Gynaecology for Postgraduates*, 3rd edn., pp. 16–33. (Oxford: Blackwell Scientific Publications)
3. Marchal, W. A. (1977). *Human Growth and its Disorders*. (London: Academic Press)
4. Dramusic, V. (1977). *Menstrual Disorders in Adolescence*. Doctoral thesis, Belgrade University
5. Dramusic, V. (1985). Gynaecology of childhood and adolescence. *Singapore J. Obstet. Gynaecol.*, **16** (2), 67–70
6. Dewhurst, J. (1980). *Practical Paediatric and Adolescent Gynaecology*. (New York: M. Decker)
7. Simpson, J. L. (1976). *Disorders of Sexual Differentiation: Etiology and Clinical Delineation*. (New York: Academic Press)
8. Kurjak, A. and Jurkovic, D. (1987). The value of ultrasound in the initial assessment of gynecological patients. *Ultrasound Med. Biol.*, **13**(7), 401–19
9. Grumbach, M., Grave, G. and Mayers, F. (1974). *The Control of the Onset of Puberty*. (New York: John Wiley and Sons)
10. Frisch, R. E. and Revelle, R. (1970). Height and weight at menarche and a hypothesis of critical body weights and adolescent events. *Science*, **169**, 397
11. Donovan and Van der Werf ten Bosch (1965). *Physiology of Puberty*, 1st edn., pp. 1–5. (Williams and Wilkins Company)
12. Tanner, J. M. (1962). *Growth and Adolescence*, 2nd edn. (Oxford: Blackwell Scientific Publications)
13. Greulich, W. W. and Pyle, S. J. (1959). *Radiographic Atlas of Skeletal Development of the Hand and Wrist*. (Stanford, California: Stanford University Press)
14. Lippe, B. M. and Sample, W. F. (1978). Pelvic ultrasonography in pediatric and adolescent endocrine disorders. *J. Pediatr.*, **92**, 897
15. Haller, J. O. and Schneider, M. (1980). *The Reproductive System, Pediatric Ultrasound*, p. 183. (Chicago: Yearbook Medical Publishers)
16. Hall, D. A., Hahn, L. E. and Fenucci, I. T. (1979). Sonographic morphology of the normal menstrual cycle. *Radiology*, **133**, 185
17. Funduk-Kurjak, B. (1988). Ultrasound diagnosis in child and adolescent gynecology. *Zdrav. Vestn.*, **57** (11), 128–31
18. Haller, J. O., Friedman, A. P. and Schaffer, R. (1983). The normal and abnormal ovary in childhood and adolescence. *Semin. Ultrasound*, **4**, 206
19. Hall, D. A. (1983). Sonographic appearance of the normal ovary, of polycystic ovary disease and of functional ovarian cysts. *Semin. Ultrasound*, **4**, 149
20. Lavery, Y. P. and Sanfilippo, J. S. (1985). *Pediatric and Adolescent Obstetrics and Gynaecology*, pp. 304–12. (New York: Springer-Verlag)
21. Sivit, C., Nussbaum-Blask, A. and Bulas, D. (1993). Pediatric pelvic sonography. *Ultrasound Q.*, **11**, (1), 59–93
22. Peters, H., Himelstein-Braw, R. and Mogens, F. (1976). The normal development of the ovary in childhood. *Acta Endocrinol.*, **82**, 617
23. Apter, D., Cacciatore, B. and Alfthan, H. (1989). Serum LH concentrations increase 100-fold in females from 7 years of age to adulthood as measured by time-resolved immunofluorometric assay. *J. Clin. Endocrinol. Metab.*, **68**, 53
24. Granberg, S. and Wikland, M. (1985). Comparison between endovaginal and transabdominal transducers for measuring ovarian volumes. *J. Ultrasound Med.*, **6**, 647–53
25. Hall, D. (1983). Sonographic appearance of the normal ovary of polycystic ovary disease and of functional ovarian cysts. *Semin. Ultrasound*, **4**, 149–65
26. Salardi, S., Orsini, L. and Caccian, E. (1985). Pelvic ultrasonography in premenarchal girls: relation to puberty and sex hormone concentration. *Arch. Dis. Child.*, **60**, 120–5
27. Morley, P. and Bennet, E. (1985). The ovarian mass. In Sanders, R. and James, A. (eds.) *The Principles and Practice of Ultrasonography in Obstetrics and Gynecology*, 3rd edn., pp. 473–515. (Norwalk, Conn: Appleton–Century–Crofts)
28. Leopold, G. (1987). Pelvic ultrasonography. In Sarti, D. (ed.) *Diagnostic Ultrasound Text and Cases*, 2nd edn., pp. 684–7. (Chicago: Year Book Medical)
29. Neiman, H. and Mendelson, E. (1988). Ultrasound evaluation of the ovary. In Callen, P. (ed.) *Ultrasonography in Obstetrics and Gynecology*, 2nd edn., p. 424. (Philadelphia: W. B. Saunders)
30. Cohen, H. L., Tice, H. M. and Mandel, F. S. (1990). Ovarian volumes measured by US: bigger than we think. *Radiology*, **177**, 189–92
31. Funduk-Kurjak, B. (1986). Ultrasound follow-up of uterine and ovarian growth at prepubertal and postpubertal age. *Arch. Mother Child Health*, **30**, 243–7
32. Muram, D. (1987). Pediatric and adolescent gynecology. In Pernol, M. L. and Benson, R. C. (eds.) *Current Gynecology and Obstetric Diagnosis and Treatment*, pp. 563–85. (Norwalk: Appleton & Lange)
33. Ivarsson, S. A., Nilson, K. O. and Persson, P. H. (1983). Ultrasonography of the pelvic organs in prepubertal and postpubertal girls. *Arch. Dis. Child.*, **58**, 352–4
34. Campbell, S., Goessens, L., Goswamy, R. and Whitehead, M. (1982). Real-time ultrasonogra-

phy for determination of ovarian morphology and volume. *Lancet*, **1**, 425–6

35. Orsini, L. F., Rizzo, N., Calderoni, P., Pilu, G. and Bovicelli, L. (1983). Ultrasound monitoring of ovarian follicular development: a comparison of real-time and static scanning techniques. *J. Clin. Ultrasound*, **11**, 207–13
36. Cicciatore, B., Apter, D. and Alfthan, H. (1991). Ultrasonic characteristics of the uterus and ovaries in relation to pubertal development and serum LH, FSH, and estradiol concentrations. *Adolesc. Pediatr. Gynaecol.*, **4**, 15–20
37. Muram, W., Emerson, D., Muram, D. and Bouldden, T. (1989). The sonographic features of the peripubertal ovaries. *Adolesc. Pediatr. Gynecol.*, **3**, 160–3
38. Sanfilippo, J. S. and Lavery, J. P. (1988). The spectrum of ultrasound: antenatal to adolescent years. *Sem. Repro. Endocrinol.*, **6**, 45
39. Salardi, S., Orsini, L. F. and Cacciari, E. (1988). Pelvic ultrasonography in girls with precocious puberty, congenital adrenal hyperplasia obesity or hirsutism. *J. Pediatr.*, **112**, 880–7
40. Stanhope, R., Adams, J. and Brook, C. G. D. (1985). The treatment of central precocious puberty using an intranasal LHRH analogue (Buserelin). *Clin. Endocrinol.*, **22**, 795
41. Brauner, R., Thibaud, E. and Bischof, P. (1985). Long-term results of GnRH analogue (Buserelin) treatment in girls with central precocious puberty. *Acta Paediatr. Scand.*, **74**, 945–9
42. Boepple, P. A., Mansfield, J. M. and Wiederman, J. M. (1986). Use of potent long-acting agonist of gonadotropin-releasing hormone in the treatment of precocious puberty. *Endocrinol. Rev.*, **7**, 24
43. Hall, D. A., Crowley, W. F. and Wierman, M. E. (1986). Sonographic monitoring of LHRH analogue therapy in idiopathic precocious puberty in young girls. *J. Clin. Ultrasound*, **14**, 331
44. Clayton, P. E., Shalet, S. M., Morris-Jones, P. H. and Price, D. A. (1988). Growth in children treated for acute lymphoblastic leukemia. *Lancet*, **1**, 460
45. Logghe, K. A., Bourguignon, J. P. and Craen, M. (1988). Factors contributing to the impairment of growth in children with acute lymphoblastic leukemia. *Horm. Res.*, **30**, 62
46. Maneschi, F., Fugardi, M. and Pagano, G. (1992). Sonographic monitoring of pelvic organs of leukemia survivors. *Adolesc. Pediatr. Gynecol.*, **5**, 177–81
47. Funduk-Kurjak, B. and Kurjak, A. (1982). Ultrasound monitoring of follicular maturation and ovulation in normal menstrual cycle and in ovulation induction. *Acta Obstet. Gynecol. Scand.*, **61**, 329–35
48. Cohen, H. L. and Haller, J. O. (1989). Pediatric and adolescent genital abnormalities. *Clin. Diagn. Ultrasound*, **24**, 187–215
49. Carrington, B. M., Hricak, M. and Nuruddin, R. (1990). Mullerian duct abnormalities. MR imaging evaluation. *Radiology*, **176**, 715–20
50. Massarano, A. A., Adams, J. A., Preece, M. A. and Brook, C. G. D. (1989). Ovarian ultrasound appearances in Turner syndrome. *J. Pediatr.*, **114**, 568–73
51. McDonough, P. G. and Byrd, J. R. (1977). Gonadal dysgenesis. *Clin. Obstet. Gynecol.*, **20**, 565–79
52. Lippe, B. M. (1979). Ambiguous genitalia and pseudohermaphroditism. *Pediatr. Clin. N. Am.*, **26**, 91–106
53. Canty, T. G. (1977). The child with ambiguous genitalia: a neonatal surgical emergency. *Ann. Surg.*, **186**, 272–81
54. Apter, D. Viinika, L. and Vihko, R. (1978). Hormonal pattern of adolescent menstrual cycles. *J. Clin. Endocrinol. Metab.*, **47**, 945
55. Yen, S. S. C. (1980). The polycystic ovary syndrome. *Clin. Endocrinol. (Oxf.)*, **12**, 177–207
56. Wakim, N. (1990). Polycystic ovarian diseases. *Adolesc. Pediatr. Gynecol.*, **3**, 183–7
57. Dramusic, V., Goh, H. H., Yang, M. and Ratnam, S. S. (1991). Menstrual dysfunction in adolescence. *Singapore J. Obstet. Gynaecol.*, **22**(2), 69–75
58. Schulz, I. R., Newton, W. A. and Clatworthy, H. W. (1963). Torsion of previously normal tube and ovary in children. *N. Engl. J. Med.*, **268**, 343–6
59. Swayne, L. C., Love, M. B. and Karasick, S. R. (1984). Pelvic inflammatory disease: sonographic–pathologic correlation. *Radiology*, **151**, 751–5
60. Timor-Tritsch, I. E. and Rotten, S. (1991). *Transvaginal Sonography*. (New York: Elsevier)
61. Timor-Tritsch, I. E., Yeh, M. N., Peisner, D. B., Lesser, K. B. and Slavik, T. A. (1989). The use of transvaginal ultrasonography in the diagnosis of ectopic pregnancy. *Am. J. Obstet. Gynecol.*, **161**, 157–61
62. Mahoney, B. S., Filly, R. A., Nyberg, D. A. *et al.* (1985). Sonographic evaluation of ectopic pregnancy. *J. Ultrasound Med.*, **4**, 221–8
63. Siegel, M. J. (1991). Pediatric gynecologic sonography. *Radiology*, **179**, 593–600
64. Neiman, H. L. and Mendelson, E. B. (1988). Ultrasound evaluation of the ovary. In Callen, P. W. (ed.) *Ultrasonography in Obstetrics and Gynecology*, 2nd edn., pp. 423–46. (Philadelphia: W. B. Saunders)
65. DeSa, D. J. (1975). Follicular ovarian cysts in stillbirths and neonates. *Arch. Dis. Child.*, **50**, 45–50
66. Carlson, D. H. and Griscom, N. T. (1972). Ovarian cysts in the newborn. *Am. J. Reprod.*, **116**, 664–72
67. Nusbaum, A., Sanders, R. and Hartman, D. (1988). Neonatal ovarian cysts: sonographic–pathologic correlation. *Radiology*, **168** (3), 818
68. Spence, J., Domingo, M. and Pike, C. (1992). The resolution of fetal and neonatal ovarian cysts. *Adolesc. Pediatr. Gynecol.*, **5**, 27–31
69. Scully, R. E. (1979). Germ cell tumors. In Hart-

mass, W. H. (ed.) *Atlas of Tumor Pathology*, pp. 226–86. (Washington D.C.: Armed Forces Institute of Pathology)

70. Surratt, J. T. and Siegel, M. J. (1991). Duplex Doppler sonography of the pediatric ovary. *Radiology*, **181**(P), 268
71. Surratt, J. T. and Siegel, M. J. (1991). Imaging of pediatric ovarian masses. *Radiographics*, **11**, 533–48
72. Wu, A. (1987). Sonography of pelvic masses in children: diagnostic predictability. *Am. J. Roentgenol.*, **148**, 1199–202

The ovary and genetics

5

L. Zergollern

There are many clinical entities in human medicine with ovarian changes, etiologically connected with abnormal quantity and quality of the human genome. These changes are primarily the result of gene or chromosome mutations. Gonadal dysgenesis and ovarian cancer are among the most important clinical and genetic problems related to the ovary which are challenging investigators and which are expected to be solved in the near future.

GONADAL DYSGENESIS

Gonadal dysgenesis is usually associated with monosomy of the X gonosome or structural abnormalities of both gonosomes. We know that the role of sex chromosomes (gonosomes) for early development of female and male gonads is important, but we still do not completely understand their action.

Our understanding of the etiology of females with an XY gonosomal pair and males with an XX gonosomal complement has increased, due to progress in human genetics, especially molecular genetics.

The discovery of testis-determining factor has facilitated our understanding of the mechanism by which most XY females and XX males originate. During male meiosis, instead of the crossover that usually occurs in the pseudoautosomal region, a crossover takes place between the X and Y chromosome-specific regions proximal to the pseudoautosomal region. Four sex chromosomes result from this meiotic event; two are normal X and Y, and two are abnormal. The abnormal X carries the testis-determining factor and for this reason, in spite of the existence of the XX gonosomal complement, the result is a phenotypically male human being, an XX-male, the product of an abnormal X–Y interchange. The complementary product is an abnormal Y that has lost testis-determining factor and the result of fertilization with such a Y gonosome will be a female with an XY complement and with dysgenic testes.

The sexual development of individuals with male (testicular) and female (ovarian) gonadal dysgenesis is very complicated and still unclear. The aim of this short survey is to try to explain some genetic facts about ovarian dysgenesis as the most common type of gonadal dysgenesis.

In the majority of patients with gonadal dysgenesis, female or male, the underlying cause is some chromosomal aberration; nevertheless, almost all types of gonadal dysgenesis may occur in individuals in whom no chromosomal aberrations are recognized. In these cases, submicroscopic chromosomal abnormalities, undetected mosaicism, abnormal inactivation of the X gonosome or some unknown etiological mechanism may play a role[1].

TURNER SYNDROME

Turner syndrome, X-monosomy, chromosome 45,X syndrome, gonadal dysgenesis of the Turner type, Ulrich–Turner syndrome, mosaic Turner syndrome, are the synonyms for a variable entity that includes many clinical features besides those originally reported by Turner in 1938 (ovarian streaks, stunted growth, webbing of the neck and cubitus valgus)[2].

Epidemiology

Turner syndrome and other conditions involving ovarian dysgenesis are considerably less common than their male counterpart, Klinefelter syndrome. This is because embryos with karyotype 45,X are very prone to abort. As we know, chromosomal abnormalities are the cause of as many as 50% of all first-trimester abortions;

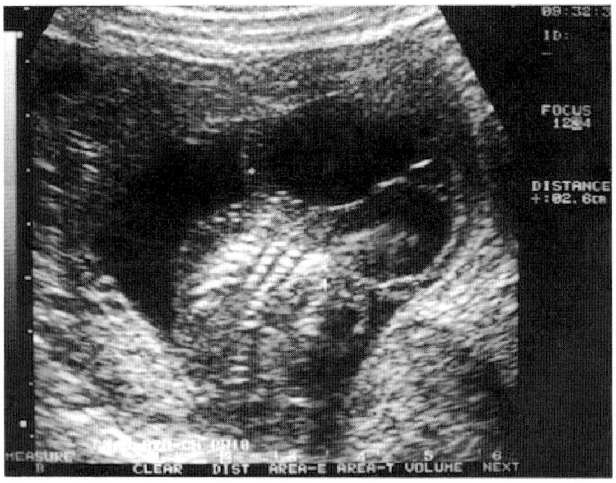

Figure 1 Cystic hygroma of the fetus with 45,X karyotype

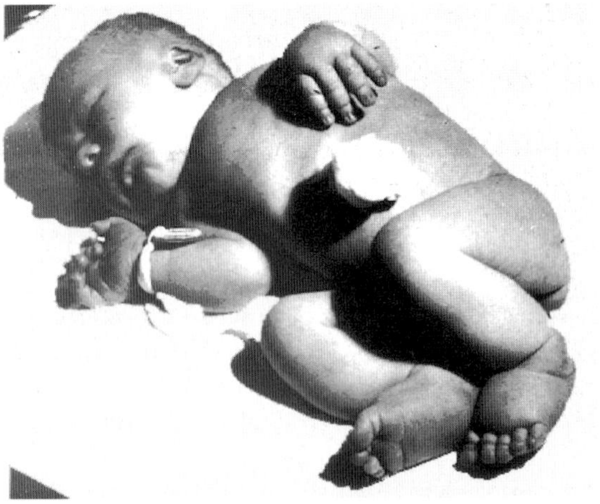

Figure 2 Lymphedema of the hands and feet in a newborn with Turner syndrome (45,X)

among these, one fifth have the 45,X chromosomal formula. If 15% of all pregnancies end in spontaneous abortion, and if one tenth of these are 45,X embryos, it means that 1.5% of all conceptuses are 45,X and that is a huge number. The minimum estimated occurrence of Turner syndrome is 1:5000 or 0.2 per 1000; in comparison, the frequency of XXX newborn females is 0.6 per 1000, the frequency of chromatin-positive newborn males is 1.3 per 1000 and of XYY males, 0.7 per 1000. The of recurrence for a sib of a patient with Turner syndrome is very low, unless it is an identical twin. There is no risk of a patient's child being affected, since 99% of patients with Turner syndrome are sterile. The reason for such a high incidence of abortion among 45,X embryos cannot be explained, especially in view of the relatively mild phenotypic anomalies in 45,X individuals.

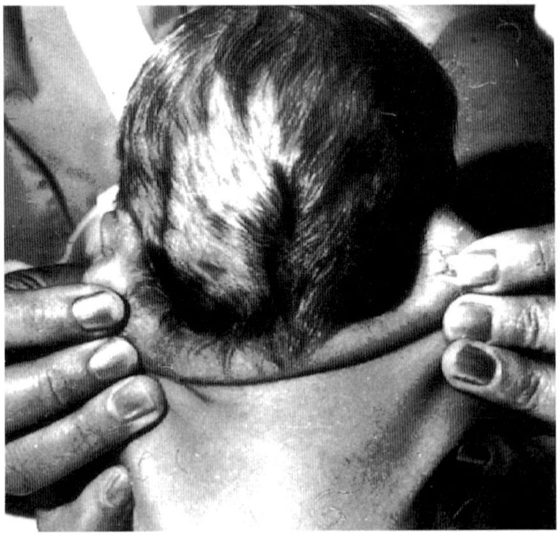

Figure 3 Pterygium colli in a newborn with the 45,X karyotype

Diagnostic criteria

Turner syndrome may be diagnosed cytogenetically in the preimplantation period. Ultrasonography offers prenatal diagnosis as well[3]. The edema seen in fetuses is frequently profound and may be detected by ultrasound as hydrops fetalis or cystic hygroma (Figure 1); the lymphedema results from atresia, hypoplasia and delayed development of the lymphatic system. After the birth, a female should be tested for the diagnosis of Turner syndrome if she has edema of the hands and feet (found in 40% of newborns with Turner syndrome) and excessive skin of the neck (webbed neck in 50% of cases) (Figures 2 and 3). The most common external features of the Turner syndrome phenotype are small stature (100%), often visible prenatally by ultrasonography and at birth; ptosis of the eyelids; hypertelorism; narrow maxilla (80%); micrognathia (>70%); malformed, most often prominent ears (80%); low posterior hairline with short neck (80%) (Figure 4); broad chest, with pectus excavatum and

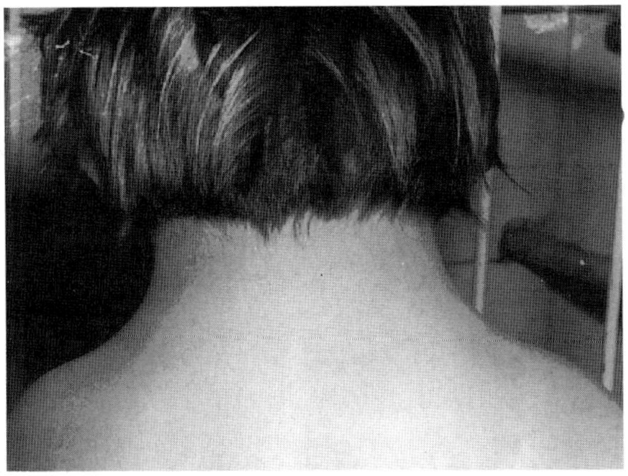

Figure 4 Pterygium colli and low posterior hairline with short neck

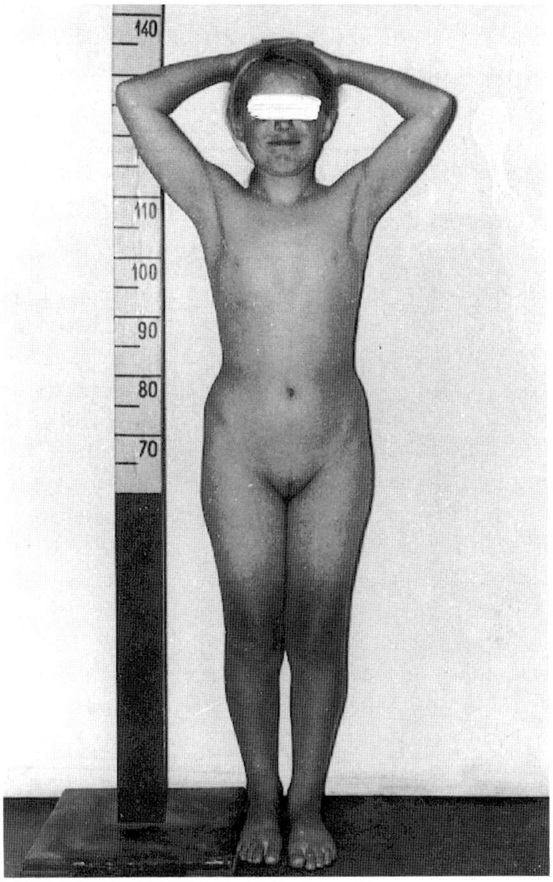

Figure 5 Thirteen-year-old girl with untreated Turner syndrome; marked pectus infundibuliforme and widely spaced hypoplastic nipples

widely spaced, hypoplastic or inverted nipples (>80%) (Figure 5); cubitus valgus (70%); narrow, hyperconvex and deeply set nails (70%); pigmented nevi (50%) and abnormal dermatoglyphic features with large hypothenar and fingertip patterns. Other clinical features are renal anomalies (horseshoe kidney and double or cleft renal pelvis in 60%); cardiac and aortic defects (bicuspid aortic valves and coarctation in 20–40% of patients, especially in those with webbing of the neck); hypertension (27%); hearing impairment (50%); short metacarpals and metatarsals of the fourth digits (50%); mental retardation (spatial inability); and primary or secondary amenorrhea[4]. Thyroiditis, diabetes mellitus and collagen-vascular disease are associated findings. Among complications, aortic dissection and gonadal neoplasia (in gonadal dysgenesis with karyotype 45,X/46,XY or with a structurally abnormal Y) have an increased lethal risk if not treated promptly.

Etiology

Etiology is connected with abnormalities (structural or numerical) of gonosomes. Structural changes may be very fine, at the molecular level. The most frequent basis for Turner syndrome is complete monosomy X. Mosaic individuals may be 45,X/46,XX in which case the effects of the monosomic cell line may be palliated by the normal cell line. Structural abnormalities of the X gonosome produce partial monosomy of either the p- or q-arms or both. When one of the short arms of the XX complement is deleted, the Turner syndrome phenotype is always present while normal gonadal development and function is usually maintained. However, the function is lost if the deletion extends to the proximal region of Xp11. The Xq monosomy creates gonadal dysgenesis when the breakpoint is at or proximal to Xq21; about 50% of patients with this type of karyotype show symptoms of Turner syndrome. Pure gonadal dysgenesis is observed when the breakpoint is at or distal to Xq22[5].

The most common finding in gonadal dysgenesis, monosomy X, may occur as a result of nondisjunction during gametogenesis in either mother or father; it may also be the consequence of errors in mitosis after fertilization. In testable cases the paternal sex chromosome (X or Y) is more often missing than the maternal X. This would suggest that a meiotic error in spermatogenesis or a loss of the paternal X or Y gonosome during abnormal mitosis is the more usual origin of Turner syndrome.

It is clear that monosomy X is very lethal prenatally; more than 95% of Turner syndrome conceptuses do not reach term. It is clear also that the early development of ovaries and oogenesis is normal in 45,X embryos and fetuses, but later on, the rate of primary oocyte degeneration appears to be increased compared with the degeneration of oocytes in normal XX females. The reason for the massive degeneration of oocytes remains unclear. Because of this event, it would be more precise to use the term gonadal degeneration instead of gonadal dysgenesis.

By puberty, girls with Turner syndrome have only a few (if any) oocytes in their ovaries. If the ovarian degeneration was not abundant, then the remaining oocytes help these females to develop secondary sexual characteristics and menses and to be fertile; the germ cell reduction is most likely less severe and oocytes persist to puberty and beyond. Mosaicism (45,X/46,XX) is another explanation for normal puberty and fertility of individuals with Turner syndrome. Earlier onset of climax is not rare in mosaic (mixoploid) Turner syndrome patients[6].

Patients with 45,X/46,XY (mixed gonadal dysgenesis) may have clitoral enlargement at birth and may virilize to some extent at puberty. Gonadoblastoma occurs very often and the gonads have to be removed early in childhood. The pathogenesis of this malignant transformation is not known[7].

Genetics

Chromosomal abnormalities

The etiology of the gonadal dysgenesis in Turner syndrome demonstrates the narrow connection between the phenotype of Turner syndrome and genotypic changes. The most frequent genotype abnormality is karyotype 45,X, i.e. complete monosomy X (80%) (Figure 6). The monosomy X may arise as a consequence of meiotic non-disjunction during gametogenesis in one parent or from loss of a sex chromosome during an early cleavage division of the zygote. Studies of X-linked genes (mainly of the Xg^a blood group antigen) in 45,X persons and their parents show that the missing sex chromosome is of paternal origin in 77% (X^m0) and maternal origin in 23% (X^p0).

Other X chromosome abnormalities have been described, all representing a less than complete absence of a second X gonosome. The variable deficiency of the sex chromosome is associated with a highly diverse modification of the classic Turner syndrome (45,X) phenotype.

Deletion of the short arm of gonosome X (Xp−) The patient's karyotype with this deletion is usually connected with short stature and typical stigmata of the Turner syndrome phenotype. Sometimes, these patients exhibit well-developed female secondary sex characteristics and have dysfunctional menstrual bleeding. Lack of the short arm, especially of the Xcen–Xp11 region (b region) may cause full-blown Turner syndrome. Since deletions of truly inactivated regions do not seem to cause any symptoms, it is supposed that the b region always stays active in a normal inactive X, but is inactivated in X chromosomes with deletions, especially in Xq− gonosomes. Patients monosomic for the Xp gonosome are always shorter than patients disomic for Xp.

Deletion of the long arm of gonosome X (Xq−) This deletion does not induce specific symptoms different from those caused by Xp deletions, although breakpoints distal to Xq25 do not give rise to any phenotypic anomalies except in a few cases of secondary amenorrhea or premature menopause. Most of the patients with 46,XXq− are taller than those with 46,XXp− karyotypes. The explanation for short stature seen in 43% of those with 46,XXq− would be that the inactivation of the deleted Xq may spread to the tip of the Xp. This event would explain the apparently variable behavior of the Xg and STS genes and the short stature of some Xq− carriers. The long arm of the X chromosome, Xq, has a 'critical region' (Xq11.2–q21), but the role of that region in ovarian development is still obscure. Cytogenetic analyses have previously shown that the critical region is retained in all structurally abnormal X

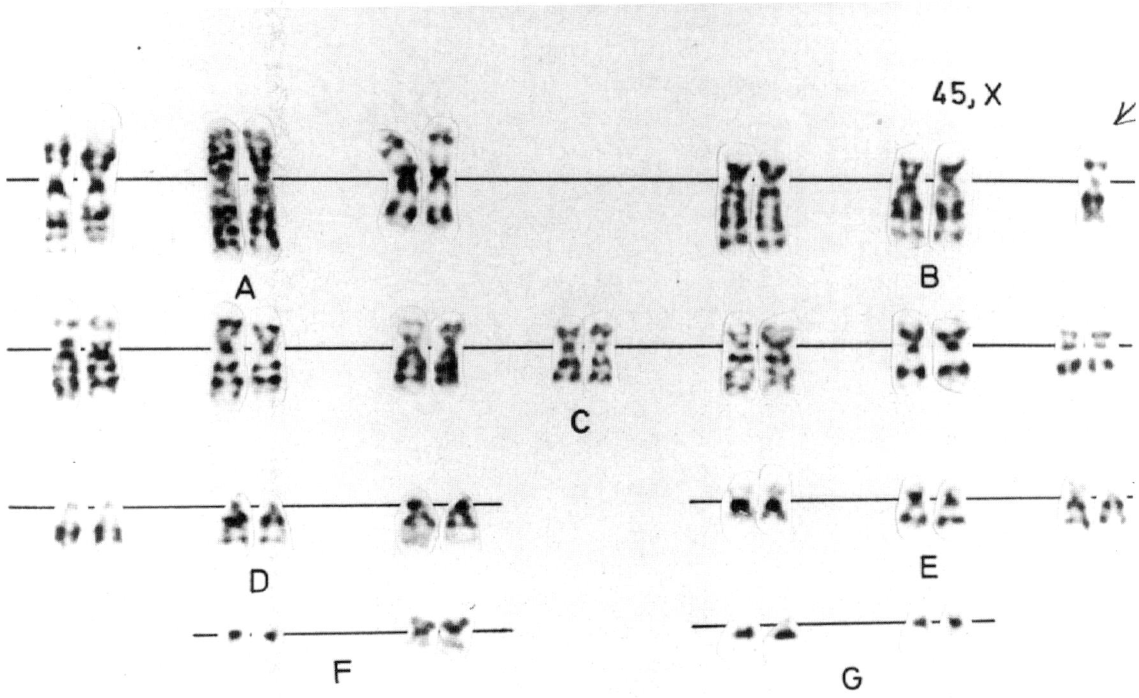

Figure 6 The most frequent karyotype in Turner syndrome (45,X)

chromosomes. From these observations the conclusion has been drawn that this critical region contains the locus controlling X inactivation. Structurally abnormal X gonosomes without the X− inactivation center would allow nullisomy, disomy or trisomy for genes on the X− gonosome and this condition is presumed to be non-viable[7].

Long arm isochromosome X – i(Xq) ± This genotype has a positive X chromatin pattern with larger Barr-bodies. The phenotype does not deviate from the typical form; some somatic anomalies such as lymphedema of the hands and feet, webbed neck, and coarctation of the aorta are obviously less frequent in persons with the 46,Xi(Xq) karyotype (Figure 7). Sterility is the norm in women with the i(Xq) karyotype.

Ring chromosome X The karyotype of persons with gonadal dysgenesis of the Turner type may include this chromosome (Figure 8). Sometimes it is impossible to differentiate between a small marker chromosome, a Y-ring chromosome (r(Y)) and an X-ring chromosome (r(X)) by conventional cytogenetic techniques, including high-resolution banding, especially if they are small. However, differentiation is now possible with new technologies – restriction fragment length polymorphism (RFLP), Southern blot and the polymerase chain reaction (PCR). Fluorescent *in situ* hybridization (FISH) may also help in identification of small markers and r-chromosomes, separating r(X) from r(Y)[8,9]. This differentiation is very important. The hypoplastic (degenerated) gonad with r(Y) in its karyotype must be removed immediately because of the high risk of malignant transformation[10,11]. The high rate of mental retardation among girls with r(X) has a hypothetical explanation, the lack of lyonization of the r(X) due to loss of the X-inactivation center[12]. Persons with the cytogenetically different types of Turner syndrome have no mental retardation.

X chromosome mosaicism Karyotypes of Turner syndrome with very rich phenotypic varieties may

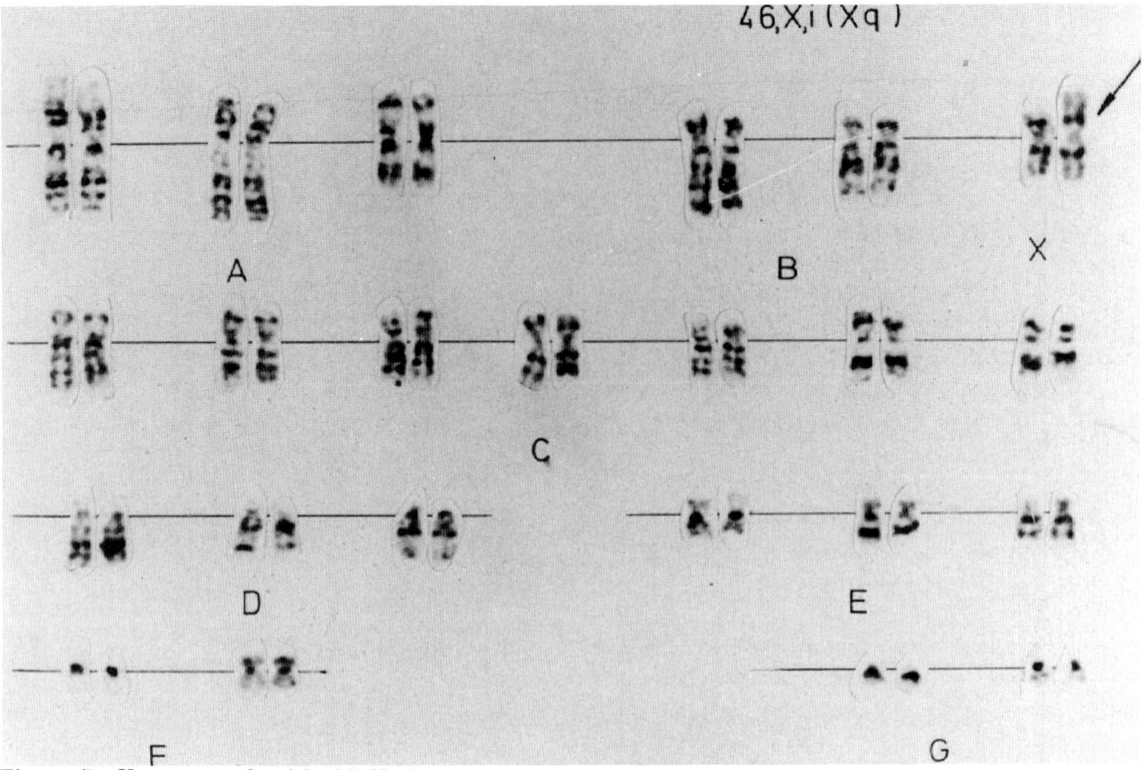

Figure 7 Karyotype of a girl with Xq isochromosome 46,Xi(Xq)

involve an X0 cell line in diverse combinations (45,X/46,XX; 45,X/46,XX/47,XXX; 45,X/46,XY) or an X0 cell line in an association with a structural abnormality of the X or Y chromosome (isochromosome X, X or Y deletion, or ring X or Y chromosome). In all cytogenetic combinations, the leading symptoms would be results of the 45,X genotype (X0 cell line) or the cell line genotype of some structural anomaly of the X chromosome.

Molecular genetics in gonadal dysgenesis

DNA analysis appears to be a useful and rapid way to screen for Turner syndrome. It could be an alternative to cytogenetic investigation in diagnosing growth retardation disorders or delayed puberty, especially when these events are not accompanied by the Turner phenotype. Diagnostic use of polymorphic DNA markers for the X chromosome could also help to reduce the time-consuming karyotype analyses needed. The M27β probe maps on the X chromosome to Xcen-Xp11–22 and detects heterozygosity with multi-allelic polymorphism in more than 83% of female subjects with Turner syndrome. Gicquel and co-workers[13] extracted genomic DNA from leukocytes of 49 Turner syndrome patients with different genotypes (45,X; 45,X/46,XX; 46,XiX(q) etc.), digested it with *Eco*RI or *Hind*III and analyzed it by the Southern blot technique. In 45,X patients, the authors found a single hybridization band of reduced intensity compared with the homozygous 46,XX control. Two hybridization bands of different intensities were seen in mosaic patients and 8% of Turner syndrome patients failed to be detected by Southern blotting.

Marker and minute chromosomes in Turner syndrome subjects, often originating from the Y chromosome, may show characteristic fluorescence and be very difficult to identify by conventional cytogenetic techniques. The fear that markers and minute chromosomes may be the parts of the Y chromosome predisposing to malignant alteration of dysgenetic gonads, was the reason that Medlej and co-workers[14] used the

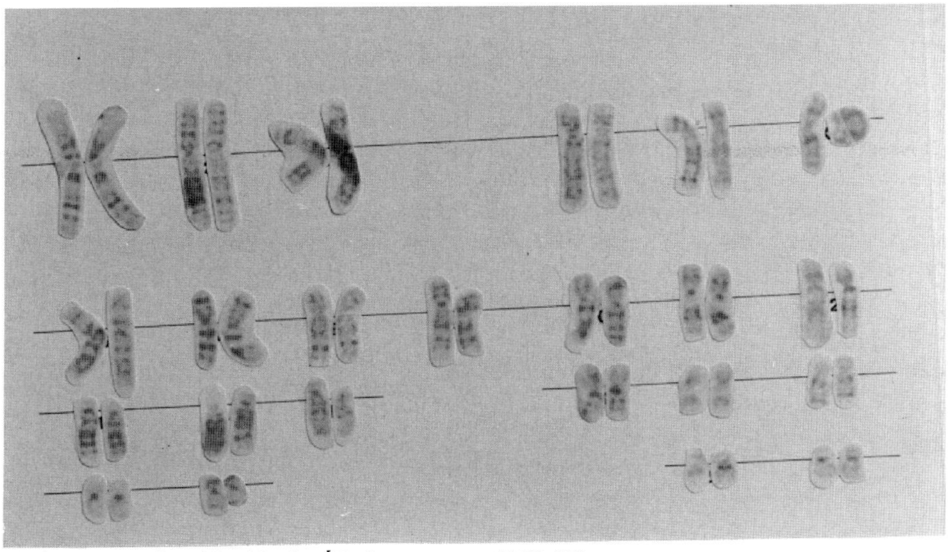

Figure 8 Karyotype of a girl with ring X chromosome 46,Xr(X)

PCR to expand the Y sex-determining region. The authors found it worth performing PCR in Turner syndrome patients with marker chromosomes, considering the potential risk of the presence and consequences of the presence of Y chromosome material in phenotypic females, which is known to increase the risk for developing gonadoblastoma. Molecular findings using the PCR technique help the differentiation between X-ring and Y-ring chromosomes, which cannot be differentiated by conventional and high-resolution banding methods[15,16]. Marker chromosomes may be identified using X and Y chromosome-specific α-satellite DNA probes and hybridizing them to locus DX23 by FISH[17,18].

Polymorphic DNA probes were also used in studies of the parental origin of the single X in 45,X Turner patients. Lorda-Sanchez and co-workers[19] found that the single X was paternal in origin in 22.2% of cases and maternal in 77.8%. Cockwell and associates[20], using a DNA RFLP technique, found very similar results in the parental origin of 45,X fetuses. Molecular genetic and cytogenetic findings suggest that *in vivo* selection of structurally altered sex chromosomes exists. Thus, the observation of apparent non-mosaic 45,X chromosomal complement in live-born individuals with Turner syndrome does not contradict the hypothesis that some degree of mosaicism is necessary for survival in early pregnancy[21]. The high fetal loss rate (greater than 95%) of 45,X embryos and fetuses has led to the hypothesis that fetal survival with the 45,X karyotype requires the presence of mosaicism[21,22]. However, mosaicism is very often not detected. Following the pregnancy of an older woman whose embryo was studied cytogenetically by the chorionic villus sampling technique, showing 45,X/46,Xr(X) mosaicism, and after the birth only showed the 45,X chromosomal complement, Kelly and co-workers[22] suggested that infants with the 45,X karyotype probably had mosaicism for a structurally abnormal X or Y chromosome during embryogenesis, but the abnormal cell line disappeared prior to birth.

Just and his group[23] performed studies on a series of fibroblasts from patients with numerical or structural aberrations of the X chromosomes. The fibroblasts were scored for the amount of mRNA for the ribosomal protein S4 gene (RPS4X). Just showed that RPS4X does not give rise to an expected type of haplo-insufficiency in Turner syndrome because it escapes inactivation even on structurally anomalous X chromosomes. They assumed that RPS4X was not the most prominent candidate gene for Turner syndrome[23].

There are many more investigations and experiments going on. Molecular genetics will surely help scientists to explain and understand the enigmas connected with Turner syndrome in the near future.

OVARIAN CANCER

Epidemiology

Ovarian cancer is the leading cause of gynecological cancer mortality in the western world. In the United States, it is the sixth most common malignancy in women; there are over 20 000 new patients with ovarian cancer detected every year[24]. Among newborn females, 1:70 will develop ovarian cancer in adulthood[24].

The highest incidence rates of ovarian cancer exist in northwestern Europe (13%). The age-specific incidence rate increases from 2:100 000 for women in their 20s to 55:100 000 for women at the age of 70 years. The highest number of new patients is found in the age group of 50–59 years[25].

The mortality for ovarian cancer is about 7.3–13:100 000. The age-adjusted mortality is 0.5:100 000 at the age of 20 and 45:100 000 at the age of 75[26]. In the last decades there has been a constant increase in the incidence and the mortality of ovarian cancer, but epidemiologic studies have not produced an adequate explanation for this.

Although there have been numerous advances in the diagnosis and treatment of ovarian cancer, the 5-year survival of patients has increased from 36% in 1975 to only 39% in 1990[27]. Over 90% of patients with Stage I cancer can be cured if the diagnosis of ovarian disease is made early, but most of the women continue to see their gynecologists for the first time with the advanced stage of disease (III–IV), when the prognosis is poor in spite of appropriate, but late start of treatment[27].

The best way to prevent ovarian cancer and reduce its mortality rate should be the use of early-stage screening methods. Today, the most effective method is the safe transvaginal sonography screening test. According to van Nagell and coworkers[28], transvaginal sonography screening should be offered to all menopausal women (over 50 years). The exceptions are women with a positive family history of ovarian cancer in first- or second-degree relatives; they should undergo screening tests at the age of 30. The odds ratios for those with ovarian cancer in first- and second-degree relatives are 3.6 and 2.9, respectively, compared with no family history of ovarian cancer[29].

Unilocular cystic ovarian tumors, less than 5 cm in diameter, have a relatively low malignancy. Tumors with a complex morphological pattern, or with papillations, are associated with a high frequency of malignancy. The finding of increased vascularity in an ovarian tumor by the use of vaginal color flow Doppler, associated with an elevated serum level of CA-125, are very suspect signs of ovarian cancer[30,31].

Etiology

Environmental factors

The hypothesis that environmental factors may play an important role in the etiology of ovarian cancer was suggested by the observation that the most industrialized countries, with the only exception of Japan, have the highest incidence. The fact that Japanese women born in Japan and emigrating to the United States have the same incidence of ovarian cancer in the postmenopausal age group as American women, and that Jewish women born in the United States or in Europe and living in Africa have a higher incidence of ovarian cancer than Jewish women born and living in Africa, might support the environmental hypothesis. There is an increased incidence of ovarian cancer among certain racial groups after migration to a country with a high incidence of the disease, possibly explained by the finding that women with higher education, higher incomes and rich alimentation (meat, animal fats, caffeine, artificial sweeteners and cream) more often have ovarian cancer than women with lower education and poor diet[32]. A decreased ingestion of vitamin A is also a risk factor in genesis of ovarian cancer[33].

The relationship between industrialization and the incidence of ovarian cancer suggested a possible connection between this tumor and products of industry, but there is yet little evidence to incriminate specific products[33]. The talc–asbestos group (hydrous magnesium silicates, talc powder) has been blamed as a promoting agent. This possible role of talc or asbestos particles in talc powder became less important from 1977 because of the decreasing inclusion of talc in cosmetics[34,35].

Because it is known that not everyone is equally susceptible to environmental factors, these variations in ovarian cancer susceptibility may be dependent on predisposition and constitution, which are genetically controlled features.

Exogenous hormones (conjugated estrogen, diethylstilbestrol) have no significant etiologic correlation with ovarian cancer. Menopausal estrogen use has no important influence in ovarian cancer, but if it is taken in a cyclic rather than continuous fashion for more than five years, then menopausal women may develop endometroid cancer of the ovary. The use of long-acting progesterones is without an increased risk for ovarian, endometrial or breast cancer[36–38]. Women using oral contraceptives have a significantly lower risk of ovarian cancer, directly related to the duration of application; this lower risk remains with long-term effect[39].

Viral infections were studied in connection with mumps virus and ovarian cancer. It seems that the mumps virus damages the ovaries causing premature depletion of oocytes in 5% of cases. A possible protective effect from mumps virus infection was suggested by West[40]. Rubella infection in girls between the ages of 12 and 18 years, however, increases the risk of ovarian cancer fourfold[32]; there is no increased risk if the infection occurs in childhood.

Irradiation of pelvic organs was associated with no increased incidence of ovarian carcinoma in a study of women who underwent radiation therapy[41].

Genetics

Human carcinogenesis is a multiphase process which results in the accumulation of a number of genetic changes within a single cell finally converting a normal cell to its malignant counterpart.

Family aggregation of ovarian cancer

Although the true etiology of ovarian cancer is still unknown, the most important known risk factor is strong family history of several cases over three or four generations. The familial occurrence of ovarian cancer has several specific features:

(1) The tendency toward earlier onset (45 years)[42];

(2) The serous type of tumor (90–97%);

(3) The trend toward poorly differentiated adenocarcinomas; and

(4) A high percentage of bilateral onset of ovarian cancer (70–80%).

According to Lynch and associates[43] there are three different hereditary syndromes:

(1) Site-specific familial ovarian cancer syndrome – the women in these families are at risk of developing ovarian cancer only. Their mothers and sisters already have ovarian cancer;

(2) Breast–ovarian cancer syndrome – the female members in the families have breast and ovarian cancer, alone or in combination; if a mother or sister had ovarian or breast cancer, the daughter or sister has a 50% risk for ovarian cancer;

(3) Cancer family syndrome (CFS) – the members of that family, males and females, are at risk of developing colon cancer and other adenocarcinomas (ovarian, endometrial); the woman from the family with CFS may be at risk for ovarian cancer if one of her close relatives had one form of cancer.

Consistent with an autosomal dominant inheritance, these three familial syndromes have a risk of 50% in the female offspring of affected first-degree relatives. The risk appears to be highest in patients who have two or more first-degree relatives or a first-degree and second-degree relative known to have ovarian cancer[37,44].

Although the exact pathogenesis of these syndromes is not yet clear, three theoretical interpretations are feasible:

(1) There is a distinct genetic susceptibility of ovarian tissue to carcinogenic influence;

(2) There is a genetic defect that influences a hormonal imbalance which may be potentially carcinogenic;

(3) There is a genetic defect causing an altered immunological response resulting in ovarian cancer[32].

In the families with ovarian cancer risk syndromes, prophylactic oophorectomy is of major preventive interest; the dilemma whether or not to remove the ovaries in a young woman from an ovarian cancer-risk family still exists and it is not easy to determine how many will benefit from such a procedure. In the absence of a genetic marker, there is no possibility of genetic proof; if the mother has an autosomal dominant ovarian cancer with the gene or chromosomal marker for ovarian cancer, the chance of her daughters inheriting the same marker is 50%.

In general, prophylactic oophorectomy appears to be justified after termination of childbearing (>35 years), although even with this procedure the women remain at risk for carcinomas of extragonadal celomic epithelium[45–47].

Among some genetic syndromes there is a higher than expected incidence of ovarian tumors; for instance Peutz–Jeghers syndrome with granulosa cell tumor and cystadenoma, multiple basal cell carcinoma with ovarian fibroma, gonadal dysgenesis (45,X/46,XY; 45,X) with dysgerminoma and gonadoblastoma[48].

In this description of the etiology of ovarian cancer, all cell types have been included, but as the large majority of ovarian cancers are of epithelial origin, the incidence of epithelial ovarian carcinoma is nearly identical to that of ovarian cancers in general.

Endocrinological factors

Endocrinological factors cannot be separated from genetic factors because of the fact that the endocrine gland functions are controlled by many genes. Compared with normal subjects, women with ovarian cancer have an increased incidence of nulliparity, miscarriages and low number of pregnancies. Married but never pregnant women, in comparison to women who never married, also have an increased risk for ovarian cancer. The possible interpretation could be that the endocrinological status in pregnancy protects against ovarian cancer and that the lack of this protection puts infertile women at a higher risk. The second explanation could be that infertility and ovarian cancer are the result of the same gonadal condition. Women with ovarian cancer have fewer full term pregnancies, less total time breast feeding and difficulties with conception. In spite of some controversy about the problem, it seems that women with a late onset of menopause do not have an increased risk of ovarian cancer[41].

Genesis of ovarian cancer

Summarizing all given facts about the possible etiology of ovarian cancer, we have to acknowledge the importance and connection of incessant ovulation[49]. The hypothesis is that the ovarian surface acquires minor injuries with each ovulation which cumulatively could contribute to the development of an ovarian tumor. Cessation of ovulation by pregnancy or oral contraceptives (connected with low gonadotropin levels) interrupts the process of repeated ovarian trauma and may consequently protect against ovarian cancer, although undesired infertility in women who ovulate regularly increases the risk. The high gonadotropin levels in menopausal women seem to be related to the development of ovarian tumors.

Pathogenesis

Ovarian cancer pathogenesis is explained by the following theory. The first risk step towards malignant growth is the formation of inclusion cysts by entrapment of surface epithelium in the ovarian stroma. The second step is direct or indirect stimulation of the included epithelium by gonadotropins and extra- or intraglandular estrogen, resulting in differentiation, proliferation and sometimes malignant transformation[50]. The final impetus to malignant transformation is still unknown, but it is obvious that all factors that cause inclusion cyst formation, high extra- or intraglandular estrogen levels and high gonadotropin levels, make women at risk for ovarian cancer. Consequently, factors that may prevent one or more of these stimuli may protect against ovarian cancer.

Biomarkers

The excess of familial ovarian cancer beyond the number that might be expected by aggregation of epidemiological factors, has inspired an investigation for the genetic origin of ovarian cancer. The exploration of genetically determined biomarkers, such as blood group antigens, some enzymes and other serum markers, was one approach. In some studies, blood group A has been associated with increased risk. The individuals with blood group A do not recognize the A antigen and because of that they may have decreased recognition of ovarian neoplasms. ABO blood group has been significant as a risk factor in a wide variety of cancers including ovarian cancer[51–53].

The enzyme galactose-1-phosphate uridyl transferase, which catalyzes a rate-limiting step in the conversion of galactose to glucose, is another biomarker for ovarian cancer risk. Low levels of this enzyme induce elevated levels of galactose. Women with very high galactose levels often show a hypogonadotropic hypogonadal state. This state can be speculated to be a consequence of ovarian toxicity from very high galactose levels which lead to disruption of the gonadal–pituitary endocrine axis following the high excretion of gonadotropin. The high levels of gonadotropin, according to the hypergonadotropic hypogonadism hypothesis, may promote cell proliferation and subsequent oncogenesis[54]. This hypothesis has been investigated further. Women with galactosemia who have hypergonadotropic hypogonadism have not been found to be at elevated ovarian cancer risk[55].

Decreased levels of the enzyme α-L-fucosidase, influential in processing glycoproteins of the ABO and Lewis blood groups, have been connected with ovarian cancer risk. In three large pedigrees, family studies showed that relatives of patients with ovarian cancer also had lower levels of the enzyme, proportionate to their relatedness to the patient. This implies a genetic connection between ovarian cancer and α-L-fucosidase levels, as opposed to the low levels being an outcome of the ovarian cancer process. Wells and co-workers[56] proposed that a significant inverse correlation between α-L-fucosidase activity and the lipid-associated sialic acid plasma concentration may be a reason for ovarian cancer susceptibility.

Peptide growth factors

The recent discovery of peptide growth factors (PGF) and cancer-causing genes (tumor supressor genes and oncogenes) has provided an exciting opportunity to understand the molecular pathology of ovarian cancer. Peptide growth factors are heat- and acid stable, with low molecular weight; they are inactivated by reducing agents due to the presence of disulfide bonds. PGF have different names (epidermal – EGF, fibroblast – FGF and platelet-derived growth factors – PDGF), but they all stimulate proliferation of a wide group of normal cells in culture. It is supposed that PGF play a role in processes of normal cell growth and differentiation and that they are secreted into the region where they interact with special cell membrane receptors on different types of cells nearby. This phenomenon is called paracrine growth stimulation. The precise role of PGF in particular organs or systems remains unknown, although it has been demonstrated that the expression and function of PGFs and their receptors usually are deranged in human cancers. The number of ovarian cell surface receptors and their affinity to epidermal growth factors are similar in ovarian cancer cells and normal ovarian cells.

PGF produced by a cell interacts with receptors on the same cell (so-called autocrine growth stimulation). Two different growth factors, transforming growth factors α and β (TGF-α and TGF-β), act synergistically and cause the loss of cancer cell growth[57]. In an experiment by Berchuck and colleagues[57], with cultures of different ovarian cancer cell lines, one cancer cell line secreted latent TGF-β, which means that TGF-β acts as an autocrine growth inhibitory factor in this cell line. This finding, according to Berchuck, has to be confirmed.

To investigate ovarian cancer growth regulation, Berchuck and co-workers[57] have examined the role of PGF in growth control of normal human ovarian epithelial cells which are usually the native cells of ovarian cancer. The authors found that proliferation of normal ovarian epithelial cells was strikingly stimulated by EGF (located on chromosome 4) while the ovarian cancer cells were resistant to EGF[57]. In addition, insulin-like growth factors 1 and 2 (very likely produced by the ovary as well as EGF), had no effect on proliferation of ovarian epithelial cells. Epidermal growth factor combined with insulin-like growth factors resulted in greater stimulation of epithelial cell proliferation than when epidermal growth factor was used alone; it is probable that these three growth factors act to stimulate regrowth of epithelium after the ovarian surface disruption at ovulation[58].

Cancer genes

Genetic changes contributing to cancer transformation include altered gene function, altered expression of genes and loss of genes[24]. The discovery of protooncogenes was made in an attempt to characterize the genes responsible for malignant transformation of cells. The protooncogenes are divided into several functional groups: growth factors, growth factor receptors, G-proteins and nuclear binding proteins. The protooncogenes are required for normal growth and differentiation of a cell, but when changed, they function as transforming oncogenes which act generally in a dominant way.

The oncogenes and tumor suppressor genes of known function seem to be involved in regulation of differentiation, division and growth of cells. Many other genes, with the later mutations in them, may be important in progression of tumors and in development of later stages. Tumors need mutations of several different genes in order to become malignant; fewer mutations are needed for benign tumors.

The most important genes involved in ovarian malignancy are oncogenes and suppressor genes; the first type activate oncogenesis, while the second type inactivate this genetic event. More than 30 existing oncogenes in the human genome can become carcinogenic by:

(1) The overexpression of normal product without amplification, e.g. by loss of a controller element or increased RNA stability, etc.;

(2) The amplification of the oncogene itself; or

(3) The mutation of the gene to produce a gene product that has a greater transforming ability[59].

The alteration in a single allele of an oncogene can alter cells when the gene is activated by overexpression, translocation or mutation; oncogenes are therefore supposed to be dominant transforming genes. Specific oncogenes appear to be activated preferentially in some types of cancer; even the cancers of different patients differ with respect to cancer-gene activation.

The oncogenes can be classified into different families on the grounds of structural and functional characteristics. A vast family of oncogenes are the tyrosine kinases. There are two types of tyrosine kinases: the first act as cell-surface PGF receptors, the second are anchored to the inner surface of the cell membrane. Both of them phosphorylate and activate cellular proteins involved in signal transduction. The first, receptor kinases, are regulated by PGF, but relatively less is known about regulation of the non-receptor tyrosine kinases. The cytoplasmic serine–threonine kinases may act as oncogenes as well as the membrane-associated G proteins[57].

It is not clear whether the majority of oncogenes play a role in growth regulation and transformation of ovarian cancer. Many authors have examined expression of some tyrosine kinases – EGF receptor (*erb-B*), HER-2/neu (*erbB-2*) and *fms* (macrophage colony-stimulating factor, M-CSF)[57–59]. The authors have found that EGF receptor (*erb-B*) is expressed in both the epithelium and underlying stroma, but in advanced-stage ovarian cancer, the EGF receptor was expressed in 77% of samples only. The *erbB-2* gene is located on chromosome 17q21. Survival of ovarian cancer EGF-receptor negative patients was significantly better than that of patients who were EGF-receptor positive. Levels of normal HER-2/neu protein, produced by an overexpressed HER-2/neu gene, are increased in ovarian cancer.

One third of patients with ovarian cancer have overexpression of HER-2/neu and they have a poor prognosis. It is unclear whether overexpression of HER-2/neu is an early sign of carcinogenesis or a later phenomenon that points to metastatic potential[57].

Some patients with ovarian cancer have elevated serum levels of M-CSF; the M-CSF receptor (fms) is expressed by cancer cells, but not by normal ovarian epithelial cells. Expression of *fms* was also associated with elevated invasiveness in endometrial cancers. Even though not demonstrated to be oncogenically mobilized in ovarian cancer, if fms was provided by cancer or nearby cells, the ability for autocrine or paracrine growth stimulation would exist[57].

Different G proteins have been activated in human cancers due to point mutations. Mutations in *ras* genes as the part of G proteins have been noted in a representative number of human malignancies (colon and pancreas carcinomas, leukemias, epithelial ovarian cancer, cystadenocarcinoma). The family of N-*ras*, Ki-*ras* and H-*ras* oncogenes is most widespread. Amplification of some *ras* genes is described in human cancers; Ki-*ras* (located on chromosome 6p) is uncommon in ovarian cancer and may be amplified in 5–10% of epithelial ovarian cancers, more often in other types; H-*ras* gene amplification is very rare. Increased levels of non-mutated protooncogene products such as *ras*, which transduce signals of growth stimulation, may lead to transformation (similarly to receptor tyrosine kinases). The *ras* family of genes are thought to be transforming in dominant mode.

Amplification of *myc* genes that are the nuclear transcription factors, is also a common finding in a number of solid tumors including epithelial ovarian cancer (c-*myc* oncogene). Because of the small number of investigated patients, it cannot be determined whether a connection exists between c-*myc* amplification and biological behavior of ovarian cancer[57].

In spite of the fact that the results of investigating the involvement of different oncogenes in the etiology of ovarian cancer are far from satisfactory, there is the hope that with a help of new technologies (RFLP, PCR, etc.) we will be able to obtain more information about the mechanism by which the oncogenes and their products act.

Tumor suppressor genes

Tumor suppressor genes function to suppress cell proliferation. Loss or inactivation of both alleles removes the normal restriction of cell growth. Tumor suppressor genes have attracted significant attention in human genetics. According to the recent investigations, they usually act as recessive genes since generally both alleles must be inactivated to produce altered gene expression. Since inactivation of genes by mutation is more frequent than activation, mutations in tumor suppressor genes may play a significant part in the development of a tumor. The loss of small specific chromosomal regions in the tumor may indicate loss of the expression of products which normally regulate cell growth and differentiation, indirectly suppressing tumor development. Tumors can develop either from an inherited mutation in a gene (intragenic) on one chromosome with subsequent loss of the normal allele on the other chromosome, or from *de novo* somatic mutation in the gene of an otherwise normal person; in such a case, the tumor arises when loss of the normal allele takes place on the other chromosome from a chromosomal pair. Allele loss may occur by a number of different genetic mechanisms, such as mitotic recombination, deletion, uniparental disomy, genetic imprinting, etc.[60].

An inherited germline mutation means that there is only one normal copy of the gene in all cells and therefore malignancy is likely to be more frequent, with an earlier occurrence in those individuals. Germline mutations are most likely the cause of ovarian cancer in families with multiple cases.

There are probably numerous examples of allele heterozygosity loss associated with tumor suppressor genes; oncogenes are activated if a heterozygosity is lost for particular loci and the result of that event may be tumorigenesis.

In a situation when a germline mutation is found, the possibility of identifying a mutant gene and helping those at risk is greater. Investigating somatic allele loss in ovarian tumors also helps research for tumor suppressor genes.

Allele-loss investigation in cells of ovarian tumors is possible thanks to the DNA technologies. It is necessary to collect DNA from tumors as well as from normal tissue samples from the same person. The DNA is digested with a suitable restriction enzyme, separated by electrophoresis and then blotted onto nitrocellulose membranes and probed with sequences from the chromosome areas of concern. The tumor tissue sample must be free of normal tissue and should be from tumors of a clarified histological type; under these conditions the procedure will be effective[61,62].

Foulkes and co-workers[60] have investigated 30 malignant tumor/normal DNA paired samples to date for allele loss. Because of cytogenetic proof of deletion of part of the long arm in a significant proportion of ovarian cancer samples, and because of specific translocations, chromosome 6 was chosen. The authors have been able to show that the allele loss is mainly on 6q rather than 6p where the major histocompatibility complex genes lie; there were no tumors if only 6p was lost without 6q, and there was no allele loss in the benign or borderline ovarian tumors[60]. Some other authors have studied loss of heterozygosity in ovarian tumor samples, analyzing chromosomes 1p, 4p, 7p, 8q, 11p, 12p, 12q, 16p, 16q, 17p, 17q, 19p, and 19q, and they found loss of heterozygosity in more than 25% of cited chromosomes[61,62]. There was no significant loss on chromosomes 1q, 2q, 5q, 6p, 7q, 11q, 12p, or 22q. The loss of alleles on both long arms on the 17 chromosome pair was found in 43% of tumors sampled. The representative of suppressor genes, the p53 tumor antigen, was found in increased amounts in a wide variety of transformed cells. The p53 is involved in cell cycle regulation and has structural and functional similarities to the *myc* family of protooncogenes. The locus of p53 is situated on the terminal band of the short arm of chromosome 17 (17p13.105–p12), probably in exons 5 or 7[63].

Chromosomes 3p, 6q, 11p, 17p and 17q show the greatest degree of allele loss, but much of the work remains preliminary and more probes in DNA technologies need to be used in attempts to localize the regions of maximum allele loss accurately[27].

Genetic linkage studies

Classic studies of genetic linkage have been undertaken with the aim of finding regions of DNA that seem to be connected with the occurrence of ovarian cancer. If a susceptibility locus is localized on a chromosome near a genetic marker such as a blood group antigen or a well typified sequence of DNA, then the marker and disease susceptibility locus are expected to segregate together in a pedigree; this type of coinheritance is called genetic linkage. Families with a history of both ovarian and breast cancers have a susceptibility locus on chromosome 1p36 near the Rh blood group locus; the Rh blood group is tightly linked to the α-L-fucosidase gene which is a biomarker of risk for ovarian cancer. The combination of these factors in the same person may be very risky[27].

Cytogenetic changes in ovarian cancer

Cytogenetic studies of tumor cells have revealed the presence of chromosomal aberrations in the majority of human malignancies; consistent deletions, translocations and duplications have provided useful information regarding the location of genetic transformation concerning human carcinogenesis. Although carcinomas represent over 80% of human malignancies, there are relatively few cytogenetic facts concerning solid tumors in adults. Trent and Salmon were the first to report on the presence of a special chromosomal abnormality in ovarian cancer[64]. The authors noted frequent deletions on the long arm of chromosome 6. Specific translocation between 6q and 14q was discovered in some serous ovarian carcinomas. In the cytogenetic study of primary epithelial ovarian carcinomas (serous cystadenocarcinoma followed by endometrioid carcinoma, and mucinous cystadenocarcinoma) Gallion and co-workers[65] found normal chromosomes in poorly differentiated tumors, in tumors of low malignant potential and in grade I tumors. There were only occasional exceptions. In a few poorly differentiated tumors, the karyotype changes were multiple and very complicated; in contrast, in some tumors of low malignant potential, simple duplications of whole chromosomes (trisomy, tetrasomy, etc.) were the only chromosomal changes. Thus in most cases a normal cytogenetic finding of tumor cells may be explained either by the overgrowth of benign stromal cells or by the presence of changes too small to be detected by conventional cytogenetic procedures (e.g. tumor specific allelic losses on chromosomal segments of 6q, 11p and 17p in ovarian cancer).

In highly differentiated and malignant tumors,

a mean of seven diverse chromosomes per tumor had recognized abnormalities, mostly deletions, translocations, and partial or complete chromosomal additions[65]. Chromosomes 1 and 11 were the most commonly involved (84%); the frequent involvement of chromosome 1 is consistent with observations in most other solid tumors (lung, breast, colon, cervix). Abnormalities of chromosome 11 (structural changes) were present in 79% of invasive tumors. Abnormalities (structural and numerical) of chromosomes 3, 5, 7 and 14 were also noted in connection with ovarian cancer[65].

In cónclusion, one has to admit that further cytogenetic and molecular genetic studies of ovarian cancer should be done. They may give insight into specific genetic alterations involved in the pathogenesis of ovarian cancer and may also be very useful in the identification of patients at high risk.

References

1. de la Chapelle, A. (1990). Sex chromosomal abnormalities. In Emery, A. E. H. and Rimoin, D. L. (eds.) *Principles and Practice of Medical Genetics*, pp. 273–82. (London: Churchill Livingstone)
2. Turner, H. H. (1938). A syndrome of infantilism, congenital webbed neck, and cubitus valgus. *Endocrinology*, **23**, 566–74
3. Nicolaides, K., Shawwa, L., Brizot, M. and Snijders, R. (1993). Ultrasonographically detectable markers of fetal chromosomal defects. *Ultrasound Obstet. Gynecol.*, **3**, 56–69
4. Davee, M. A. and Weaver, D. D. (1990). Turner syndrome. In Buyse, M. L. (ed.) *Birth Defects Encyclopedia*, pp. 1717–19. (Oxford: Blackwell Scientific Publications)
5. Passarge, P. and Schmidt, A. (1983). Functional consequence of X-chromosome loss in the human female. In Sandberg, A. (ed.) *Cytogenetics of Mammalian X-chromosome*, Part B, pp. 301–20. (New York: Alan R. Liss)
6. Therman, E. and Susman, B. (1990). The similarity of phenotypic effects caused by Xp and Xq deletions in the human female: a hypothesis. *Hum. Genet.*, **85**, 175–83
7. Pettitgrew, A. L., McCabe, E. R., Elder, F. F. and Ledbetter, D. H. (1991). Isodicentric X chromosome in a patient with Turner syndrome – implications for localisation of the X-inactivation center. *Hum. Genet.*, **87**, 498–502
8. Jacobs, P. A., Betts, P. R., Cockwell, A. E., Crolla, C. A., Mackenzie, M. J., Robinson, D. O. and Youings, S. A. (1990). A cytogenetic and molecular reappraisal of a series of patients with Turner's syndrome. *Ann. Hum. Genet.*, **54**, 209–23
9. Cooper, C., Crolla, J. A., Laister, C., Johnston, D. I. and Cooke, P. (1991). An investigation of ring and dicentric chromosomes found in three Turner's syndrome patients using DNA analysis and *in situ* hybridisation with X and Y chromosome specific probes. *J. Med. Genet.*, **1**, 6–9
10. Krasna, I. H., Lee, M. L., Smilow, P., Sciorra, L. and Eierman, L. (1992). Risk of malignancy in bilateral streak gonads: the role of the Y chromosome. *J. Pediatr. Surg.*, **11**, 1376–80
11. Hassold, T., Oettay, D., Robinson, A. and Uchida, I. (1992). Molecular studies of parental origin and mosaicism in 45,X conceptuses. *Hum. Genet.*, **89**, 647–52
12. Fryns, J. P., Kleczkowska, A. and Van Den Berghe, H. (1990). High incidence of mental retardation in Turner syndrome patients with ring chromosome X formation. *Genet. Couns.*, **1**, 161–5
13. Gicquel, C., Carbol, S., Schneid, H., Girard, F. and Le Bouc, Y. (1992). Molecular diagnosis of Turner's syndrome. *J. Med. Genet.*, **29**, 547–51
14. Medlej, R., Lobaccaro, J. M., Berta, P., Belon, C., Leheup, B., Toublanc, J. E., Weill, J., Chevalier, C., Dumas, R. and Sultan, C. (1992). Screening for Y-derived sex determining gene SRY in 40 patients with Turner syndrome. *J. Clin. Endocrinol. Metab.*, **75**, 1289–92
15. Wegner, R. D., Scherer, G., Pohlschmidt, M., L'Allemand, D. and Gal, A. (1992). Ring Y chromosome: cytogenetic and molecular characterization. *Clin. Genet.*, **42**, 71–5
16. Lodie, E., Nemeti, M., Torfi, H., Poskanzer, L. B., Anderson, F. R. and Johnson, J. P. (1991). Identification of Y-chromosomal DNA in a Turner syndrome mosaic by polymerase chain reaction. *Ann. Genet. (Paris)*, **34**, 252–5
17. Tharapel, S. A., Wilroy, R. S., Keath, A. M., Rivas, M. L. and Tharapel, A. T. (1992). Identification of the origin of ring/marker chromosomes in patients with Ullrich–Turner syndrome using X and Y specific alpha satellite DNA probes. *Am. J. Med. Genet.*, **42**, 720–3
18. Koch, J., Kolvraa, S., Hobolt, N., Petersen, G. B., Willard, H. F., Waye, J. S., Gregersen, N. and Bolund, L. (1990). A case of 46,XX,r(X) (p1q1) diagnosed by *in situ* hybridization. *Clin. Genet.*, **37**, 216–20
19. Lorda-Sanchez, I., Binkert, F., Maechler, M. and

Schinzel, A. (1992). Molecular study of 45,X conceptuses: correlation with clinical findings. *Am. J. Med. Genet.*, **42**, 487–90

20. Cockwell, A., MacKenzie, M., Youings, S. and Jacobs, P. (1991). A cytogenetic and molecular study of series of 45,X fetuses and their parents. *J. Med. Genet.*, **28**, 152–5
21. Held, K. R., Kerber, S., Kaminsky, E., Singh, S., Goetz, P., Seemanova, E. and Goedde, H. W. (1992). Mosaicism in 45,X Turner syndrome: does survival in early pregnancy depend on the presence of two sex chromosomes? *Hum. Genet.*, **88**, 288–94
22. Kelly, T. E., Ferguson, J. E. and Golden, W. (1992). Survival offetuses with 45,X: an instructive case and an hypothesis. *Am. J. Med. Genet.*, **42**, 825–6
23. Just, W., Geerkens, C., Held, K. R. and Vogel, W. (1992). Expression of RPS4X in fibroblasts from patients with structural aberrations of the X chromosome. *Hum. Genet.*, **89**, 240–2
24. Editorial (1992). Genetic changes in epithelial ovarian neoplasia. *Gynecol. Oncol.*, **47**, 135–6
25. Greene, M. H., Clark, J. W. and Blayney, D. W. (1984). The epidemiology of ovarian cancer. *Semin. Oncol.*, **11**, 209–26
26. Amos, C. I. and Struewing, J. P. (1993). Genetic epidemiology of epithelial ovarian cancer. *Cancer*, **71**, 566–72
27. Cutler, S. J. and Young, J. L. (eds.) (1975). Third National Cancer Survey: Incidence data. *National Cancer Institute Monograph no 41*, pp. 775–82. (Bethesda: DHEW Publication (NIH))
28. Van Nagell, J. R. Jr, De Priest, P. D., Puls, L. E., Donaldson, E. S., Gallion, H. H. and Pavlick, E. J. (1991). Ovarian cancer screening in asymptomatic postmenopausal women by transvaginal sonography. *Cancer*, **68**, 452–62
29. McKusic, V. A. (1990). *Mendelian Inheritance in Man*, p. 701. (Baltimore: Johns Hopkins University Press)
30. Kurjak, A., Zalud, I. and Alfirevic, Z. (1991). Evaluation of adnexal masses with transvaginal color ultrasound. *J. Ultrasound. Med.*, **10**, 295
31. Kurjak, A. and Predanic, M. (1992). New scoring system for prediction of ovarian malignancy based on transvaginal color Doppler sonography. *J. Ultrasound Med.*, **11**, 631–8
32. Heintz, A. P. M., Hacker, N. F. and Lagasse, L. D. (1985). Epidemiology and etiology of ovarian cancer: a review. *Obstet. Gynecol.*, **66**, 127–35
33. Lingeman, C. M. (1983). Environmental factors in the etiology of carcinoma of the human ovary. *Am. J. Indust. Med.*, **4**, 365
34. Longon, D. L. and Young, R. C. (1979). Cosmetic talc and ovarian cancer. *Lancet*, **2**, 349
35. Roe, F. J. C. (1979). Controversy: cosmetic talc and ovarian cancer. *Lancet*, **2**, 744
36. Venter, P. F. (1981). Ovarian epithelial cancer and chemical carcinogenesis. *Gynecol. Oncol.*, **12**, 281
37. Centers for Disease Control Cancer and Steroid Hormone Study (1983). Oral contraceptive use and the risk of ovarian cancer. *J. Am. Med. Assoc.*, **249**, 1596
38. Piver, M. S., Baker, T. R., Jishi, M. F., Sandecki, A. M., Tsukada, Y., Natarajan, N., Mettlin, Cj. and Blake, C. A. (1993). Familial ovarian cancer. *Cancer*, **71**, 582–8
39. Hulka, B. S. (1983). Oral contraceptives: the good news. Editorial. *J. Am. Med. Assoc.*, **12**, 1624
40. West, R. O. (1966). Epidemiologic study of malignancies of the ovary. *Cancer*, **19**, 1001
41. Lingeman, C. M. (1974). Etiology of cancer of the human ovary. A review. *J. Natl. Cancer. Inst.*, **53**, 1603
42. Lynch, H. T., Watson, P., Lynch, J. F., Conway, T. A. and Fili, M. (1993). Hereditary ovarian cancer. *Cancer*, **71**, 573–81
43. Lynch, H. T., Guinis, M. A. and Albert, S. (1974). Familial association of carcinoma of the breast and ovary. *Surg. Gynecol. Obstet.*, **138**, 717
44. Lynch, H. T., Conway, T. and Lynch, J. F. (1991). Hereditary ovarian cancer: pedigree studies, part II. *Cancer Genet. Cytogenet.*, **53**, 161–3
45. Schweppe, K. W. and Beller, F. K. (1979). Prophylactic oophorectomy. *Geburtsh. Frauenheilk. D*, **39**, 1024
46. Fribourg, S. (1993). Should women with familial ovarian cancer undergo prophylactic oophorectomy? *Obstet. Gynecol.* **81**, 315
47. Kerlikowske, K., Brown, J. S. and Grady, D. G. (1993) Letters reply. *Obstet. Gynecol.*, **81**, 315
48. Bachman, G. A. (1990). Hysterectomy. A critical review. *J. Reprod. Med.*, **35**, 839–62
49. Fathalla, M. R. (1971). Incessant ovulation: a factor in ovarian neoplasia? *Lancet*, **2**, 163
50. Cramer, D. W. and Welch, W. R. (1983). Determinants of ovarian cancer risk. II. Interferences regarding pathogenesis. *J. Natl. Cancer Inst.*, **71**, 717
51. Bjorkholm, E. (1984). Blood group distribution in women with ovarian cancer. *Int. J. Epidemiol.*, **13**, 15–17
52. Osborne, R. H. and De George, F. V. (1963). The ABO blood groups in neoplastic disease of ovary. *Am. J. Hum. Genet.*, **15**, 380–8
53. Lynch, H. T., Schuelke, G. S., Wells, I. C., Cheng, S. C. and Kimberling, W. J. (1985). Hereditary ovarian carcinoma: biomarker studies. *Cancer*, **55**, 410–15
54. Cramer, D. W., Harlow, B. L., Willet, W. C., Welch, W. R., Bell, D. A., Sully, R. E. *et al.* (1989). Galactose consumption and metabolism in relation to the risk of ovarian cancer. *Lancet*, **2**, 66–77
55. Reichlin, S. (1989). Galactose consumption and risk of ovarian cancer (letter). *Lancet*, **2**, 565
56. Wells, I. C., Lynch, T. H. and Lynch, J. F. (1987). Alfa-1-fucosidase variant and lipid associated sialic acid in hereditary ovarian cancer. *Cancer Genet. Cytogenet.*, **25**, 247–51

57. Berchuck, A., Kohler, M. F., Boente, M. P., Rodrigez, G. C., Whitaker, R. S. and Bast, R. C. Jr. (1993). Growth regulation and transformation of ovarian epithelium. *Cancer*, **71** (suppl. 2), 545–51
58. Rodrigez, G. C., Berchuck, A., Whitaker, R. S., Schlossman, D., Clarke-Pearson, D. L. and Bast, R. C. Jr. (1991). Epidermal growth factor receptor expression in normal ovarian epithelium and ovarian cancer. *Am. J. Obstet. Gynecol.*, **164**, 745–50
59. Hunter, T. (1991). Cooperation between oncogenes. *Cell*, **64**, 249–70
60. Foulkes, W., Stamp, G. and Trowsdale, J. (1992). Molecular genetics of ovarian cancer. In Sharp, F., Mason, W. P. and Creasman, W. (eds.) *Ovarian Cancer: Biology, Diagnosis and Management*, pp. 17–22. (London, Glasgow, New York, Tokyo, Melbourne, Madras: Chapman & Hall Medical)
61. Lee, J. H., Kavanagh, J. J., Wildrick, D. M., Wharton, J. T. and Blick, M. (1990). Frequent loss of heterozygosity in chromosome 6q, 11, and 17q in human ovarian carcinomas. *Cancer Res.*, **50**, 2724–8
62. Ehlen, T. and Dubeau, L. (1990). Loss of heterozygosity on chromosomal segments 3p, 6q, and 11p in human ovarian carcinomas. *Oncogene*, **5**, 219–23
63. McKusic, V. A. (1990). Tumor protein p53 (TP53; p53). In McKusic, V. A. (ed.) *Mendelian Inheritance in Man*, 9th edn., pp. 952. (Baltimore: Johns Hopkins University Press)
64. Trent, J. M. and Salmon, S. E. (1981). Karyotypic analysis of human ovarian carcinoma cells cloned in short term agar culture. *Cancer Genet. Cytogenet.*, **3**, 279–91
65. Gallion, H., Powell, D., Smith, L., Morrow, J. K., Martin, A., van Nagell, J. R. and Donaldson, E. (1990). Chromosome abnormalities in human epithelial ovarian malignancies. *Gynecol. Oncol.*, **38**, 473

The ovary and assisted reproduction 6

F. G. Balen, A. H. Balen and S.-L. Tan

The advancement and wider availability of assisted conception therapies have occurred to a large extent as a result of developments in ultrasonography. Not only has the use of ultrasonography simplified the technique of oocyte retrieval, enabling transvaginal ultrasound-directed procedures to be performed under sedation instead of laparoscopic oocyte collection under general anesthesia, but ultrasound has also become the mainstay of monitoring follicular growth. Indeed the accuracy that is provided by ultrasound monitoring has led some centers to virtually abandon endocrine monitoring of ovarian stimulation by gonadotropins[1] (and unpublished observations). *In vitro* fertilization (IVF) is a successful therapy with cumulative conception rates that compare favorably with spontaneous conception in women of the same age[2,3]. We have recently analyzed the results of 5055 consecutive IVF cycles undertaken on 2735 patients and found that the cumulative conception and livebirth rates after five cycles were 54% and 45%, respectively, for women under the age of 35 years[2]. Ovulation induction therapies for anovulatory infertility also produce very favorable success rates. We have shown, in a series of 200 women who underwent 1227 consecutive cycles of induction of ovulation, that the overall cumulative conception and livebirth rates were approximately 62% and 54%, respectively, after six cycles of treatment[4]. Assisted reproduction has completed its formative years and should now be made more widely available to the large numbers of infertile couples who would benefit from it. Pelvic ultrasonography provides a reliable form of monitoring and is helping to simplify these successful treatments and to make them more cost effective[1].

In this chapter we shall outline the use of ultrasound in monitoring the ovarian response to stimulation and aiding oocyte retrieval procedures. The importance of correctly identifying ovarian morphology will be discussed. We shall touch upon some of the complications that might be encountered, such as ovarian cysts and the ovarian hyperstimulation syndrome and, finally, discuss some of the promising areas of ongoing research and development.

Transvaginal ultrasound examination of the pelvic organs is preferred to the transabdominal approach, as it not only obviates the need for a full bladder with its associated discomfort, but also allows high-frequency probes to be used, producing higher resolution and greater precision in measurements of the pelvic structures, follicular diameters and endometrial thickness[5]. It is especially advantageous in patients who are undergoing assisted conception as they commonly have lower abdominal scars, which impair the penetration of ultrasound. Furthermore, periadnexal adhesions tend to immobilize the ovaries deep into the pelvis and limit the elevation of these structures that normally occurs when the bladder is filled for a transabdominal scan. A recent study comparing transabdominal with transvaginal scanning demonstrated that the margins of the follicles were more sharply defined in 90% of cases when the transvaginal approach was used, compared with only 41% with a transabdominal approach[5]. The same study found that the numbers and sizes of the dominant follicles correlated better with the serum estradiol concentrations when transvaginal scanning was used[6].

OVARIAN MORPHOLOGY

We recognize in the ovary three distinct morphological appearances: normal (Figure 1), polycystic (Figure 2) and multicystic (Figure 3). Multi-

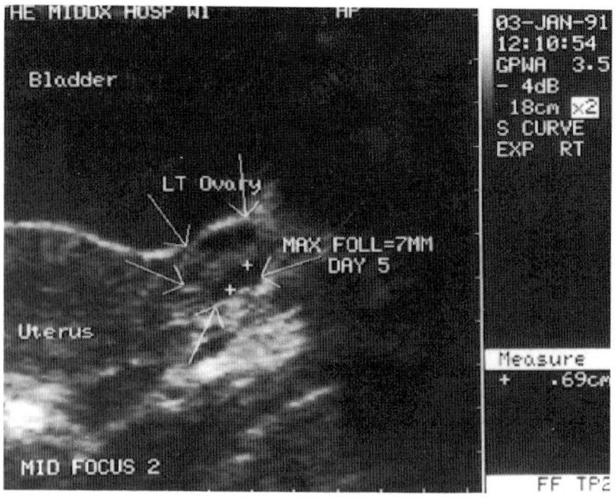

Figure 1 Transabdominal ultrasound scan of a normal ovary in the early follicular phase of the cycle. Arrows outline the ovary

cystic ovaries are characteristically observed in pubertal girls and women with amenorrhea related to weight loss[7]. These multicystic (or multifollicular) ovaries are normal in size or slightly enlarged, and contain six or more cysts that are 4–10 mm in diameter. In contrast to women with polycystic ovaries, the stroma is not increased. The multicystic ovary appears to develop as a consequence of reduced hypothalamic secretion of gonadotropin-releasing hormone (GnRH) which results in subnormal stimulation of the ovaries by the gonadotropins. The multicystic ovary has a normal response to exogenous stimulation, by either pulsatile GnRH or gonadotropins, and the ultrasound appearance of the ovary usually reverts to normal[7].

Polycystic ovaries are a separate entity and have a distinct response to induction of ovulation and ovarian stimulation for IVF. The association of enlarged, sclerocystic ovaries with amenorrhea, infertility and hirsutism was first described by Stein and Leventhal in 1935[8], now described as the polycystic ovary syndrome (PCOS). Since then, it has become apparent that polycystic ovaries may be present in women who are non-hirsute and who have regular menstrual cycles. Thus, a clinical spectrum exists between the typical Stein–Leventhal picture on the one hand (PCOS), and the symptomless situation on the other. Even patients described as having the PCOS exhibit considerable heterogeneity[9].

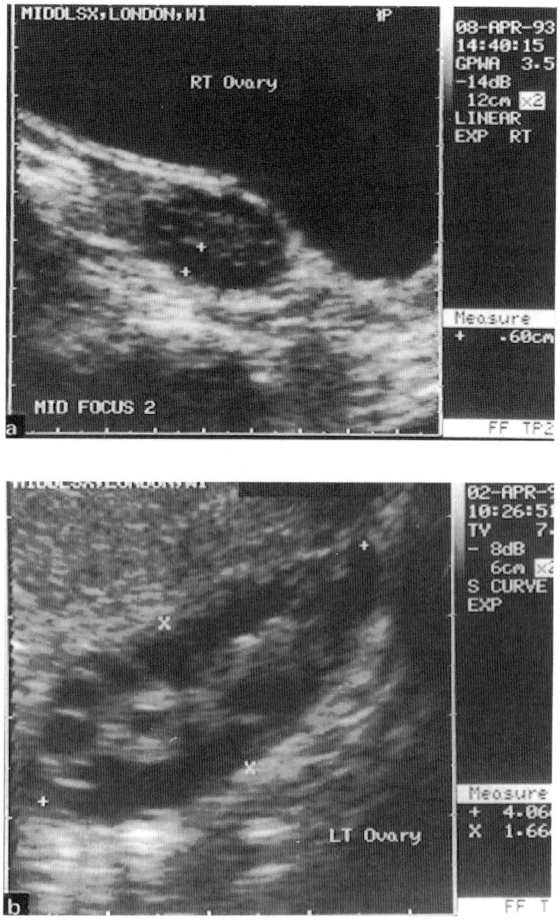

Figure 2 (a) Transabdominal; and (b) transvaginal ultrasound scans of a polycystic ovary

Therefore, the diagnosis of polycystic ovaries is best made, not on the clinical presentation, but rather on the ovarian morphology. With the advent of high-resolution ultrasound, identification of polycystic ovaries is simple, and ovarian biopsy, which is invasive and possibly damaging to future fertility because it can cause adhesions, is unnecessary. Ovaries are described as polycystic if there are 10 or more cysts, 2–8 mm in diameter, arranged around a dense stroma or scattered throughout an increased amount of stroma[7].

It is important to differentiate between polycystic ovaries and the PCOS. The former term describes the morphological appearance of the ovary, whereas the latter term is only appropriate when polycystic ovaries are found in association with a menstrual disturbance (amenorrhea or,

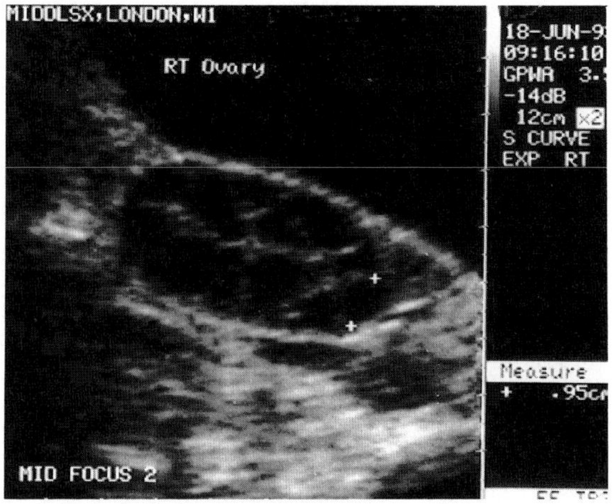

Figure 3 Transabdominal ultrasound scan of an unstimulated multicystic ovary. Note the absence of a thickened stroma, in contrast to the polycystic ovary

more commonly, oligomenorrhea), the complications of hyperandrogenization (seborrhea, acne and hirsutism) and obesity. The PCOS is also associated with endocrinological abnormalities and in particular with elevated serum concentrations of luteinizing hormone (LH), prolactin, estrogens and androgens. In about 40% of cases, plasma concentrations of LH are raised[9] and there is an increased ratio of LH to follicle-stimulating hormone (FSH). As with the clinical picture, these changes are variable and patients with PCOS may have normal endocrine parameters. Thus their measurement is not as helpful as ultrasound in making the diagnosis.

The prevalence of polycystic ovaries in women with ovulatory disorders has been well documented. Franks and colleagues[10] described a greater than 50% prevalence in patients presenting with oligo- or amenorrhea. With the use of high resolution ultrasound, it is nowadays apparent that as many as 87% of patients with oligomenorrhea and 26% with amenorrhea have polycystic ovaries[11]. We have also identified polycystic ovaries in women with hypogonadotropic hypogonadism who attended our ovulation-induction clinic[12]. Whilst these patients had no endogenous production of gonadotropins, they responded to stimulation in a characteristically 'polycystic' fashion, with a sudden growth of multiple follicles[12,13]. Polson and associates[14] found the prevalence of polycystic ovaries to be 22% in a volunteer 'normal' population. The prevalence in patients referred for IVF is not well known. We have studied over 500 patients who underwent IVF and found 34% to have ultrasound-detected polycystic ovaries[15].

Polycystic ovaries with or without clinical symptoms are therefore a common finding in patients referred for ovulation induction or IVF. Indeed, the patient's primary diagnosis often is not the PCOS but rather another cause of subfertility that necessitates assisted conception therapy[15]. It is of the utmost importance to make a careful assessment of the morphological appearance of the ovary prior to commencing ovarian stimulation as the presence of polycystic ovaries should alert one to the risks and complications that might occur (see below).

OVARIAN CYSTS

Besides making a careful assessment of ovarian morphology, it is necessary to perform a baseline ultrasound scan of the ovaries prior to commencing ovarian stimulation, in order to detect the presence of ovarian cysts[16]. There remains some controversy as to the significance of ovarian cysts with respect to their effect on the treatment cycle. None the less, it is obviously necessary to record the presence of any cystic structures prior to commencing ovarian stimulation, in order to monitor accurately the development of new follicles. Although it has been suggested that the presence of ovarian cysts reduces the success of the subsequent IVF cycle[17], other studies have failed to confirm this[18]. It also is necessary to distinguish between cysts that are present before the administration of hormonal agents and those which might arise as a result of hormonal stimulation, because of the exaggerated release of gonadotropins that occurs when GnRH agonist therapy is commenced[19].

We recently performed a study in which ovarian cysts encountered during IVF were divided into two categories: those present before and those present after GnRH agonist therapy was commenced[19]. The outcome of IVF was studied in both groups of patients who were randomized to either having cyst aspiration or having their cysts left alone[19]. In the patients who had a baseline cyst, unrelated to hormonal stimulation, the ovaries in which the cysts were aspirated developed a greater number of follicles and hence eggs, but there was no difference in the total number of follicles or eggs between the two patient groups. On the other hand, the patients who developed cysts as a result of GnRH agonist therapy had a comparable response to treatment in either ovary, irrespective of whether or not cyst aspiration was performed prior to ovarian stimulation[19]. Thus the aspiration of a unilateral cyst does not appear to improve either folliculogenesis or oocyte recovery rates.

If the patient is known to have endometriosis it is important to avoid aspirating the cyst, if possible, either before ovarian stimulation is commenced or during the oocyte retrieval procedure itself, because of the risk of infection. An endometrioma has the characteristic hazy, echodense appearance of blood in the cyst. Inadvertent, or unavoidable, aspiration of an endometrioma necessitates full antibiotic cover.

The situation is slightly different in patients who are undergoing ovulation induction for anovulatory infertility. In such patients, cysts are functional and secrete estrogens and progesterone. If a cyst is seen in these patients on a baseline ultrasound scan, the usual policy is to commence ovarian stimulation only after the patient has had a spontaneous menstrual bleed, which indicates that the endogenous secretion of ovarian hormones has reached baseline levels (unpublished observations). Further confirmation of this is provided by a thin (less than 7 mm) endometrium.

The baseline ultrasound scan also permits inspection of the other pelvic structures and might reveal the presence of hydrosalpinges, submucous fibroids (Figure 4) or even an elusive intrauterine contraceptive device – which on removal should cure the patient's subfertility!

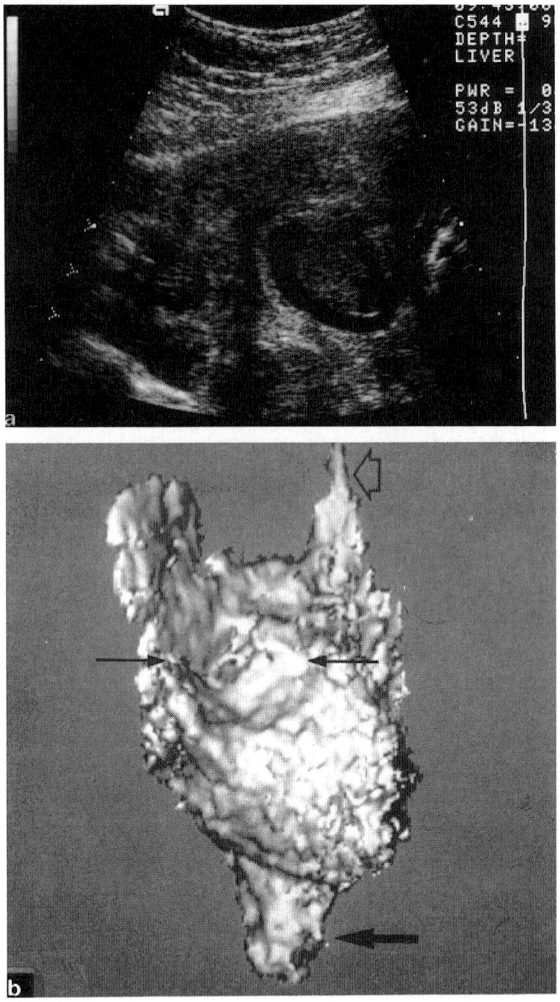

Figure 4 Submucous fibroid. (a) Plain transabdominal ultrasound after introduction of normal saline into the uterine cavity. The hypoechoic saline is shown surrounding the submucosal fibroid; (b) three-dimensional reconstruction of the saline-filled uterine cavity, illustrating the fundal filling defect (small arrows) caused by the submucosal fibroid. The cervical canal is delineated by the large arrow and the left cornu by the open arrow. Reproduced by kind permission of *The British Journal of Radiology*[79]

UNSTIMULATED CYCLES AND OVULATION INDUCTION CYCLES (Figure 5)

The first successful IVF pregnancies were achieved in spontaneous, unstimulated cycles[20]. The limitations of a natural cycle are the development of only one follicle, the possibility of not collecting an oocyte on the day of the retrieval procedure and the necessity for intensive monitoring in order to detect a spontaneous preovulatory LH surge. As pregnancy rates are higher with the transfer of several embryos[21] superovulation stra-

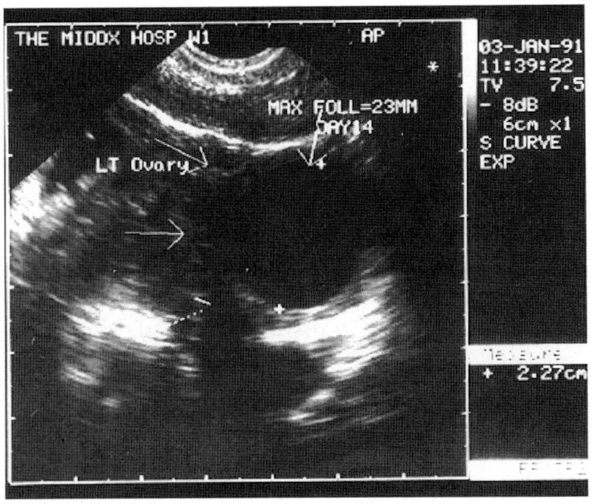

Figure 5 Transvaginal ultrasound scan of unifollicular development on day 14 of ovulation induction in a normal ovary, with a single 23 mm follicle. Arrows outline the edge of the ovary

tegies have been developed in order to increase the total number of oocytes available. There has, however, been a slight resurgence of interest in natural cycle IVF in recent years[22,23] because of a desire to avoid some of the complications of superovulation, such as multiple pregnancy and the ovarian hyperstimulation syndrome.

The resolution of transvaginal and transabdominal scans is 2–3 mm and 3–5 mm, respectively, and so small follicles can be visualized easily as echo-free structures, which are usually towards the periphery of the more echogenic ovarian tissue. The internal diameter of the follicle should be measured in three planes and the mean value calculated. The intraobserver standard deviation of transabdominal follicular measurement was reported in one study to be 0.6 mm and the interobserver standard deviation 1.2 mm, irrespective of the follicular diameter[24]. The 95% confidence limits for any particular measurement would therefore be ± 2.4 mm[24]. One would expect transvaginal measurements to confer even greater accuracy[25]. In spontaneous cycles, therefore, the small follicles can generally be visualized about 10 days before the day of ovulation (day − 10). By day − 5 there is usually a dominant follicle which then grows at a rate of approximately 2–3 mm daily until the day of ovulation.

Plasma estradiol concentrations correlate well with follicular diameter in natural cycles[26], although not in superovulated cycles[2]. The increase in circulating estrogen levels results in an increase in the overall uterine size and a thickening of the endometrium[27], which serves as a useful bioassay for follicular estradiol production.

Foulot and colleagues[23] reported a 22.5% pregnancy rate per cycle of natural-cycle IVF. They monitored the patients with daily ultrasound scans from day 9 or 10, depending on the length of the menstrual cycle. Human chorionic gonadotropin (hCG) was administered when the dominant follicle was > 18 mm, unless the daily assays of serum LH indicated the onset of a spontaneous surge, in which case the oocyte retrieval operation was brought forward[23].

In ovulation-induction cycles for *in vivo* fertilization, that is, either timed intercourse, donor insemination or intrauterine insemination with husband or donor semen, the first ultrasound scan is scheduled for day 8 of ovarian stimulation, that is, 1 week after the baseline scan. The result of this scan determines whether the dose of stimulatory drugs should be increased and when the next scan should be performed. In practice, it is only necessary to scan a patient every 2–4 days if clomiphene citrate or pulsatile GnRH is used (unpublished observations). If gonadotropins are used, hCG should be administered when the dominant follicle is 17–18 mm in diameter in order to be able to indicate to the patient when best to have intercourse. If a spontaneous LH surge should occur, it should be augmented with hCG, as the surge in superovulated cycles is often attenuated[28] and might be insufficient to trigger ovulation. We believe that hCG should not be administered for *in vivo* fertilization if there are more than three follicles that are greater than 16 mm in diameter, or more than six follicles that are greater than 14 mm, because of the respective risks of multiple pregnancy and the ovarian hyperstimulation syndrome. An endometrial thickness of greater than 7–8 mm on the day of administration of hCG is suitable for implantation, although pregnancies are more likely to occur if the endometrial thickness is at least 9 mm[4].

SUPEROVULATION INDUCTION CYCLES

The initial experience in ovulation induction for IVF was with human menopausal gonadotropin (hMG) with or without clomiphene citrate[29]. Although good results can be obtained, close monitoring of follicular growth is necessary and despite this, 15–30% of cases have a spontaneous LH surge. The move towards pituitary desensitization with a GnRH agonist[30] has become increasingly popular in assisted conception clinics. The reversible hypogonadotropic hypogonadism so produced permits unimpeded control over follicular development[31] and improved pregnancy rates in IVF programmes[32,33]. The practical advantage of such a regimen is that detailed endocrine monitoring for the detection of the onset of the preovulatory LH surge is no longer required. When GnRH agonists are used in the long protocol there is virtually no risk of an LH surge occurring and so ovarian stimulation may be continued until the optimal number of follicles have developed[34]. Once the largest follicle has attained a diameter of at least 18 mm, there is a window of at least 3 days during which hCG can be given without affecting the rates of fertilization and pregnancy[26,30].

The regimen we have most commonly used involves daily administration of buserelin (500 μg daily by subcutaneous injection) commencing on day 1 or 2 of the menstrual cycle. Once pituitary suppression has been confirmed (serum estradiol less than 150 pmol/l and LH less than 5 IU/l) the dose of buserelin is decreased to 200 μg daily and ovarian stimulation started, with an initial daily intramuscular dose of 2 ampules hMG for women up to the age of 34 years. This standard dose is adjusted upwards in older women or in previous poor responders and downwards in patients with polycystic ovaries because of the increased risk of the ovarian hyperstimulation syndrome[35]. Previously, it was our practice to monitor follicular development by daily ultrasonography and estradiol measurements from day 8 of ovarian stimulation[15]. Nowadays, we would only perform two or three ultrasound scans if the long protocol of GnRH agonist is used. No hormonal monitoring at all is performed unless the patient has polycystic ovaries, in which case one or two estradiol assays are performed when the follicles are deemed to have reached a size suitable for hCG administration.

Ultrasound monitoring of follicular growth during superovulation regimens provides more accurate information of follicular development and number than can be obtained by measurement of serum estradiol concentrations[36]. Follicles of different sizes secrete estradiol at widely differing rates and there is a wide range of estradiol levels for any given ultrasound picture[4]. Ultrasonography also demonstrates the location of the follicles for aspiration and it has been found that follicular dimensions, based on the volume of aspirated fluid, correlate well with the ultrasonic measurements[37]. In the same study, it was found that there was no correlation between the diameter of the largest follicle and the serum concentration of estradiol.

Ultrasound monitoring is sufficiently accurate for it to be used alone in monitoring gonadotropin therapy for both *in vivo* (unpublished observations) and *in vitro* fertilization[38], particularly when GnRH agonists are used in IVF cycles[34]. Estradiol measurements do, however, provide additional information which is of particular relevance when it comes to predicting the likelihood of a patient developing the ovarian hyperstimulation syndrome. Also, if there are only one or two follicles, the serum estradiol concentration provides an additional guide as to whether the cycle should be cancelled – the serum estradiol concentration on the day of hCG administration should be at least 2500 pmol/l.

During ovarian stimulation for IVF, a scan should be performed 1 week after the baseline scan, that is on day 8 of ovarian stimulation. The subsequent frequency of ultrasound monitoring depends both on the individual clinic's policy and on the treatment regimen that is being used. Regimens that involve clomiphene citrate or gonadotropins alone require more frequent monitoring than those in which GnRH agonists are used, and daily ovarian scans are necessary once a dominant follicle is formed. Such close monitoring is less vital in GnRH agonist cycles, because there is minimal risk of a spontaneous LH surge. As timing of hCG administration remains critical

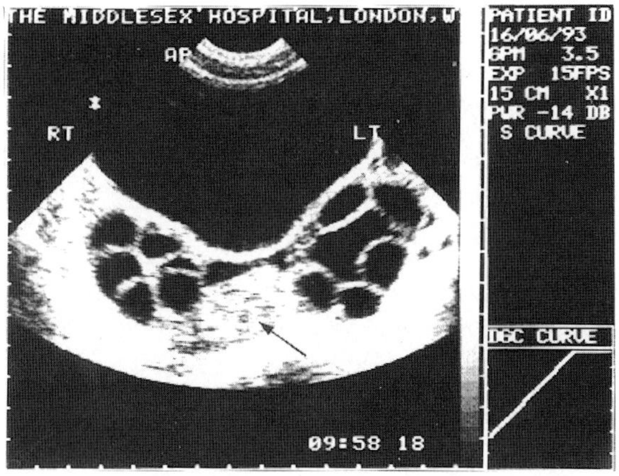

Figure 6 Transabdominal ultrasound scan of multifollicular development during superovulation induction for *in vitro* fertilization. Axial scan through uterine fundus (arrow) and both ovaries

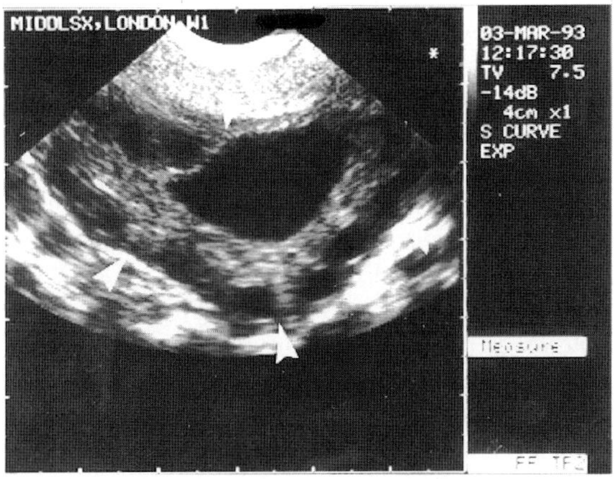

Figure 7 Transvaginal scan of unifollicular development in a polycystic ovary, with the edges of the ovary delineated by arrows

when the short protocol of GnRH agonist is used, however, close monitoring of follicular growth is necessary. If pituitary desensitization has been achieved, however, the number of ultrasound scans can be drastically reduced.

There have been a number of retrospective studies that demonstrated that hCG administration can be safely delayed for 1 or 2 days beyond the standard time of administration[39–41]. We recently performed a prospective study in which 247 patients, all of whom were on the long protocol of buserelin, were randomized into three groups[34]. Patients in group 1 ($n=79$) had hCG administered when the mean diameter of the largest follicle had reached 18 mm and at least two other follicles were greater than 14 mm. Patients in group 2 ($n=84$) and group 3 ($n=84$) had hCG administered 1 day and 2 days, respectively, after the above criteria had been reached. Whilst there was a significantly progressive increase in the mean diameter of the largest follicle and the number of days in rise of serum estradiol concentrations among the three groups, there were no differences in the mean number of preovulatory or medium-sized follicles, number of oocytes collected or embryos transferred. There were also no significant differences in the oocyte recovery, fertilization or cleavage rates, and the pregnancy rates were similar in the three groups. Thus there is no significant advantage in the precise timing of hCG administration when GnRH agonists are used to desensitize the pituitary during IVF cycles and this enables greater flexibility and simplicity in programming the workload of the clinic.

At each scan, the number and size of the follicles are documented and plotted graphically so that one can see at a glance the rate of follicular growth in each ovary. When multiple folliculogenesis occurs, the follicles are rarely spherical and it is therefore important to measure three orthogonal diameters in two planes for each follicle and then to calculate the mean diameter (Figure 6).

THE RESPONSE OF THE POLYCYSTIC OVARY TO STIMULATION

The response of the polycystic ovary to stimulation in the context of ovulation induction aimed at unifollicular ovulation is well documented and differs significantly from that of normal ovaries. The response tends to be slow initially, but may become 'explosive', with a significant risk of ovarian hyperstimulation and/or cyst formation. The therapies that are used aim for unifollicular development (Figure 7) in order to achieve a singleton pregnancy by either timed intercourse, donor insemination or intrauterine insemination.

The simplest methods of ovulation induction

involve short courses of an anti-estrogen (clomiphene citrate, cyclofenil or tamoxifen) administered in the early follicular phase. The cumulative conception rate is about 80% by 12 months[42]. Women with the PCOS who do not respond to oral therapy may succeed in having ovulation induced by gonadotropins, either combined with hMG or by FSH alone[4].

Regimens have been developed which, by a gradual stepwise increase in dose, reduce the risk of hyperstimulation[43]. A proposed scheme is one ampule of hMG daily for up to 14 days, until a response is seen with ultrasound monitoring; the daily dose is then increased by half an ampule every 7 days until a response is seen[44].

Conventional IVF nowadays depends on inducing multifollicular recruitment. It is thus to be expected that the response of the polycystic ovary within the context of an IVF program should also differ from the normal. Jacobs and associates[45] described an increase in follicular production in patients with polycystic ovaries and others[46] refer to the 'explosive' nature of the ovarian response. There are several possible explanations for this explosive response. There are many partially developed follicles present in the polycystic ovary and these are readily stimulated to give rise to the typical multifollicular response. Thecal hyperplasia provides large amounts of androstenedione and testosterone which act a substrates for estrogen production. Granulosa cell aromatase, although deficient in the 'resting' polycystic ovary, is readily stimulated by FSH. Therefore, normal quantities of FSH act on large amounts of substrate (testosterone and androstenedione) to produce large amounts of intraovarian estrogen. Ovarian follicles, of which there are too many, are increasingly sensitive to FSH (receptors for which are stimulated by high local concentrations of estrogen) and as a result there is multiple follicular development associated with very high levels of circulating estrogen. In some cases, this may result in the ovarian hyperstimulation syndrome, to which patients with polycystic ovaries are particularly prone, because they exhibit greater sensitivity than women with normal ovaries to exogenous stimulation[47].

In a comparison of 76 patients with polycystic ovaries and 76 consecutive controls (matched for age, diagnosis and stimulation regimen) undergoing *in vitro* fertilization, the number of follicles (14.9 ± 0.7 compared to 9.8 ± 0.6 in the controls, $p<0.001$) and peak serum estrogen level (5940 ± 255 compared to 4370 ± 240 pmol/l, $p<0.001$) were significantly increased in the polycystic ovary group[35]. Both groups of patients received similar total amounts of hMG.

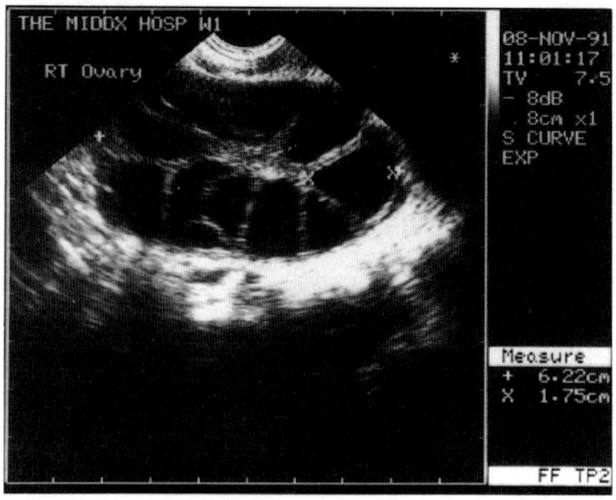

Figure 8 Transvaginal scan of an overstimulated ovary

We now recommend the long protocol of pituitary desensitization for the majority of women undergoing IVF. It is also particularly advantageous to women identified as having polycystic ovaries, as these patients often hypersecrete LH, which is both detrimental to fertilization rates and increases the risk of subsequent miscarriage[48]. It has indeed been shown that the rate of miscarriage in these patients is decreased following pituitary desensitization[15,49,50], presumably as a result of the suppression of serum LH levels.

THE OVARIAN HYPERSTIMULATION SYNDROME

The ovarian hyperstimulation syndrome (OHSS) is a well recognized complication of ovulation induction (Figure 8). In its severe form, it is characterized by ascites, ovarian enlargement with cyst formation, pleural effusion and electrolyte disturbances[51]. Oliguria and vascular complications may ensue and there have been fatalities. It is believed to be relatively rare in patients undergoing ovarian stimulation for IVF despite the multiple follicular development and high estrogen levels that commonly occur, and it has been suggested that the protective mechanism is mediated through aspiration of ovarian follicular fluid at the time of oocyte collection[52]. However, it does occur in IVF[46,53,54] and, when severe, is the only life-threatening condition associated with ovarian stimulation in IVF.

It has been apparent for some time that patients with polycystic ovaries undergoing straightforward ovulation induction are particularly at risk of developing OHSS[51,55]. Recently this has been confirmed in IVF as well[46,54]. In a total population of 1302 patients, we recently identified 15 patients who underwent ovarian stimulation for IVF or other assisted conception techniques and developed OHSS of sufficient severity to merit hospital admission (prevalence of 1.2% with 0.6% having severe OHSS). Of these patients, 53% had ultrasonically diagnosed polycystic ovaries and 87% were undergoing their first attempt at IVF. All had received luteal support in the form of hCG. Although the pregnancy rate in this group was very high (93.3%), the multiple pregnancy rate was 57% with a miscarriage rate of 14.3%[54]. As a result of our analysis of the results in these patients, we now recommend that if polycystic ovaries are identified on the baseline scan, the dose of gonadotropins should be reduced.

Careful monitoring of estrogen levels and numbers of follicles by ultrasound scan during stimulation for IVF can also help to identify those at risk. In patients thought to be at risk of OHSS, luteal support in the form of hCG should be withheld and progesterone should be administered instead. Transfer of a maximum of two embryos in this group will reduce the multiple pregnancy rate with its attendant obstetric and neonatal problems. The safest approach to preventing the OHSS in those who are thought to be at risk, is the elective freezing of all embryos at the pronuclear stage and their subsequent replacement in a non-stimulated natural or artificial (that is, hormone replacement) cycle. The reason for this is that the endogenous hCG produced by a pregnancy continues to stimulate the ovaries and worsens the OHSS and the patient's condition.

OOCYTE RETRIEVAL

As assisted conception techniques have evolved, so have the methods for collecting oocytes. Steptoe and Edwards first described the technique of laparoscopic oocyte collection[56]. The disadvantages of this method are the invasiveness of the protocol and the need for general anesthesia, which are important considerations, since many patients undertake repeated attempts before conceiving[2]. Moreover, many patients who undergo IVF have severe pelvic adhesions, and in 5–10% of patients this makes laparoscopic oocyte collection impossible[57]. Laparoscopic oocyte retrieval should be now confined to gamete intrafallopian transfer (GIFT) procedures, since laparoscopy remains the preferred approach for transfer of the gametes into the Fallopian tubes. It is our experience, however, that even for GIFT the oocyte retrieval is most easily and successfully performed by transvaginal ultrasound-directed follicle aspiration prior to GIFT, to reduce the duration of the laparoscopic procedure.

Ultrasound-directed follicle aspiration for oocyte recovery was pioneered by Lenz and colleagues[58], using the transcutaneous, transvesical route. A number of other transabdominally visualized routes were employed, including transvaginal–transvesical[59] and perurethral[60]. These techniques were not easy to learn and so it was not until the advent of the direct transvaginal approach[61] that ultrasound-directed follicle aspiration took over from the laparoscopic methods. Direct transvaginal oocyte collection permits easy access to the ovaries, which might be bound by dense adhesions. The procedure usually takes less than 20–30 min, can be performed under sedation (oral lorazepam combined with intramuscular pethidine) and is acceptable to the majority of patients.

An ultrasound machine that provides a clear image is essential for follicular aspiration (Figure 9). High ultrasound frequencies are required (5–7.5 MHz). The biopsy probe should lie flush with the transducer and be securely attached so that the needle is stable and in the centre of the image throughout the procedure. With the patient in the lithotomy position, the vagina is first cleansed and the needle is then introduced

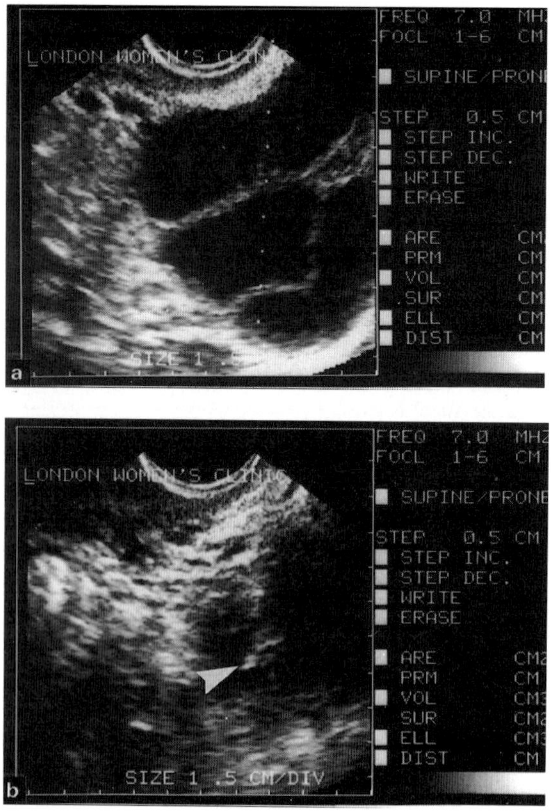

Figure 9 Transvaginal ultrasound-guided oocyte retrieval. (a) Dotted line indicates guideline for passage of the needle into a stimulated ovary; (b) after follicular aspiration, the needle can be seen (arrow) in a collapsed follicle

through the lateral fornix of the vagina into the ovary. Suction is applied when the needle is in the centre of the follicle and the needle is rotated gently whilst the follicle collapses. The embryologist examines the follicular fluid for the presence of an oocyte. It is our practice not to flush the follicle more than once with culture medium as we have found, in a prospective study, that the quality of any oocytes collected at flushing rapidly declines with the number of successive flushes[62] and oocytes that are collected in the initial aspirate have better fertilization and cleavage rates and form the embryos that are most likely to achieve pregnancies. When the follicle has been completely emptied, often shown by the presence of a little blood-stained fluid in the collection tubing, the needle is quickly moved to the adjacent follicle. The needle is not withdrawn from the ovary until every follicle is empty and the procedure is then repeated for the opposite ovary. The pelvis should be inspected before finally withdrawing the ultrasound probe to ensure that there is no excessive collection of fluid/blood in the pouch of Douglas, especially if repeated flushing has been attempted.

Vaginal bleeding is the commonest intraoperative complication and almost always responds to pressure on the bleeding point. Sometimes it is necessary to provide extra analgesia during the procedure. It is also mandatory to have easy access to resuscitation equipment in the event of a vasovagal faint or an apneic attack. Pelvic sepsis occasionally occurs after aspiration of ovarian cysts, particularly if they are endometriotic and antibiotic prophylaxis is advised in such cases[63].

Occasionally the ovaries are inaccessible through the lateral fornices and it becomes necessary to pass the needle directly through the myometrium to reach a posteriorly fixed ovary or to use the transabdominal route for ovaries that are fixed high above the pelvis. Such cases are rare.

LUTEAL PHASE

It is important to perform an ultrasound scan in the mid-luteal phase in both natural and stimulated cycles for *in vivo* fertilization. The corpus luteum may have a number of appearances, either ovoid or irregular in outline, with a cystic, echo-free interior, or it may have a hazy, echodense appearance because of the presence of cellular debris and blood[64] (Figure 10). The combination of a corpus luteum seen on ultrasound examination and an elevated serum progesterone concentration confirms ovulation. Occasionally there is no follicular rupture and a cystic structure persists in the luteal phase of the cycle associated with an elevated serum progesterone concentration. This is referred to as 'luteinized unruptured follicle' (LUF) (Figure 11). There is some debate about the incidence of the LUF syndrome, in which the follicle fails to rupture but changes in function to secrete progesterone in normal quantities[65–67]. In our experience the LUF occurs in less than 5% of cycles of patients undergoing ovulation induction therapy and does not tend to be a recurrent phenomenon (unpublished observations).

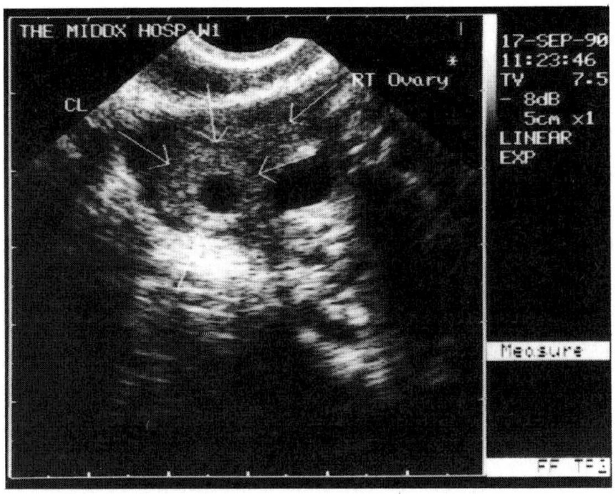

Figure 10 Transvaginal scan of a corpus luteum (arrowed)

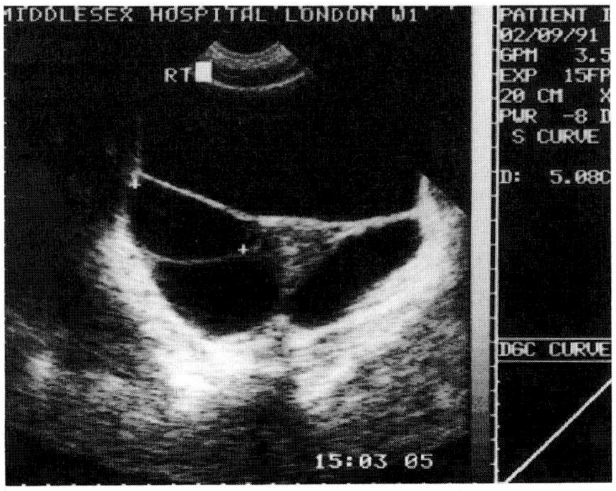

Figure 11 Several large corpus luteal cysts

DOPPLER ULTRASOUND IN ASSISTED CONCEPTION

The combination of transvaginal ultrasound with color Doppler measurements is beginning to provide a detailed picture of follicular events around the time of ovulation[68], and it allows assessment of the uterine blood flow to predict endometrial receptivity[69,70]. The precise uterine requirements for successful implantation are yet to be elucidated fully. The probability of a pregnancy occurring during assisted conception procedures depends both on embryo quality and uterine receptivity. In order to improve the chance of conception it has become customary to transfer two, three or four pre-embryos – and in some centers even more. In the United Kingdom it is now illegal to transfer more than three pre-embryos in any one cycle and many centers are turning to the routine transfer of two pre-embryos, particularly in women under the age of 35 years, who have a higher chance of a multiple pregnancy and a reduced rate of miscarriage[14,71,72]. Methods to improve our ability to assess endometrial receptivity for implantation might help prevent the transfer of precious pre-embryos in cycles that are virtually doomed to failure. The embryos could then be frozen and transferred later, in a cycle that is judged to be optimal for implantation – perhaps following hormonal manipulation of the endometrial response. Until recently, the only way to assess endometrial receptivity was by way of an endometrial biopsy. Doppler ultrasound is proving to be a valuable, non-invasive method which provides an instantaneous picture of uterine blood flow (Figure 12).

Blood flow through the uterine and ovarian arteries has been extensively investigated in both spontaneous[69,70] and stimulated cycles[71]. Steer and colleagues[70] were the first to use transvaginal color Doppler to study the uterine arteries in 23 normally cycling women, and they found that the lowest pulsatility index (PI) occurred 9 days after the LH peak. This indicates that the maximum uterine perfusion occurs at about the time of expected implantation. Another index of blood flow, the resistance index, was measured on the day of embryo transfer in a series of women undergoing IVF[73] and it was found to be lower in those who subsequently became pregnant. A similar study was performed by Steer and colleagues[74] in 82 patients undergoing IVF. They measured the PI on the day of embryo transfer, classified it as being low (1–1.99) ($n = 27$), medium (2–2.99) ($n = 36$) or high (3+) ($n = 19$) and related pregnancy rates to the PI. There were no pregnancies in the high PI group. The pregnancy rate, implantation rate and multiple pregnancy rate in the low PI group were 41%, 15.5% and 27.3%, respectively, compared with 47%, 22.2% and 47.1% in the medium PI group. They suggested that the PI on the day of embryo transfer could be used to alter the management, such that a high

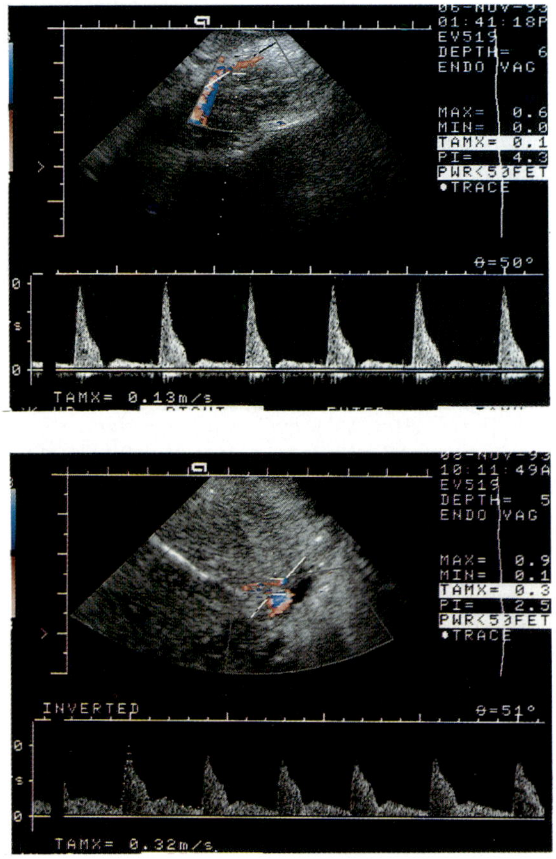

Figure 12 Doppler studies of uterine blood flow in a frozen embryo replacement cycle, during which a regimen of estrogen and progesterone is administered. (a) The pulsatility index (4.39) indicates resistance to flow and so estrogen therapy is continued for 2 more days until (b) the pulsatility index is more favorable

value (>3) would lead to elective freezing of the embryos for transfer at a later date in a more favorable cycle. If the PI was normal, the number of embryos transferred could be reduced to minimize the risk of a multiple pregnancy.

Doppler studies of the ovarian circulation are still very much at the research stage. It has been reported in one study in natural cycles that resistance to arterial flow was lower on the side containing the dominant follicle[75] and in gonadotropin-stimulated cycles it was reported that ovarian impedance was inversely proportional to the number of follicles larger than 15 mm[76]. It has also been reported that, in IVF cycles, there was a lower ovarian impedance 3 days after embryo transfer in those patients who conceived compared with those who did not[77]. Bourne and colleagues[78] found that the first signs of perifollicular blood flow could only be detected after the mid-cycle LH surge. They found that there was a rapid increase in the number of small vessels around the preovulatory follicle in the few hours preceding ovulation, which was accompanied by an increase in the blood flow velocity. Immediately after follicular rupture the blood flow velocity to the corpus luteum rose even further, suggesting a process of rapid angiogenesis at this time. The significance of these findings and possible clinical applications remain to be seen. The future might hold the possibility of timing the administration of hCG to coincide with optimal ovarian blood flow for either the release or collection of the highest quality oocytes.

CONCLUSIONS

Ultrasound examination of the ovaries and other pelvic structures is a vital adjunct to the successful management of the subfertile patient. It not only provides essential information about the patient's ovarian morphology and natural menstrual cycle but also enables the programming of safe and effective treatment, whether it be ovulation induction for anovulatory infertility or superovulation regimens for assisted conception procedures. It is important to diagnose polycystic ovaries at the time of the baseline scan so that appropriate stimulation regimens are administered and the patient and clinician are alerted to the possible risks of the ovarian hyperstimulation syndrome and multiple pregnancy. Ultrasound monitoring of follicular growth provides a reliable assessment of ovulation induction therapy and enables appropriate scheduling for the administration of the preovulatory injection of hCG. In assisted conception cycles, when GnRH agonists are used to achieve pituitary desensitization, there is at least a 3-day window for the effective administration of hCG once the largest follicle has reached a diameter of 18 mm. Thus, assisted conception procedures can be simplified and made more cost-effective, with expensive endocrine monitoring being reserved for difficult cases – for example, those patients thought to be at particular risk of developing the ovarian hyperstimulation syndrome. New techniques, such as color Doppler imaging, are providing interesting insights into ovarian and uterine blood flow and might have a future clinical role in optimizing the timing of hCG administration and embryo transfer. Ultrasound-guided follicular aspiration has replaced laparoscopy as the optimal method for collecting oocytes as it is a quick, safe and efficient procedure. An ultrasound scan in the luteal phase helps to confirm that ovulation has occurred and, hopefully, a few weeks later, can be used to visualize the gestational sac of an early pregnancy.

ACKNOWLEDGEMENT

We would like to thank Miss Anita Patel DCR, DMU, Senior Ultrasonographer, The Middlesex Hospital, for kindly providing the ultrasound pictures.

References

1. Tan, S. L. (1993). Simplification of IVF therapy. *Proceedings of The VIIIth World Congress of Human Reproduction*, Bali. (Carnforth, UK: Parthenon Publishing)
2. Tan, S. L., Royston, P., Campbell, S., Jacobs, H. S., Betts, J., Mason, B. and Edwards, R. G. (1992). Cumulative conception and livebirth rates after *in-vitro* fertilisation. *Lancet*, **339**, 1390–4
3. Hull, M. G. R., Eddowes, H. A., Fahy, U., Abuzeid, M. I., Mills, M. S., Cahill, D. J., Fleming, C. F., Wardle, P. G., Ford, W. C. L. and McDermott, A. (1992). Expectations of assisted conception for infertility. *Br. Med. J.*, **304**, 1465–9
4. Balen, A. H. *et al.* (1993). *J. Obstet. Gynaecol.*, **13**, 397–8
5. Yee, B., Barnes, R. B., Vargyas, J. M. and Marrs, R. P. (1987). Correlation of transabdominal and transvaginal ultrasound measurements of follicle size and number with laparoscopic findings for *in-vitro* fertilisation. *Fertil. Steril.*, **47**, 828–32
6. Andreotti, R. F., Thompson, G. H., Janowitz, W., Shapiro, A. G. and Zusmer, N. R. (1989). Endovaginal and transabdominal sonography of ovarian follicles. *J. Ultrasound Med.*, **8**, 555–60
7. Adams, J., Polson, D. W., Abdulwahid, N., Morris, D. V., Franks, S., Mason, H. D., Tucker, M., Price, J. and Jacobs, H. S. (1985). Multifollicular ovaries: clinical and endocrine features and response to pulsatile gonadotrophin releasing hormone. *Lancet* **2**, 1375–8
8. Stein, I. F. and Leventhal, M. L. (1935). Amenorrhoea associated with bilateral polycystic ovaries. *Am. J. Obstet. Gynecol.*, **29**, 181–91
9. Conway, G. S., Honour, J. W. and Jacobs, H. S. (1989). Heterogeneity of the polycystic ovary syndrome: clinical, endocrine and ultrasound features in 556 patients. *Clin. Endocrinol.*, **30**, 459–70
10. Franks, S., Adams, J., Mason, H. and Polson, D. (1985). Ovulatory disorders in women with polycystic ovary syndrome. In Jacobs, H. S. (ed.) *Reproductive Endocrinology*, pp. 605–32. *Clin. Obstet. Gynaecol.*, **12**. (Philadelphia: W. B. Saunders)
11. Adams, J., Polson, D. W. and Franks, S. (1986). Prevalence of polycystic ovaries in women with anovulation and idiopathic hirsutism. *Br. Med. J.*, **293**, 355–8
12. Shoham, Z., Conway, G. S., Patel, A. and Jacobs, H. S. (1992). Polycystic ovaries in patients with hypogonadotrophic hypogonadism: similarity of ovarian response to gonadotrophin stimulation in patients with polycystic ovary syndrome. *Fertil. Steril.*, **58**, 37–45
13. Schachter, M., Balen, A. H., Patel, A., Jacobs, H. S. (1993). Hypogonadotrophic patients with ultrasonographically diagnosed polycystic ovaries have aberrant gonadotropin secretion when treated with pulsatile gonadotrophin releasing hormone – a new insight into the pathophysiology of polycystic ovary syndrome. *Fertil. Steril.*, in press
14. Polson, D. W., Wadsworth, J., Adams, J. and Franks, S. (1988). Polycystic ovaries: a common finding in normal women. *Lancet*, **2**, 870–2
15. Balen, A. H., Tan, S. L., MacDougall, J. and Jacobs, H. S. (1993). Miscarriage rates following *in vitro* fertilisation are increased in women with polycystic ovaries and reduced by pituitary desensitisation with buserelin. *Hum. Reprod.*, **8**, 959–64
16. Hornstein, M. D., Barbieri, R. L., Ravnikar, V. A. and McShane, P. M. (1989). The effects of baseline ovarian cysts on the clinical response to controlled ovarian stimulation in an *in-vitro* fertilisation program. *Fertil. Steril.*, **52**, 437–40
17. Thatcher, S. S., Jones, E. and DeCherney, A. H. (1989). Ovarian cysts decrease the success of controlled ovarian stimulation and *in-vitro* fertilisation. *Fertil. Steril.*, **52**, 812–16
18. Karande, V. C., Scott, R. T., Jones, G. S. and

Muasher, S. J. (1990). Non-functional ovarian cysts do not affect ipsilateral or contralateral ovarian performance during *in-vitro* fertilisation. *Hum. Reprod.*, **5**, 431–3

19. Rizk, B., Tan, S. L., Kingsland, C., Steer, C., Mason, B. A. and Campbell, S. (1990). Ovarian cysts aspiration and the outcome of *in-vitro* fertilisation. *Fertil. Steril.*, **54**, 661–4
20. Edwards, R. G., Steptoe, R. G. and Purdy, J. M. (1980). Establishing full-term human pregnancies using cleaving embryos grown *in vitro*. *Br. J. Obstet. Gynaecol.*, **87**, 737
21. Tan, S. L., Doyle, P., Campbell, S., Beral, V., Risk, P., Brinsden, P., Mason, B. A. and Edwards, R. G. (1992). Obstetric outcome of pregnancies resulting from *in-vitro* fertilisation compared with normally occurring pregnancies. *Am. J. Obstet. Gynaecol.*, **167**, 778–84
22. Paulson, R. J., Sauer, M. V. and Lobo, R. A. (1989). *In vitro* fertilization in unstimulated cycles: a new application. *Fertil. Steril.*, **51**, 1059–60
23. Foulot, H., Ranoux, C., Dubuisson, J.-B., Rambaud, D., Aubriot, F.-X. and Poirot, C. (1989). *In-vitro* fertilisation without ovarian stimulation: a simplified protocol applied to 80 cycles. *Fertil. Steril.*, **52**, 617–21
24. Eissa, M. K., Hudson, K., Docker, M. F., Sawers, R. S. and Newton, J. R. (1985). Ultrasound follicle diameter measurement: an assessment of interobserver and intraobserver variation. *Fertil. Steril.*, **44**, 751–4
25. Gonzalez, C. J., Curson, R. and Parsons, J. (1988). Transabdominal versus transvaginal ultrasound screening of ovarian follicles: are they comparable? *Fertil. Steril.*, **50**, 65–74
26. Hackeloer, B. J., Fleming, R., Robinson, H. P., Adam, A. H. and Coutts, J. R. T. (1979). Correlation of ultrasonic and endocrinologic assessment of human follicular development. *Am. J. Obstet. Gynecol.*, **135**, 122–8
27. Adams, J., Tan, S. L., Wheeler, M. J., Morris, D. V., Jacobs, H. S. and Franks, S. (1988). Uterine growth in the follicular phase of spontaneous ovulatory cycles and during luteinising hormone-releasing hormone-induced cycles in women with normal or polycystic ovaries. *Fertil. Steril.*, **49**, 52–5
28. Balen, A. H. and Jacobs, H. S. (1991). Gonadotrophin surge attenuating factor – a missing link in the control of LH secretion? *Clin. Endocrinol.*, **35**, 399–402
29. Fleming, R. and Coutts, J. R. T. (1990). Induction of multiple follicular development for *in-vitro* fertilisation. In Edwards, R. G. (ed.) *Assisted Human Conception, Br. Med. Bull.*, **46**, 596–615. (Edinburgh: Churchill Livingstone)
30. Porter, R. N., Smith, W., Craft, I. L., Abdulwahid, N. A. and Jacobs, H. S. (1984). Induction of ovulation for *in-vitro* fertilisation using buserelin and gonadotrophins. *Lancet*, **2**, 1284–5
31. Fleming, R., Haxton, M. J., Hamilton, M. P. R., McCune, G. S., Black, W. P., McNaughton, M. C. and Coutts, J. R. T. (1985). Successful treatment of infertile women with oligomenorrhoea using a combination of a luteinising hormone releasing hormone agonist and exogenous gonadotrophins. *Br. J. Obstet. Gynaecol.*, **92**, 369–74
32. Rutherford, A. J., Subak-Sharpe, R. J., Dawson, K. J., Margara, R. A., Franks, S. and Winston, R. M. L. (1988). Improvement of *in-vitro* fertilisation after treatment with buserelin, an agonist of luteinising hormone releasing hormone. *Br. Med. J.*, **296**, 1765–8
33. Frydman, R., Fries, N., Testart, J., Belaisch-Allart, J. C., Forman, R., Hazout, A. and Testart, J. (1988). Luteinising hormone releasing hormone agonists in *in-vitro* fertilisation: different methods of utilization and comparison with previous ovulation stimulation treatments. *Hum. Reprod.*, **3**, 559–61
34. Tan, S. L., Balen, A. H., Hussein, E. E., Mills, C., Campbell, S., Yovich, J. and Jacobs, H. S. (1992). A prospective randomised study of the optimum timing of human chorionic gonadotrophin administration after pituitary desensitisation in *in vitro* fertilisation. *Fertil. Steril.*, **57**, 1259–64
35. MacDougall, M. J., Tan, S. L., Balen, A. H. and Jacobs, H. S. (1993). A controlled study comparing patients with and without polycystic ovaries undergoing *in-vitro* fertilisation. *Hum. Reprod.*, **8**, 233–7
36. Haning, R. V., Austin, C. W., Kuzma, D. L., Shapiro, S. S. and Zweibel, W. J. (1982). Ultrasound evaluation of estrogen monitoring for induction of ovulation with menotropins. *Fertil. Steril.*, **37**, 627–32
37. Montzavinos, T., Garcia, J. E. and Jones, H. W. (1983). Ultrasound measurement of ovarian follicles stimulated by human gonadotrophins for oocyte recovery and *in-vitro* fertilisation *Fertil. Steril.*, **40**, 461–5
38. Bordt, J., Hander, J. P. and Schneider, H. P. G. (1986). Ultrasound controlled gonadotrophin therapy of anovulatory infertility. *Fertil. Steril.*, **46**, 818–22
39. Conaghan, J., Dimitry, E. S., Mills, M., Margara, R. A. and Winston, R. M. L. (1989). Delayed human chorionic gonadotrophin administration for *in-vitro* fertilisation. *Lancet* **1**, 1323–4
40. Abdalla, H., Baber, R., Leonard, T., Kirkland, A., Power, M., Mitchell, A., Owen, E. and Studd, J. (1989). Timed oocyte collection in an assisted conception programme using GnRH analogue. *Hum. Reprod.*, **4**, 927–30
41. Tan, S. L., Kingsland, C., Rizk, B., Campbell, S. and Mason, B. (1989). Timing of hCG administration after pituitary down-regulation with LHRH analogue in IVF. *Proceedings of the XIIth Asian and Oceanic Congress of Obstetrics and Gynaecology*, Taiwan
42. Hull, M. G. R., Savage, P. E. and Bromham, D. R.

(1982). Anovulatory and ovulatory infertility: results with simplified management. *Br. Med. J.*, **284**, 1681–5

43. Franks, S., Mason, S., Polson, D. W., Winston, R. M. L., Margara, R. and Reed, M. J. (1988). Mechanism and management of ovulatory failure in women with polycystic ovary syndrome. *Hum. Reprod.*, **3**, 531–4
44. Hamilton-Fairley, D. and Franks, S. (1990). Common problems in induction of ovulation. *Bailliere's Clin. Obstet. Gynaecol.*, **4**, 609–26
45. Jacobs, H. S., Porter, R., Eshel, A. and Craft, I. (1987). Profertility uses of luteinising hormone releasing hormone agonist anologues. In Vickery, B. H. and Nestor, J. J. (eds.) *LHRH and its Analogs*, pp. 303–22. (Lancaster: MTP Press)
46. Smitz, J., Camus, M., Devroey, P., Evard, P., Wisanto, A. and Van Steirteghen, A. C. (1991). Incidence of severe ovarian hyperstimulation syndrome after gonadotrophin releasing hormone agonist/HMG superovulation for *in-vitro* fertilisation. *Hum. Reprod.*, **6**, 933–7
47. Salat-Baroux, J. and Antoine, J. M. (1990). Accidental hyperstimulation during ovulation induction. *Bailliere's Clin. Obstet. Gynaecol.*, **4**, 627–37
48. Balen, A. H., Tan, S. L. and Jacobs, H. S. (1993). Hypersecretion of luteinising hormone – a significant cause of subfertility and miscarriage. *Br. J. Obstet. Gynaecol.*, **100**, 1082–9
49. Johnson, P. and Pearce, J. M. (1990). Recurrent spontaneous abortion and polycystic ovarian disease: comparison of two regimens to induce ovulation. *Br. Med. J.*, **301**, 154–6
50. Abdalla, H. I., Ahuja, K. K., Leonard, T., Morris, N. N., Honour, J. W. and Jacobs, H. S. (1990). Comparative trial of luteinising hormone releasing hormone analogue/HMG and clomiphene citrate/HMG in an assisted conception programme. *Fertil. Steril.*, **53**, 473–8
51. Schenker, J. G. and Weinstein, D. (1978). Ovarian hyperstimulation syndrome: a current survey. *Fertil. Steril.*, **30**, 255
52. Friedman, C. I., Schmidt, G. E., Chang, F. E. and Kim, M. H. (1984). Severe ovarian hyperstimulation following follicular aspiration. *Am. J. Obstet. Gynecol.*, **150**, 436–7
53. Golan, A., Ron-el, R., Herman, A., Weinraub, Z., Soffer, Y. and Caspi, E. (1989). Ovarian hyperstimulation syndrome: an update review. *Obstet. Gynaecol. Surv.*, **44**, 430–40
54. MacDougall, M. J., Tan, S. L. and Jacobs, H. S. (1992). *In-vitro* fertilization and the ovarian hyperstimulation syndrome. *Hum. Reprod.*, **7**, 597–600
55. Lunenfeld, B. and Insler, V. (1974). Classification of amenorrhoeic states and their treatment by ovulation induction. *Clin. Endocrinol.*, **3**, 223–37
56. Steptoe, P. and Edwards, R. G. (1970). Laparoscopic recovery of preovulatory human oocytes after priming of ovaries with gonadotrophins. *Lancet*, **2**, 683–9
57. Daniell, F., Pittway, D. E. and Maxton, W. S. (1983). The role of laparoscopic adhesiolysis in an *in-vitro* fertilisation program. *Fertil. Steril.*, **40**, 49–52
58. Lenz, S., Lauritsen, J. G. and Kjellow, M. (1981). Collection of human oocytes for *in-vitro* fertilisation by ultrasonically guided follicular puncture. *Lancet*, **1**, 1163–4
59. Dellenbach, P., Nisand, I., Moreu, L. *et al.* (1984). Transvaginal, sonographically controlled ovarian follicle puncture for egg retrieval. *Lancet*, **1**, 1467
60. Parsons, J., Riddles, A. and Booker, M. (1985). Oocyte retrieval for *in-vitro* fertilisation by ultrasonically guided needle aspiration via the urethra. *Lancet*, **1**, 1076
61. Wikland, M., Lennart, E. and Hamberger, L. (1985). Transvesical and transvaginal approaches for the aspiration of follicles by the use of ultrasound. *Ann. NY Acad. Sci.*, **442**, 184–92
62. Hussein, E. E., Balen, A. H. and Tan, S. L. (1992). A prospective study comparing the outcome of eggs retrieved in the aspirate to those retrieved in the flush during transvaginal ultrasound directed oocyte recovery for *in-vitro* fertilisation. *Br. J. Obstet. Gynaecol.*, **99**, 841–4
63. Howe, R. S., Blasco, L., Wheeler, C., Tureck, R. and Mastroianni, L. (1988). Pelvic infection after transvaginal ultrasound-guided ovum retrieval. *Fertil. Steril.*, **49**, 726–8
64. Deichert, U., Hackelöer, B. J. and Daume, E. (1986). The sonographic and endocrinologic evaluation of the endometrium in the luteal phase. *Hum. Reprod.*, **1**, 219
65. Marik, J. and Hulka, J. (1978). Luteinized unruptured follicle syndrome: a subtle cause of infertility. *Fertil. Steril.*, **29**, 270
66. Daly, D. C., Soto-Albors, C., Walters, C. *et al.* (1985). Ultrasonographic assessment of luteinized unruptured follicle syndrome in unexplained infertility. *Fertil. Steril.*, **43**, 62
67. Ritchie, W. G. M. (1985). Ultrasound in the evaluation of normal and induced ovulation. *Fertil. Steril.*, **43**, 167
68. Bourne, T. H., Jurkovic, D., Waterstone, J., Campbell, S. and Collins, W. P. (1991). Intrafollicular blood flow during human ovulation. *Ultrasound Obstet. Gynecol.*, **1**, 53–9
69. Scholtes, M. C. W., Wladimiroff, J. W., van Rijen, H. J. M. *et al.* (1989). Uterine and ovarian flow velocity waveforms in the normal menstrual cycle: a transvaginal Doppler study. *Fertil. Steril.*, **52**, 981–5
70. Steer, C., Campbell, S., Pampiglione, J., Kingsland, C., Mason, B. A. and Collins, W. (1990). Transvaginal colour flow imaging of the uterine arteries during ovarian and menstrual cycles. *Hum. Reprod.*, **5**, 391–5

71. Balen, A. H., MacDougall, J. and Tan, S. L. (1993). The influence of the number of embryos transferred during *in-vitro* fertilization on pregnancy outcome. *Hum. Reprod.*, **8**, 1324–8
72. Tan, S. L. *et al.* (1994). *Am. J. Obstet. Gynecol.*, in press
73. Sterzik, K., Grab, D., Sasse, S., Hutter, H., Rosenbusch, B. and Torinde, R. (1989). Doppler sonographic findings and their correlation with implantation in an *in-vitro* fertilisation program. *Fertil. Steril.*, **52**, 825–8
74. Steer, C., Campbell, S., Tan, S. L., Crayford, T., Mills, C., Mason, B. A. and Collins, W. P. (1992). The use of transvaginal color flow imaging after IVF to identify optimum uterine conditions before embryo transfer. *Fertil. Steril.*, **57**, 372–6
75. Taylor, K., Burns, P., Wells, P., Conway, D. and Hull, M. (1985). Ultrasound Doppler flow studies of the ovarian and uterine arteries. *Br. J. Obstet. Gynaecol.*, **92**, 240–6
76. Deutinger, J., Reinthaller, A. and Bernaschek, G. (1989). Transvaginal pulsed Doppler measurement of blood flow velocity in the ovarian arteries during cycle stimulation and after follicle puncture. *Fertil. Steril.*, **51**, 466–70
77. Barber, R. J., McSweeney, M. B., Gill, R. W. *et al.* (1988). Transvaginal pulsed Doppler ultrasound assessment of blood flow to the corpus luteum in IVF patients following embryo transfer. *Br. J. Obstet. Gynaecol.*, **95**, 1226–30
78. Bourne, T. H., Jurkovic, D., Waterstone, J., Campbell, S. and Collins, W. P. (1991). Intrafollicular blood flow during human ovulation. *Ultrasound Obstet. Gynecol.*, **1**, 53–9
79. Balen, F. G., Allen, C. M., Gardener, J. E., Siddle, M. and Lees, W. R. (1993). 3-dimensional reconstruction of ultrasound images of the uterine cavity. *Br. J. Radiol.*, **66**, 588–91

The corpus luteum

7

I. Žalud, A. Kurjak and Z. Weiner

INTRODUCTION

The corpus luteum forms in the ovary at the site of the ruptured follicle immediately after ovulation. It is colored by a golden pigment, from which it derives its name, which means 'yellow body'. The first description comes, probably, from de Graaf:

> Those structures, which thought normal, are only at certain times found in the testes of women, are globular bodies in the form of conglomerate glandulae which are composed of many particles, extending from the center to the circumference in straight rows, and are enveloped by a special membrane. We assert that these globules do not exists at all times in the testicles of females; on the contrary, they are only detected in them after coitus, (being) one or more in number according as the animal brings forth one or more fetuses from that congress.

Probably, de Graaf concluded that coitus brought about the appearance of the corpus luteum because of comparisons he made with anatomical findings in animals that are induced ovulators, such as the rabbit.

The corpus luteum is a morphologically very well studied structure, while functional aspects, specially during pregnancy, still remain controversial. By advanced imaging techniques, it is possible to observe ovarian cyclic changes non-invasively with great accuracy. High-frequency ultrasound has brought ovarian morphology into the range of routine clinical work-up. The use of ultrasound in the detection of ovarian pathology has been widespread over a number of years. With transabdominal sonography, the ovaries are often easily seen and ovarian abnormalities identified, although only with a moderate amount of accuracy. Patients with suspected ovarian masses can be reassured that no significant mass is present. Obese patients who have had an inadequate pelvic examination can also be screened with ultrasound. With the introduction of transvaginal sonography, the ability to identify the ovary and evaluate specific ovarian pathology has been greatly enhanced. Routine use of transvaginal ultrasound in screening for ovarian abnormalities and pelvic masses has been started in some European centers. More sophisticated ultrasound techniques employing transvaginal color and pulsed Doppler capabilities, have recently enabled the precise study of ovarian blood flow. Ultrasound is now capable of visualizing ovarian morphology and vascularization simultaneously. With blood flow studies ultrasound has added some functional aspects to the traditionally anatomical diagnostic approach. Although we are able to visualize more of the ovary, at the same time we face new controversies. The corpus luteum has added greatly to this confusion. The variety of morphological appearances and blood flow patterns are the reason for more false-positive and false-negative findings when searching for ovarian pathology. 'The great imitator' is indeed the right name for the corpus luteum. This chapter deals with these diagnostic challenges.

MORPHOLOGICAL ASPECTS

Rupture of the mature follicle is attended by extrusion of the egg and, with it, the zona pellucida, the corona radiata and a considerable number of the cells of the cumulus. It is difficult to distinguish between a mature follicle and an early corpus luteum, since the lutein changes in granulosa and theca cells are not abrupt but very gradual in their evolution. The collapse of the follicle, with the subsequent crumpled, festooned pattern, is probably the most reliable index of ovulation.

With the collapse of the follicle and escape of

the follicular fluid, the second or corpus luteum phase of the menstrual cycle begins, reaching its maximum several days before the onset of the next cycle. The gross appearance of a mature corpus luteum is not always the same, nor is its size, which varies from 10 to 20 mm in diameter. Its yellowish color can often be seen shimmering through the surface of the ovary, above which it may project as a more-or-less conspicuous mound that at times is actually polypoid. In other cases, the corpus luteum may seem to lie beneath the surface, being revealed only by cutting into the ovary. The cavity may be small with only a scant amount of fluid, or it may be very large and distended, with a yellowish liquid.

Microscopically, it has been observed that the corpus luteum undergoes four stages of development and demise: proliferation, vascularization, maturity, and regression. In the proliferative stage, when the mature Graafian follicle ruptures, the ovum, follicular fluid, and a considerable portion of the surrounding granulosa, are discharged. The collapsed walls of the empty follicle form convolutions about the blood-filled cavity. There are many large lacunae that contain extravasated blood but, initially, no blood vessels. The cells of the formed follicular wall begin structural and functional transformation into cells that will make up the corpus luteum. It appears that following approximately 60% of ovulations in women, there is slight hemorrhage into the evacuated follicle. Endothelial sprouts from the vessels penetrate the granulosa and the hemorrhagic cavity of the ruptured follicle.

Over the 48–72 h following ovulation, the walls of the evacuated follicle become profoundly vascularized. This is the stage of vascularization. Blood and lymphatic vessels follow angiogenic factors and colonize the developing corpus luteum. The cells of the former follicular wall become luteinized and greatly increase in size. Progesterone secretion increases during this time. Four days following ovulation, the cells of the corpus luteum have attained maximal size and have completed the transformation to luteal cells[1]. This marks the next stage in corpus luteum development: maturity. A discernible layer of connective tissue typically lines the cavity of the corpus luteum if a central cavity is present. In the absence of a central cavity, a thin, highly echogenic line is usually seen in the center of the corpus luteum. There is typically a pronounced ring of vascularity that appears to follow the path of the vascular supply surrounding the former preovulatory follicle and which becomes even more apparent as the corpus luteum matures.

Regressive changes occur in the corpus luteum, occasionally as early as the 23rd day of the menstrual cycle. These changes become progressively more marked, up to the onset of menstruation, until the central coagulum has been obliterated by connective tissue, and blood pigment has been removed by leukocytes. The regression of the corpus luteum is marked by fatty degeneration, fibrosis and, later, hyalinization of the lutein zone with increase of the cicatricial tissue within the cavity. The yellowish color may persist for a long time, even several months, but ultimately it disappears. The end product is the corpus albicans, appearing as a whitish, hyalinized, convoluted structure that slowly decreases in size. It is not difficult to 'date' the corpus luteum of the present cycle; to ascertain whether it is 2 or 6 months old may be more of a problem.

Although, as a rule, only one follicle each month reaches full maturation, many others advance to various stages of incomplete maturation and then are blighted (atresia folliculi). The oocyte dies, and this is followed by degeneration and later disappearance of the granulosa with not infrequent distension of the cavity with fluid. Such small follicular cysts are found in all normal ovaries during reproductive life, but under some conditions, they may be so numerous that they produce the so-called cystic ovary. The process of atresia is also exaggerated during pregnancy. The cystic stage is followed by cicatricial obliteration proceeding slowly from the periphery toward the center. The end result is the corpus fibrosum, a convoluted zone of hyalinized tissue surrounding a small central cicatrix. Its much smaller size and the narrow and usually less hyalinized fibrous wall make it easy to distinguish the corpus fibrosum from the corpus albicans.

In the event of fertilization of the ovum, the corpus luteum does not undergo regression but continues to develop, becoming considerably larger than the corpus luteum of menstruation and comprising sometimes one-third or even one-half of the ovarian volume. The large size is often due to cystic distension, but there is considerable variation in this respect, with some corpora lutea of pregnancy being of rather solid structure. The lutein cells are large and tile-like in appearance, and paralutein cells are often conspicuous. Maximum histological development is reached at about 10–12 weeks. The corpus luteum in pregnancy increases in size until approximately the 12th week of gestation. A large, anechoic (fluid-filled) central cavity typically develops in concert with the earliest detection of pregnancy until the end of the 16th week of gestation. By the end of the 16th week of pregnancy, the central cyst of the corpus luteum begins to regress. There is usually no luteal cavity observed at term. However, the corpus luteum may still be recognizable[1,2].

FUNCTIONAL ASPECTS

The main function of the corpus luteum is secretion of hormones to prepare the uterus for pregnancy and maintain pregnancy in the early stage if fertilization occurs. The duration and the function of the corpus luteum of pregnancy are the subjects of much speculation and investigation. The scientific validity of hormonal therapy in the prevention of early abortion after surgical removal of the corpus luteum is dependent on an understanding of the function of this structure.

Numerous human pregnancies have succeeded despite early ablation of the corpus luteum. Pratt reported continuation of pregnancy after an operation was performed as early as the 20th day after the last menstrual period to remove the corpus luteum, or about the time of implantation[3]. In a review of cases in which the corpus luteum had been removed early in pregnancy, Hall reported a rate of abortion of a little more than 20%[4]. He believed that such a rate was not higher than expected after any abdominal surgery that is conducted in the first trimester of pregnancy. In a well designed study, Tulsky and Koff removed the corpora lutea from 14 women who requested sterilization and therapeutic abortion[5]. Spontaneous abortion occurred in only two; in the remainder, the pregnancies were terminated by dilatation and curettage; 10 of the 14 women continued to excrete normal quantities of pregnanediol until the conceptus was removed.

The degenerative changes in the corpus luteum of an infertile cycle are delayed by the administration of chorionic gonadotropin. The corpus luteum secretes progesterone; soon after implantation, however, the human placenta apparently produces enough progesterone to maintain pregnancy. Thus, the corpus luteum, while necessary (in the human) for implantation is not required for pregnancy in women beyond the earliest stages.

To maintain a level of progesterone sufficient to support a developing pregnancy, it is necessary for the conceptus to prevent the luteal regression usually associated with impending menstruation. Maternal recognition of pregnancy is the mechanism by which the conceptus signals the maternal host to maintain luteal secretion of progesterone. In women, the mechanism for maternal recognition of pregnancy is the production of a chorionic gonadotropin (hCG). The embryo initiates production of hCG at approximately the time of implantation. Increased circulation levels of β-hCG are observed as early as 8–12 days following conception, that is approximately 4–8 days before the gestational sac may be visualized with high-frequency ultrasonography[1,6–8]. The syncytiotrophoblastic cells of the developing embryonic vesicle are responsible for the production of hCG and thus for the enhanced secretion of progesterone. Peak levels of hCG are reached at approximately the 14th week of gestation, and the levels then begin to decline. Although the human placenta begins to elaborate progesterone by the sixth week following conception, quantities sufficient to maintain the pregnancy are not available until approximately the tenth week. Morphological regression of the corpus luteum is observed beyond approximately the 20th week of gestation[9].

ULTRASOUND APPEARANCE

As opposed to transabdominal ultrasound, where the ovary is identified typically by its position and shape, with the transvaginal approach, ovaries are identified by the presence of small developing follicles. The internal architecture is distinct and

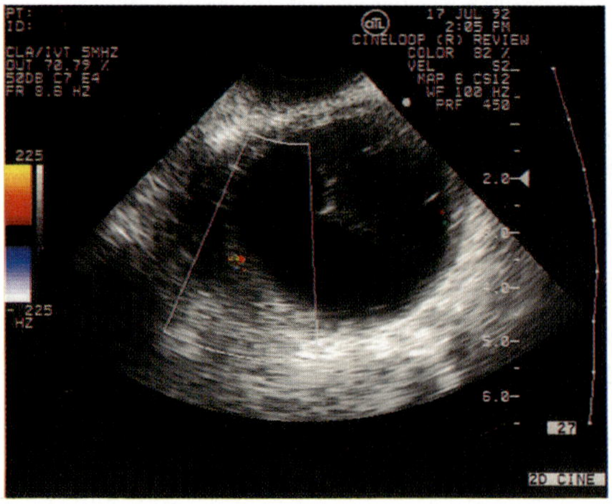

Figure 1 Cystic appearance of the corpus luteum

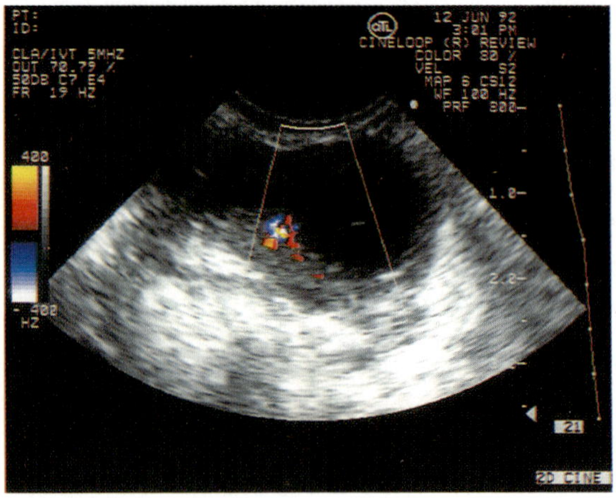

Figure 3 Typical semilunar appearance of corpus luteum blood flow on the periphery of cystic structure

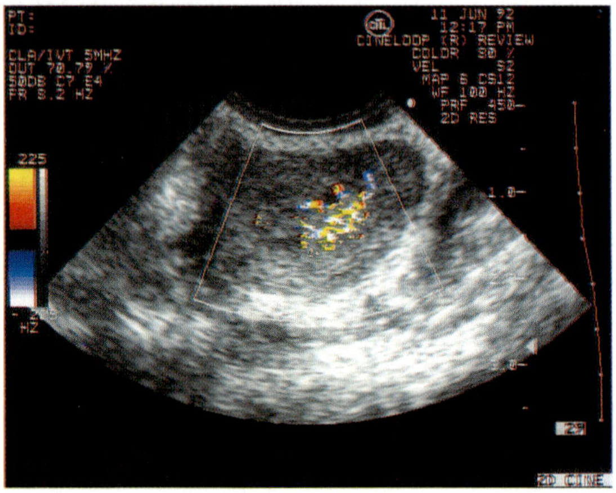

Figure 2 Collapsed corpus luteum is similar morphologically to the surrounding ovarian tissue. Color Doppler indicates the area of neovascularization. Randomly dispersed small intraovarian vessels are visualized

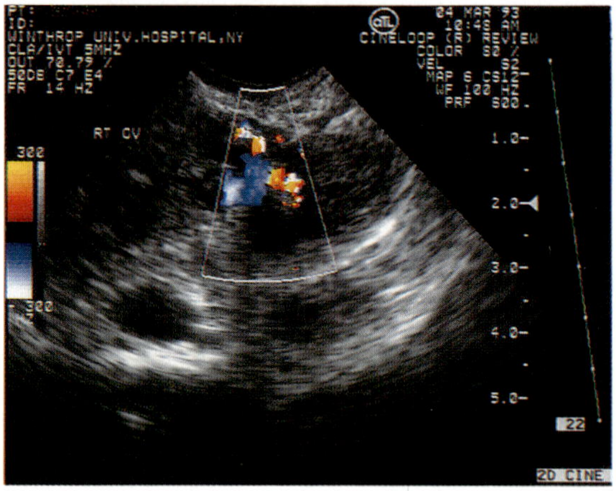

Figure 4 Very intense intraovarian color flow detected 48 h after spontaneous ovulation

can be separated from that of the uterus and myometrial masses that can simulate the ovary occasionally. Ovarian size can vary significantly, depending upon age. Ovaries as large as 3–4 cm in the long axis can be seen in normal menstruating women and if morphologically appropriate, can be considered normal.

The corpus luteum may confuse even the experienced ultrasonographer because of the high variability of its ultrasound characteristics. The corpus luteum can imitate much of ovarian pathology. The natural progression and regression of the corpus luteum involve significant macroscopic changes readily revealed by transvaginal ultrasound. After ovulation the follicular wall becomes irregular and the follicle becomes 'deflated'. De Crespigny and associates[10] observed follicular collapse in less than 1 min in two patients. In two other patients there was a rapid initial release of fluid followed by a slower release of the remaining fluid over 7 and 35 min, respectively. A corpus hemorrhagicum developed within 1 h of ovulation. Rottem and colleagues[11] were able to define clearly these textual changes after having performed more than 100 scans. The combination of clotted blood and liquid content may appear as a scalloped, irregular echogenic area within a seemingly large cyst, as a spherical multilocular cyst extending across the ovarian surface, or as tiny septa crossing the cyst. All these findings represent normal evolution of the corpus luteum in women of childbearing age and should not be mistaken for other ovarian pathology. It may be necessary to rescan the patient during the follicular phase of the next menstrual cycle, when the object should have decreased in size, thus confirming the diagnosis.

The fresh corpus luteum usually appears as a hypoechoic structure with an irregular wall and may contain some internal echoes corresponding to hemorrhage. As the corpus luteum develops some 4–8 days after ovulation, it appears as an echogenic area approximately 15 mm in size. However, this corpus luteum varies markedly in size and echo texture. Hemorrhage within the corpus luteum may simulate a solid or complex mass. Unlike the correlation between follicle size and estradiol levels during the follicular phase, no relationship has been shown between corpus luteum size and structure and progesterone levels during the luteal phase of the menstrual cycle.

Free fluid in the cul-de-sac is evidence of ovulation, particularly when a previously seen follicle has collapsed. However, the amount of fluid observed within the cul-de-sac significantly exceeds the amount of fluid actually released by follicular rupture[12]. Also, anovulatory women may demonstrate similar degrees of peritoneal fluid on sonography to ovulating women. This and other evidence support the hypothesis that peritoneal fluid is formed predominantly by hormonally stimulated secretions from the ovary and not by the follicular fluid itself[13].

DOPPLER ULTRASOUND

The development of high-resolution real-time B-mode ultrasound has provided a method for the non-invasive study of the reproductive structural changes of the ovarian tissue. In addition, Doppler ultrasound offers the possibility of studying blood flow patterns and hence allows identification of functional changes. Transvaginal ultrasound produces images of better resolution than transabdominal ultrasound, primarily through better preservation of the beam pattern and utilization of higher frequencies. It was expected that the transvaginal approach to Doppler ultrasound would offer the same benefits as for imaging alone and this approach is now utilized (Figures 1–10). The use of transvaginal color Doppler allows accurate placement of the sample volume for pulsed Doppler measurement. Using Doppler waveform analysis, it is possible to distinguish the ovary containing the active corpus luteum from the inactive ovary. The technique is simple to use and the results are available immediately. Vascular changes can usually be observed as a fluctuating area of color (with a typically semilunar appearance) and the different indexes (resistance index, pulsatility index, S/D ratio, etc.) derived from the flow velocity waveform provide a quantitative estimation of blood flow impedance.

It is known that the ovarian arterial compliance changes during normal menstrual cycles[14,15]. During the follicular phase, both ovaries show high-impedance Doppler waveforms with virtual absence or very small diastolic component of intraovarian blood flow. These high-impedance signals of an inactive ovary persist through the cycle. In an active ovary there is a marked diastolic component and consequently low-impedance Doppler signals as ovulation approaches and particularly during corpus luteum formation. Angiogenesis in the corpus luteum occurs in physiological circumstances in each menstrual cycle and functionally is probably important to maintain early pregnancy. The use of transvaginal color Doppler allows simple and precise recognition of the active ovary containing the corpus luteum[16–19]. Intensity of color corresponds with velocity of blood flow in newly formed intraovarian vessels. Color is an essential guide for pulsed Doppler exploration of such small and randomly dispersed vessels inside ovarian tissue. Without color flow, Doppler analysis would be time-consuming and potentially inaccurate.

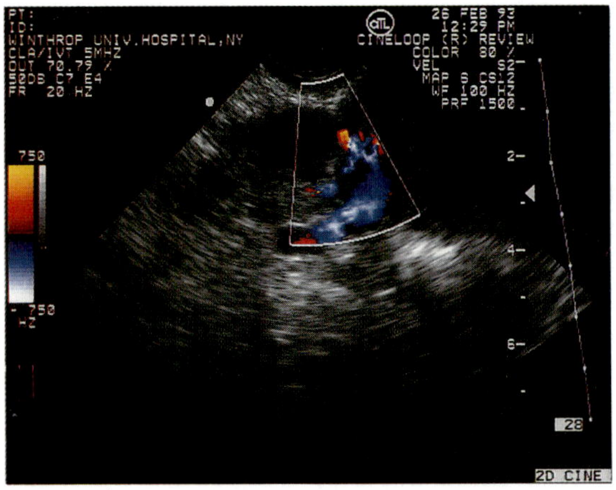

Figure 5 Intraovarian blood flow tends to be reduced at the end of the regular menstrual cycle. Blood flow shown on the figure presents mostly extraovarian venous flow

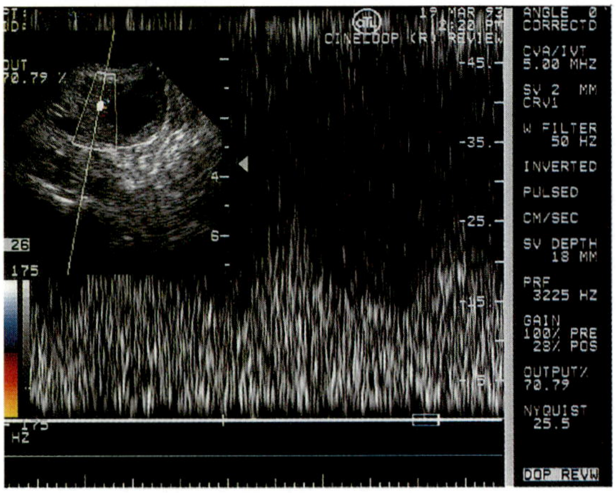

Figure 7 Pulsed Doppler waveform analysis in the luteal part of the menstrual cycle. Very high diastolic flow and low resistance are characteristic features

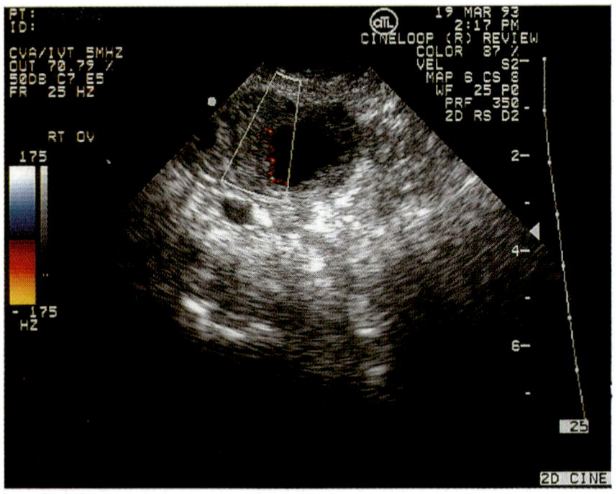

Figure 6 Typical morphology and color Doppler finding of the corpus luteum

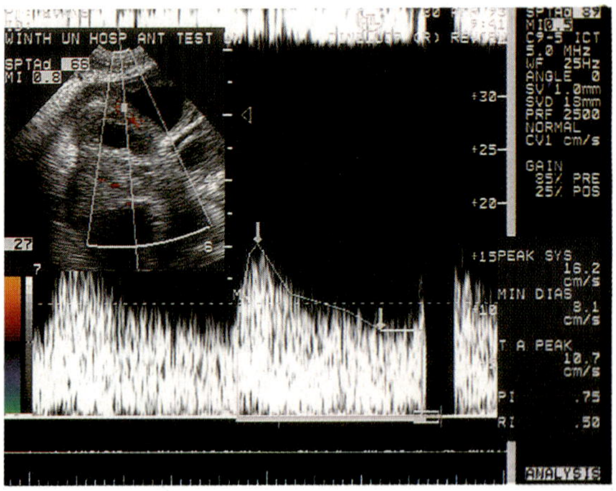

Figure 8 Multiple corpora lutea after induced ovulation

CLINICAL ASPECTS

Normal menstrual cycle

Ovarian blood flow in the normal menstrual cycle differs somewhat from the changes described in the uterine vasculature. The intraovarian vessels are usually not seen before day 8–10 of the 28-day cycle. Kurjak and colleagues[19] studied intraovarian vascular changes through an entire normal menstrual cycle. In this study, the resistance index was measured and was approximately 0.54 ± 0.04 until ovulation approached. A decline in impedance began 2 days before ovulation and reached its nadir at ovulation, 0.44 ± 0.04. It remained at this level for 4 to 5 days then gradually climbed to a level of 0.50 ± 0.04, still lower than that seen in the early follicular phase (Figure 11). The authors concluded that changes in ovarian blood flow occurred before ovulation, implying that these changes are complex and not purely secondary to progesterone action. However, the still-unanswered questions were raised: could inadequate vascularization play a role in the luteal phase defect? Similarly, could failure of adequate

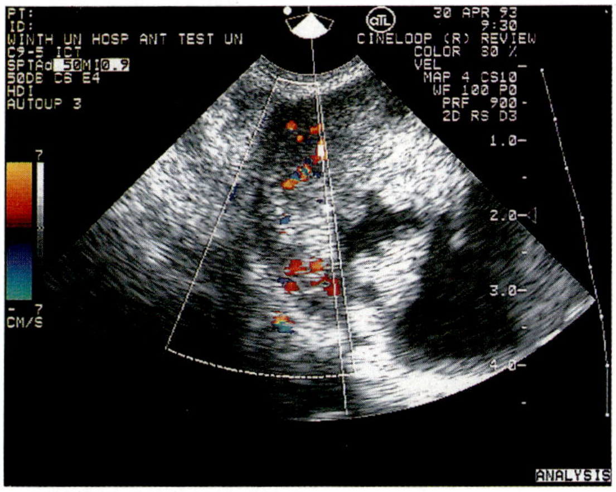

Figure 9 Corpus luteum in pregnancy. Cystic and solid components of the ovarian tissue are mixed. Color indicates blood flow

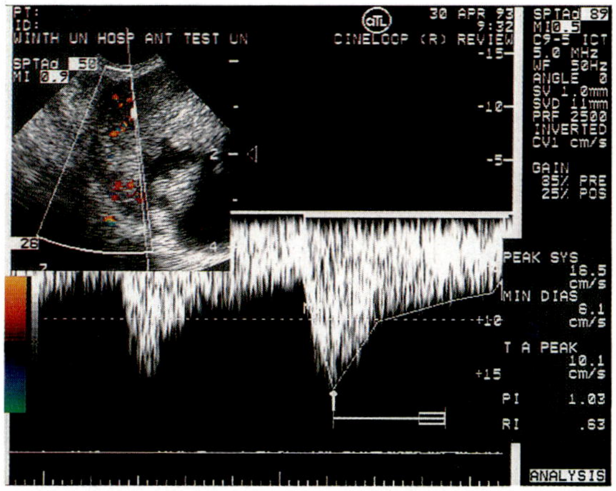

Figure 10 Pulsed Doppler analysis from the same pregnant patient as in Figure 9, at 10 weeks of gestation

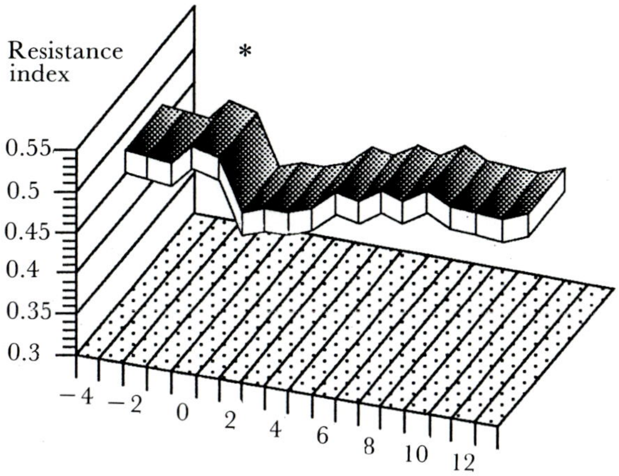

Figure 11 Doppler flow velocity in the ovary during the menstrual cycle. The day before ovulation (ovulation day 0), there is a significant (*) drop in the intraovarian blood flow resistance, which remains lower for the remainder of the cycle (modified from reference 19)

flow result in early pregnancy loss and could such blood flow changes play a role in infertility?

Hata and colleagues[15] studied the transition of ovarian arterial compliance during the human menstrual cycle and correlated their ultrasound findings with serum hormone levels. Seventy-one examinations were performed on nine healthy women with regular menstrual cycles. The change in ovarian arterial compliance was based on the calculation of the pulsatility index (PI). In the active ovary carrying a dominant follicle or corpus luteum, the PI in the early follicular phase (6.97 ± 2.01) was significantly higher than that in the late follicular phase (2.36 ± 0.31), and the PI in the early luteal phase (0.68 ± 0.09) was significantly lower than that in the late follicular phase. The PI became significantly higher in the late luteal phase (0.93 ± 0.16) than in the early luteal phase. In the inactive ovary without a follicle or corpus luteum, no changes were seen among the values for the PI, in any menstrual phase. The authors noted a significant difference between the values for the PI in the active ovary and the inactive ovary in the late follicular (2.36 vs. 6.29), the early (0.68 vs. 6.18) and the late luteal phase (0.93 vs. 6.57), respectively. The PI values for the active ovary correlated with the serum progesterone levels but not with the estradiol levels. These findings might provide a useful foundation for assessing ovarian hemodynamics during the normal menstrual cycle.

Early pregnancy

In the corpus luteum, very low-impedance blood flow can be found during the first trimester of pregnancy[16,17,20]. The failure of corpus luteum neovascularization has not been widely studied. It has been speculated that this corpus luteum failure could contribute to early pregnancy pathology. Taylor and co-workers[21] suggested that absence of luteal flow is inconsistent with a viable normotopic as well as ectopic pregnancy. Since an increasing resistance index (RI) reflects some reduction in the blood flow distal to the point at which the Doppler recording was made, namely in the corpus luteum, one might postulate that this reflects a reduction in corpus luteum function that is incompatible with pregnancy. Other authors opposed this[22]. One experimental study tested the hypothesis that estrogen and hCG can modify blood flow in the rabbit corpus luteum[23]. Radioactively labelled microspheres were used to measure luteal blood flow in pseudopregnant rabbits in which estrogen had been withdrawn to initiate premature luteal regression and in pseudopregnant rabbits injected with hCG. Removal of estradiol-filled Silastic capsules on day 10 of pseudopregnancy caused an 80% decrease in the serum progesterone concentration within 24 h. Despite the decline in progesterone secretion, luteal blood flow remained at very high levels and was not different from that in control rabbits treated continuously with estradiol. Replacement of estradiol-filled capsules for 3 h did not change the high rate of blood flow to the corpus luteum, but blood flow in the uterus, vagina, and ovarian stroma was increased. The injection of hCG on day 10 of pseudopregnancy caused a three-fold increase in the serum progesterone concentration, but luteal blood flow did not change. The author of this study concluded that the acute actions of estradiol or hCG in the rabbit corpus luteum are not mediated by changes in luteal blood flow. Further, the results suggest that the luteal vasculature is regulated differently from the vasculature of other estrogen-responsive tissues and that blood flow in the non-luteal tissue of the ovary can be regulated independently of blood flow in the corpus luteum. Oda and associates[24] studied the role of corpus luteum function in embryo implantation. Six patients with tubal infertility were studied, with a total of 27 fresh embryos being replaced following controlled ovarian hyperstimulation and *in vitro* fertilization. The data from this study suggest that a pregnancy can be achieved in spite of low circulating estradiol and progesterone levels during the luteal phase, which are generally indicative of the luteal phase defect.

The aim of our recent study[25] was to investigate the difference in intraovarian luteal blood flow in women with normal and abnormal early pregnancy. The study involved 170 pregnant women; 113 (66.5%) women had normal intrauterine pregnancies ranging from 6 to 12 weeks of gestation (confirmed by ultrasound measurement). These pregnancies were terminated due to sociomedical reasons. Fifty-seven (33.5%) patients were admitted to the hospital due to clinically suspected abnormal early pregnancy. Dilatation and curettage were done on all women and materials were sent to the pathologist for a final diagnosis. Diagnosis of ectopic pregnancy was made on laparoscopy.

Six out of 113 (5.3%) normal early pregnant women were excluded from the study because of the following reasons: two women had previously had unilateral oophorectomy; one had a multiple pregnancy; one showed the corpus luteum activity in both ovaries; and two women were without detectable corpus luteum blood flow. The mean age was 29.2 years and there was no statistically significant age difference among subgroups of normal early pregnant women. Nulliparity was present in 14 (13.1%) of 107 pregnant women. The overall detection rate of corpus luteum blood flow was higher on the left ovary (62.6%) in comparison to the right ovary (37.4%) (Fisher test, $p<0.01$) (Table 1). The mean RI and PI from corpus luteum blood flow were not influenced by gestational age in normal pregnancy (Table 2). The overall mean value for the RI was 0.452 ± 0.04 and for the PI 0.636 ± 0.09. In the group of 57 abnormal early pregnancies, six (10.5%) women were excluded from the study because of: one anembryonic pregnancy detected at 15 weeks of gestation, one molar pregnancy at 16 weeks, two cases of threatened abortion at 13 weeks, one missed abortion at 14 weeks and one woman with residual trophoblast tissue after unsuccessful artificial abortion. The patients' data and corpus luteum detection rate in 51 abnormal early pregnancies are shown in Table 3. Again, the overall detection rate of the corpus luteum was higher on the left ovary (56.7%) than on the right ovary (43.4%) (Fisher test, $p<0.01$). The mean RI from corpus luteum blood flow in patients with

Table 1 Detection rate of corpus luteum blood flow in 107 normal early pregnancies

Gestational age (weeks)	*Women* (*n*)	*Mean age* (years)	*Left luteal flow*		*Right luteal flow*	
			n	%	*n*	%
6	15	31.6	13	86.6	2	13.4
7	16	29.7	4	25.0	12	75.0
8	16	30.3	8	50.0	8	50.0
9	15	28.9	9	60.0	6	40.0
10	15	27.4	10	66.6	5	33.3
11	15	27.8	12	80.0	3	20.0
12	15	28.3	11	73.3	4	26.7
Total	107	29.2	67	62.6*	40	37.4*

Fisher test: $t=7.08$; $*p<0.01$

Table 2 The mean resistance index (RI) and pulsatility index (PI) with two standard deviations (2 SD) from corpus luteum blood flow in 107 normal early pregnancies

Gestational age (weeks)	*RI*	*2 SD*	*PI*	*2 SD*
6	0.448	0.05	0.607	0.10
7	0.444	0.04	0.614	0.09
8	0.451	0.04	0.633	0.06
9	0.451	0.03	0.671	0.10
10	0.464	0.06	0.665	0.15
11	0.458	0.05	0.654	0.09
12	0.450	0.02	0.611	0.04
Total	0.452	0.04	0.636	0.09

Statistics: one-way ANOVA and Tukey HSD type A test showed no significant differences; coefficient of variation for RI = 9.48%; coefficient of variation for PI = 15.29%

missed abortion was higher than in women with normal pregnancy ($p<0.01$) (Table 4). Both RI and PI were higher in patients with incomplete or threatened abortion in comparison with normal pregnancy ($p<0.01$). There was no statistically significant difference in the case of anembryonic pregnancy, molar or ectopic pregnancy. The RI and PI were correlated in all groups of patients ($r=0.71$).

In this study, we included pregnant women only when corpus luteum blood flow was visualized by color Doppler. We tried to define subtle differences in impedance to blood flow in such small intraovarian vessels. As a first step in this evaluation, corpus luteum blood flow was studied in normal intrauterine pregnancy with confirmed gestational age ranging from 6 to 12 weeks of pregnancy. There was no significant influence of gestational age on measured parameters such as the RI and PI. Gradual increase in gestational age was not followed by decrease or, as we expected, with increase of impedance to blood flow. Both RI and PI showed constant values. One would presume that blood flow in the corpus luteum is related to its activity. As corpus luteum activity progressed, color flow would be more intense, impedance to flow might decrease, and vice versa. However, this speculation was not confirmed in our study. Reports on corpus luteum activity during pregnancy are controversial[22,26]. There is no general agreement as to when this activity starts to decline and how long the corpus luteum can be observed at all[26]. An interesting observation from our study is that corpus luteum blood flow was more often detected on the left ovary (62.6%). The reason for this is unknown.

It was suggested in a previous report that the absence of luteal blood flow might be inconsistent with a normal pregnancy[21]. Results from our study partially support this hypothesis. Impedance to intraovarian blood flow was significantly higher in patients with abnormal early pregnancy (missed, incomplete and threatened abortion) than in women with normal pregnancy. However, this was not confirmed in patients with blighted ovum, molar and ectopic pregnancy. The impedance to lutal blood flow was almost the same as in normal pregnancy. This difference among subgroups of abnormal early pregnancy may be due to differences in natural history of the disease. Missed and incomplete abortion represent failed early pregnancy with no prospects for further development. Threatened abortion is potentially

Table 3 Detection rate of corpus luteum blood flow in normal ($n=107$) and abnormal early pregnancies ($n=51$)

Pregnancies	*Women* (*n*)	*Mean age* (years)	*Left luteal flow*		*Right luteal flow*	
			n	%	*n*	%
Normal pregnancy	107	29.2	67	62.6	40	37.4
Missed abortion	10	24.2	6	60.0	4	40.0
Blighted ovum	10	30.5	7	70.0	3	30.0
Molar pregnancy	8	26.2	3	37.5	5	62.5
Ectopic pregnancy	10	27.0	6	60.0	4	40.0
Incomplete abortion	7	29.4	3	42.8	4	57.2
Threatened abortion	6	25.2	4	66.7	2	33.3
Total	158	28.5	96	60.8*	62	39.2*

Fisher test: $t=6.89$; $*p<0.01$

Table 4 The mean resistance index (RI) and pulsatility index (PI) with two standard deviations (2 SD) from corpus luteum blood flow in 107 normal and 51 abnormal early pregnancies

Pregnancies	*RI*	*2 SD*	*Statistics*	*PI*	*2 SD*	*Statistics*
Normal pregnancy	0.452	0.04		0.636	0.09	
Missed abortion	0.536	0.06	$p<0.01$	0.782	0.05	NS
Blighted ovum	0.488	0.04	NS	0.745	0.08	NS
Molar pregnancy	0.449	0.05	NS	0.646	0.10	NS
Ectopic pregnancy	0.485	0.07	NS	0.735	0.06	NS
Incomplete abortion	0.539	0.05	$p<0.01$	0.806	0.14	$p<0.01$
Threatened abortion	0.532	0.05	$p<0.01$	0.837	0.12	$p<0.01$

Statistics: one way ANOVA and Tukey HSD type A test; NS = non-significant

a similar condition. Is decreased corpus luteum blood flow a potential cause or consequence of the disease? This remains unclear. The other possibility is anembryonic (blighted ovum), molar or ectopic pregnancy. These pathologic conditions are usually progressive and not self limited. Corpus luteum blood flow and probable activity are consistent with such conditions. This can explain why impedance to luteal blood flow in these women is similar to that in women with normal progressing pregnancy.

Baber and co-workers[20] showed that no pregnant patient after *in vitro* fertilization–embryo transfer (IVF–ET) had the RI from corpus luteum neovascularization greater than 0.50. They presumed normal corpus luteum activity to be indicated by an RI to blood flow below 0.50. Zalud and Kurjak[16] described corpus luteum blood flow in pregnant and non-pregnant women. This study included 58 women with normal early pregnancy, 73 women with proven ectopic pregnancy and 75 non-gravid normal menstruating women. Typical luteal low-impedance flow was detected in 82.8% of cases of early pregnancy, 80.8% of cases of ectopic pregnancy and 69.3% of non-pregnant women. The lowest resistance index (0.42 ± 0.12) of luteal flow was seen in non-pregnant women, and the highest resistance index (0.53 ± 0.09) was obtained in cases of early normotopic pregnancy. The corpus luteum was seen as early as a few days after ovulation in non-pregnant women and was present until about the 11th week of amenorrhea in pregnant women. Jurkovic and colleagues[18] did not find any difference in corpus luteum blood flow between normal intrauterine and ectopic pregnancy. One of our previous studies showed gradual increased impedance to blood flow in the corpus luteum if pregnancy did not occur[19]. This gradual increase in the resistance index was most prominent after the 25th day of the normal menstrual cycle. The lowest resistance index was observed within 48 hours after ovulation. These findings were explained by short activation and deactivation of the corpus luteum if there was no pregnancy. Some other reports presented similar findings[27,28].

Ectopic pregnancy

Potential difficulties arise from overlap between luteal blood flow and color flow in the case of ectopic pregnancy. Using high quality B-mode transvaginal sonography and superimposed color Doppler flow it should be possible to distinguish luteal and ectopic pregnancy blood flow. Only ovarian pregnancy can produce a diagnostic challenge. Kurjak and co-workers[29] showed that corpus luteum flow proved to be significantly different from ectopic trophoblastic flow. There was a higher RI, the mean value being dependent on a coexisting pregnancy. The RI averaged 0.48 in pregnancy, but was significantly lower (0.44 ± 0.03) in the non-pregnant state. Corpus luteum flow was not always present in cases of ectopic pregnancy. In fact, the Fisher exact test, when used, demonstrated that the presence or absence of corpus luteum flow was not an effective discriminator. The practical application of using measurements of luteal blood flow to dicriminate between intra- and extrauterine pregnancies seems limited. Jurkovic and colleagues[18] concluded that there were no significant hemodynamic differences either in the corpus luteum, uterine arteries or trophoblast when comparing intrauterine to ectopic pregnancies. The only difference was a reduction in blood flow velocity in the uterine arteries of women with ectopic pregnancy, perhaps suggesting an overall reduction in uterine blood supply. Whilst this difference was statistically significant and of academic interest, it has little, if any, clinical relevance. Although these data may suggest a limited diagnostic role for color Doppler, this is not necessarily the case. Our impression is that the most clinically helpful role of color Doppler in this context is in reliably identifying the side of the corpus luteum (on the same side as the ectopic pregnancy in over 86.4% cases) such that it can be used as a guide to direct the search for the ectopic gestational sac, specially in non-specific ultrasound features. Unfortunately, the low impedance blood pattern that can be observed in and around the corpus luteum is similar to that of the blood supply to the ectopic sac and can cause confusion. However, with care, the vascular branches to both corpus luteum and ectopic sac can be identified separately. It is this capability that can be particularly helpful in trying make a definitive diagnosis in the presence of an adnexal mass. Vessels are often seen at the periphery of the ectopic sac and are usually confined to one segment of the trophoblast ring. Reports showing the presence of low-impedance flow on the side of most ectopics are not surprising given the ipsilateral presence of the corpus luteum in most cases. The blood supply to the ectopic sac must be demonstrated as separate from that to the ovary for its recognition to be diagnostically useful. This enhances our ability to make a definitive ultrasound diagnosis of ectopic pregnancy.

Stimulated ovulation

The purpose of hormone stimulation is to induce ovulation in infertile patients, or to prepare women for oocyte retrieval for *in vitro* fertilization. The ovarian response to hormone stimulation is different from physiological changes that characterize normal menstrual cycles. The normal menstrual cycle is characterized by formation of only one corpus luteum which involves only one ovary. In ovarian stimulated cycles, a number of follicles are recruited, proceeding through the process of maturation and giving origin to the corpus luteum. Both ovaries are usually involved in this process.

Transvaginal sonography is one of the most important tools in monitoring the ovarian response to hormone stimulation[30]. Adjustment of hormonal treatment and determination of the appropriate day for oocyte retrieval is usually based on follicular measurements performed by transvaginal sonography. However, from the moment the ultrasound-guided oocyte retrieval is performed, the clinical application of ultrasonography is very limited throughout the rest of the cycle. Pregnancy can be diagnosed by transvaginal sonography as early as the 5th week of gestation[31].

The introduction of Doppler sonography gives us the opportunity to study the peculiar vascular changes which characterize the stimulated ovaries. The ovarian or uterine arteries can easily be studied with transvaginal Doppler sonography[15,32]. It is difficult, however, to recognize the intraovarian vessels without using color flow

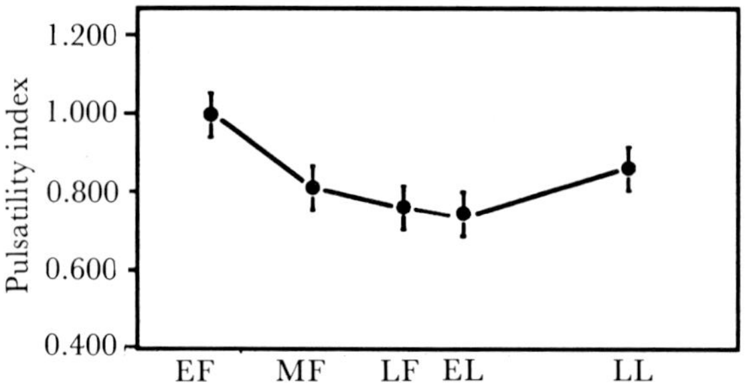

Figure 12 Intraovarian pulsatility index throughout stimulated cycles. Phases: EF, early follicular; MF, middle follicular; LF, late follicular; EL, early luteal; LL, late luteal

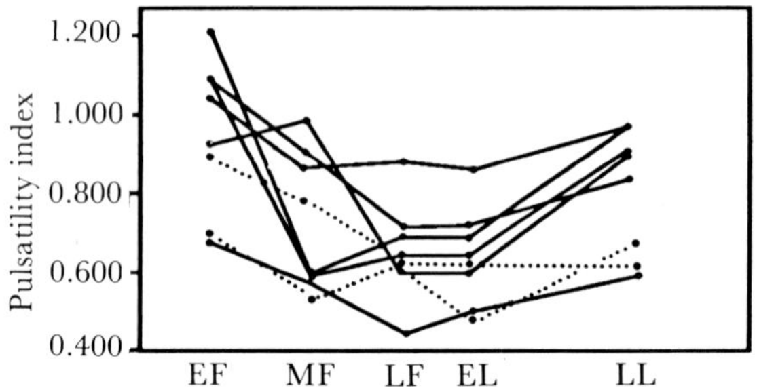

Figure 13 Intraovarian pulsatility index in eight women with successful ovarian stimulation. The dotted lines represent measurements obtained from two women who conceived following embryo transfer. Phases: EF, early follicular; MF, middle follicular; LF, late follicular; EL, early luteal; LL, late luteal

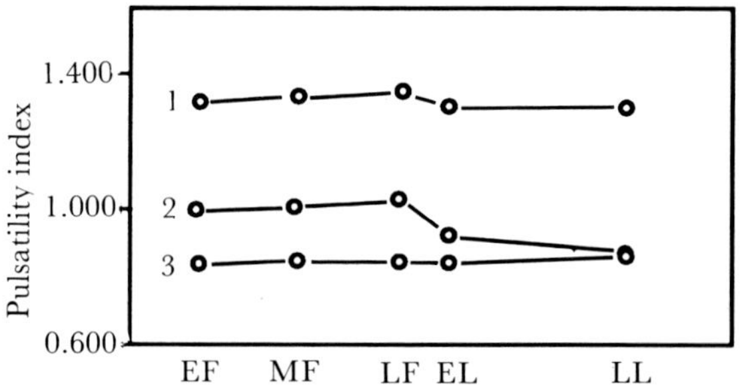

Figure 14 Three women in whom the intraovarian pulsatility index did change significantly throughout the cycle. Patients 1 and 3 failed to respond to ovarian stimulation. Phases EF, early follicular; MF, middle follicular; LF, late follicular; EL, early luteal; LL, late luteal

imaging. The color flow imaging, in particular, gives us the possibility to observe the angiogenic process which accompanies the formation of the corpus luteum[16,33]. Intraovarian blood flow changes throughout hormone stimulated cycles are similar to those changes observed throughout normal menstrual cycles[34]. These changes are characterized by a decreased impedance to blood flow during the follicular and early luteal phase (Figure 12). When patients do not become pregnant, impedance to blood flow in the intraovarian vessels returns to basal level during the late luteal phase (Figure 13).

It has been demonstrated that ovarian blood flow correlates with the number of follicles (> 15 mm) on each stimulated ovary[34,35]. The pulsatility index of the ovarian artery and intraovarian vessels decreases as the number of follicles increases. This correlation was found even during the early follicular phase when follicular recruitment and development had just started[34]. The very early vascular changes observed in hormone-stimulated women suggest that the process of vascularization guides the follicular growth from the very beginning of the cycle. Moreover, as shown by using color flow imaging, the appearance of blood vessels within the ovaries changes throughout the stimulated cycles. The number and size of blood vessels that can be detected inside the ovaries increase during the development of the follicles. In the late follicular phase most of the intraovarian vessels are arranged around one or a few leading preovulatory follicles[34]. This typical growth and arrangement of intraovarian vessels, which characterize the growing follicles, gives us extra support for the hypothesis that follicular growth and maturation is guided by its blood supply. In patients who fail to respond to hormone stimulation, intraovarian vascularization is very poor and resistance to blood flow in these vessels is persistently high (Figure 14).

Recently, it has been shown that intraovarian blood flow correlates with serum estradiol level throughout stimulated cycles[34] (Figure 15). There is a great deal of controversy related to the functional relationship between luteal blood flow and luteal steroidogenesis. Studies in the rabbit suggest that blood flow in the corpus luteum is not acutely dependent on normal rates of steroidogenesis[36]. Infusion of estradiol increases ovarian stromal blood flow but fails to alter the high level

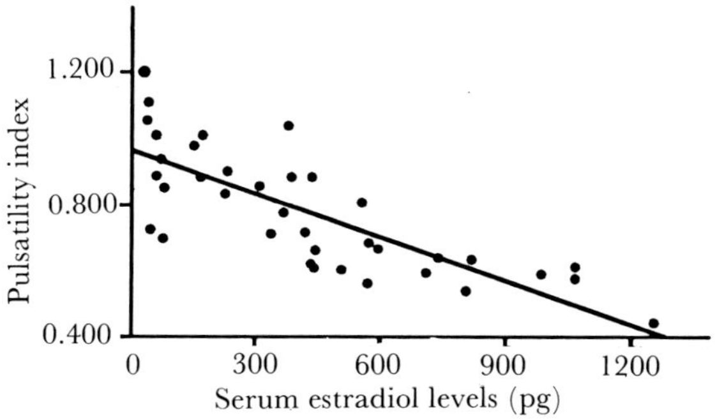

Figure 15 Correlation between intraovarian pulsatility index and serum estradiol levels

of blood flow in the corpus luteum[23], supporting the concept that the blood vessels in the corpus luteum are maximally dilated and incapable of autoregulation.

As we have just mentioned, a number of corpora lutea are usually formed during the luteal phase in hormone-stimulated cycles. Their appearance can be clearly observed by transvaginal sonography. By using color flow imaging, we are able to identify abundant blood vessels around the corpus luteum. Doppler studies of these vessels demonstrate a very low impedance to blood flow, during the early stage of the luteal phase. When women fail to become pregnant, the rich vascularization of the corpus luteum gradually disappears, and their resistance gradually increases throughout the late luteal phase[20,34]. However, when women become pregnant, the corpus luteum maintains its vascularity and the impedance to blood flow in these vessels remains low[20,34]. As shown in one study, by measuring the ovarian artery flow velocity waveforms during the second half of the luteal phase, we may identify those women who failed to become pregnant. According to this study, no patient who became pregnant had an RI greater than 0.5 during the second half of the luteal phase[20]. However, the corpus luteum may remain highly vascularized during the late luteal phase for other reasons (e.g. hyperstimulation of the ovaries).

Adnexal pathology

Previous studies with transabdominal and transvaginal sonography have shown that the corpus luteum is 'a great imitator'[37]. It may have morphological characteristics similar to other ovarian structures. The dimensions of a persistent corpus luteum may exceed 10 cm and its inner structure may appear as liquid, solid, or both[37]. It may have thin or thick septa and even papillae. All these different sonographic images of the corpus luteum make it difficult to distinguish from other benign or malignant ovarian tumors. Fortunately, this problem exists only during the premenopausal period when the incidence of malignant ovarian cancer is low. During the postmenopausal period, the differential diagnosis of an ovarian mass does not include the corpus luteum.

The use of color flow imaging, together with Doppler sonography, does not improve our ability to differentiate between the corpus luteum and other ovarian masses[38]. On the contrary, ovarian scanning with color flow imaging and Doppler sonography may even increase our confusion. Diagnosis of ovarian malignancy, by color flow imaging and Doppler, is based on the detection of low-resistance blood vessels within the ovarian mass[39]. The origin of these vessels is an angiogenic activity of the tumoral cells. The corpus luteum, however, also has an angiogenic activity which controls the formation of abundant low-resistance blood vessels. These vessels are usually well demonstrated by color flow imaging and Doppler[16,34]. It seems, therefore, that the corpus luteum appears more similar to malignant than to benign tumors, on color flow imaging.

Several guidelines are necessary in order to avoid an incorrect diagnosis of the corpus luteum. Premenopausal women should be scanned for ovarian masses at the beginning of the menstrual cycle when the corpus luteum practically does not exist. If the patient was not instructed to arrive at the beginning of the cycle, information about her last menstrual period is required. In this way we are able to estimate the probability that this patient has a functional ovarian structure. Any sonographic finding of ovarian mass which does not need an immediate intervention should be rescanned within the following 6 weeks. Disappearance or any significant decrease (> 50%) in size, compared to the previous sonographic finding, suggests a functional ovarian cyst or mass. In these cases, no surgical intervention is recommended, but simply sonographic follow-up.

CONCLUSION

Transvaginal ultrasound with color Doppler imaging provides a non-invasive tool to study the morphology and specific blood flow changes in the ovary during the luteal part of the menstrual cycle. The process of increased vascularization reaches its maximal level during the formation of the corpus luteum. It seems that this process of vascularization is more pronounced in hormone-stimulated women. When patients become pregnant, the increased intraovarian blood flow persists, in order to support the corpus luteum. The corpus luteum may present a great variety of sonographic features which may also include the appearance of a malignant ovarian tumor. Whereas, from the scientific point of view, the presented data on corpus luteum studies are promising, their practical clinical values are yet to be evaluated.

References

1. Niswender, G. D. and Nett, T. M. (1988). The corpus luteum and its control. In Knobil, E. and Neil, J. (eds.) *The Physiology of Reproduction*, pp. 489–525. (New York: Raven Press)
2. Hodgen, G. D. and Itskowitz, J. (1988). Recognition and maintenance of pregnancy. In Knobil, E. and Neil, J. (eds.) *The Physiology of Reproduction*, pp. 1995–2021. (New York: Raven Press)
3. Pratt, J. P. (1927). Corpus luteum in its relation to menstruation and pregnancy. *Endocrinology*, **11**, 195–204
4. Hall, R. E. (1955). Removal of the corpus luteum in early pregnancy: a review of the literature and report of 2 cases. *Bull. Sloane Hosp. Women*, **1**, 49–59
5. Tulsky, A. S. and Koff, A. K. (1957). Some observation on the role of the corpus luteum in early human pregnancy. *Fertil. Steril.*, **8**, 118–22
6. Solomon, S. (1988). The placenta as an endocrine organ: steroids. In Knobil, E. and Neil, J. (eds.) *The Physiology of Reproduction*, pp. 2085–92. (New York: Raven Press)
7. Timor-Tritsch, I. E., Peisner, D. B. and Raju, S. (1990). Sonoembryology: an organ-oriented approach using a high-frequency vaginal probe. *J. Clin. Ultrasound*, **18**, 286–98
8. Peisner, D. B. and Timor-Tritsch, I. E. (1990). The discriminatory zone of beta-hCG for vaginal probes. *J. Clin. Ultrasound*, **18**, 280–5
9. Lenz, S. (1985). Ultrasonic study of follicular maturation, ovulation and development of corpus luteum during normal menstrual cycles. *Acta Obstet. Gynecol. Scand.*, **64**, 15–19
10. De Crespigny, L., O'Herlihy, C. and Robinson, H. P. (1981). Ultrasonic observation of the mechanism of ovulation. *Am. J. Obstet. Gynecol.*, **139**, 636–9
11. Rottem, S., Timor-Tritsch, I. E. and Thaler, I. (1993). Assessment of pelvic pathology by high frequency transvaginal sonography. In Chervenak, F. A., Isaacson, G. C. and Campbell, S. (eds.) *Ultrasound in Obstetrics and Gynecology*, pp. 1629–41. (Boston, Toronto, London: Little, Brown and Co.)
12. Davis, J. A. and Gosink, B. B. (1986). Fluid in the female pelvis: cyclic patterns. *J. Ultrasound Med.*, **5**, 75–9
13. Hill, L. M. (1992). Infertility and reproductive assistance. In Nyberg, D. A., Hill, L. M., Bohm-Velez, M. and Mendelson, E. B. (eds.) *Transvaginal Ultrasound*, pp. 43–64. (St. Louis, Baltimore, Boston, Chicago, London, Philadelphia, Sydney, Toronto: Mosby Year Book)
14. Taylor, K. J. W., Burns, P. N., Wells, P. N. E., Conway, D. I. and Hull, M. G. R. (1985). Ultrasound Doppler flow studies of the ovarian and uterine arteries. *Br. J. Obstet. Gynaecol.*, **92**, 240–3
15. Hata, K., Hata, T., Senot, D., Makihara, K., Aoki, S., Takamiya, O. and Kitao, M. (1990). Change in ovarian arterial compliance during the human menstrual cycle assessed by Doppler ultrasound. *Br. J. Obstet. Gynaecol.*, **97**, 163–6
16. Zalud, I. and Kurjak, A. (1990). The assessment of luteal blood flow in pregnant and non-pregnant women by transvaginal color Doppler. *J. Perinat. Med.*, **18**, 215–21
17. Kurjak, A. and Zalud, I. (1991). Ectopic pregnancy. In Kurjak, A. (ed.) *Transvaginal Color Doppler*, pp. 83–95. (Carnforth, UK: Parthenon Publishing)
18. Jurkovic, D., Bourne, T. H., Jauniaux, E., Campbell, S. and Collins, W. P. (1992). Transvaginal color Doppler study of blood flow in ectopic pregnancies. *Fertil. Steril.*, **57**, 68–72
19. Kurjak, A., Kupesic-Urek, S., Schulman, H. and Zalud, I. (1991). Transvaginal color flow Doppler in the assessment of ovarian and uterine blood flow in infertile women. *Fertil. Steril.*, **56**, 870–4
20. Baber, R. J., McSweeney, M. B., Gill, R. W., Porter, R. N., Picker, R. H., Warren, P. S., Kossoff, G. and Saunders, D. M. (1988). Transvaginal pulsed Doppler ultrasound assessment of blood flow to the corpus luteum in IVF patients following embryo transfer. *Br. J. Obstet. Gynaecol.*, **95**, 1226–9

21. Taylor, K. J. W., Ramos, I. M., Feyock, A. N., Snower, D. P., Carter, D., Shapiro, B. S., Meyer, W. R. and DeCherney, A. H. (1989). Ectopic pregnancy: duplex Doppler evaluation. *Radiology*, **173**, 93–7
22. Csapo, A. I. and Pulkkinen, M. (1978). Indispensability of the human corpus luteum in the maintenance of early pregnancy. *Obstet. Gynecol. Surv.*, **33**, 69–74
23. Wiltbank, M. C., Gallagher, K. P., Dysko, R. C. and Keyes, P. L. (1989). Regulation of blood flow to the rabbit corpus luteum: effects of estradiol and human chorionic gonadotropin. *Endocrinology*, **124**, 605–11
24. Oda, T., Aoki, R., Yoshimura, S., Yoshida, J., Kobayashi, T., Nakamura, Y., Nozawa, S. and Ohno, T. (1992). Role of corpus luteum function in embryo implantation. *Horm. Res.* **37** (Suppl. 1), 75–8
25. Salim, A., Zalud, I., Farmakides, G., Schulman, H., Kurjak, A. and Latin, V. (1994). Corpus luteum blood flow in normal and abnormal early pregnancy: evaluation with transvaginal color Doppler. *J. Clin. Ultrasound*, in press
26. Cunningham, F. G., MacDonald, P. C. and Gant, N. F. (1989). *William's Obstetrics*, pp. 915–19. (East Norwalk: Appleton & Lange)
27. Steer, C. W., Campbell, S., Papiglione, J., Kingsland, C. R., Mason, B. A. and Collins, W. P. (1990). Transvaginal color flow imaging of the uterine arteries during the ovarian and menstrual cycles. *Hum. Reprod.*, **5**, 391–5
28. Fleischer, A. C. (1991). Assessment of utero-ovarian blood flow with transvaginal color Doppler sonography. *Fertil. Steril.*, **53**, 684–6
29. Kurjak, A., Zalud, I. and Schulman, H. (1991). Ectopic pregnancy: transvaginal color Doppler of trophoblastic flow in questionable adnexa. *J. Ultrasound Med.*, **10**, 685–9
30. Itskovitz, J., Boldes, R., Levron, J. and Thaler, I. (1990). Transvaginal sonography in the diagnosis and treatment of infertility. *J. Clin. Ultrasound*, **18**, 249–53
31. Goldstein, S. (1988). Very early pregnancy detection with endovaginal ultrasound. *Obstet. Gynecol.*, **72**, 200–6
32. Scholtes, M. C. W., Wladimiroff, J. W., van Rijen, H. J. M. and Hop, W. C. J. (1989). Uterine and ovarian flow velocity waveforms in the normal menstrual cycle: a transvaginal Doppler study. *Fertil. Steril.*, **52**, 981–7
33. Bourne, T. H., Jurkovic, D., Waterstone, J., Campbell, S. and Collins, W. P. (1991). Intrafollicular blood flow during human ovulation. *Ultrasound Obstet. Gynaecol.*, **1**, 53–9
34. Weiner, Z., Thaler, I., Levron, J., Lewit, N. and Itskovitz-Eldor, J. (1993). Assessment of ovarian and uterine blood flow by transvaginal color Doppler in ovarian-stimulated women: correlation with the number of follicles and steroid hormone levels. *Fertil. Steril.*, **59**, 743–9
35. Deutinger, J., Reinthaller, A. and Bernaschek, G. (1989). Transvaginal pulsed Doppler measurement of blood flow velocity in the ovarian arteries during cycle stimulation and after follicle puncture. *Fertil. Steril.*, **51**, 466–70
36. Wiltbank, M. C., Gallagher, K. P., Christensen, A. K., Brabec, R. K. and Keyes, P. L. (1990). Physiological and immunocytochemical evidence for a new concept of blood flow regulation in the corpus luteum. *Biol. Reprod.*, **42**, 139–44
37. Rottem, S. and Timor-Tritsch, I. (1991). *Transvaginal Sonography*, pp. 155–6. (New York: Elsevier Science)
38. Weiner, Z., Thaler, I., Beck, D., Rottem, S., Deutsch, M. and Brandes, J. M. (1992). Differentiating malignant from benign ovarian tumors with transvaginal color flow imaging. *Obstet. Gynecol.*, **79**, 159–64
39. Bourne, T. W., Campbell, S., Steer, C., Whitehead, M. I. and Collins, W. P. (1989). Transvaginal color flow imaging: a possible new screening technique for ovarian cancer. *Br. Med. J.*, **299**, 1367–71

Morphological evaluation of the ovary using transvaginal sonography

8

J. P. Lerner and I. E. Timor-Tritsch

Transvaginal sonography has revolutionized the evaluation of the ovary and its conditions, both benign and malignant. Sonographic imaging of small structural details is essentially due to the improved resolution of higher-frequency vaginal probes operating in close proximity to the ovary itself. Both normal and abnormal conditions can be identified with reliability. Even during the postmenopausal years, the small but normal ovaries are sometimes imaged. In this chapter, we concentrate on the morphological description of the normal and the pathological ovary, using conventional 'black and white' (gray scale) transvaginal ultrasonography. The experience gathered by color Doppler studies, reflecting physiological changes within the ovary (resistance to flow), both normal and abnormal, will be discussed in other chapters.

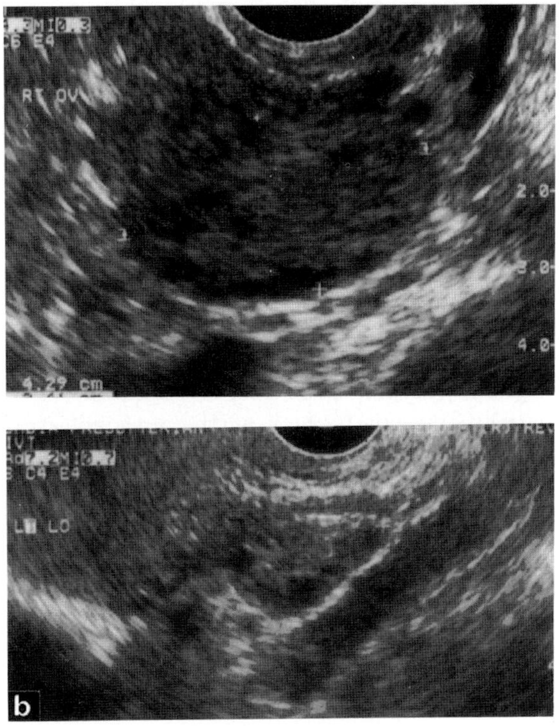

Figure 1 Two normal ovaries, both from patients in their reproductive years; (a) a normal right ovary with several follicles located in the periphery, near the ovarian cortex; (b) a normal left ovary, with its proximity to the iliac vein visible

THE NORMAL OVARY

In the reproductive years, the normal ovary is relatively easy to detect using transvaginal sonography. Characteristic small sonolucencies, representing follicles or the presence of a corpus luteum, are the sonographic markers of the ovaries and allow their rapid identification during the reproductive years (Figure 1). The ovaries are usually located lateral to the uterus, above and medial to the hypogastric vessels. Occasionally, they cause a slight depression of the hypogastric vein which has been termed 'Waldeyer's fossa' in the descriptive anatomy. At times, the healthy, mobile ovary may 'fall' into the cul-de-sac, or be found in other locations within the pelvis. Of course, previous pelvic surgery or the presence of adhesions can fix the ovaries in abnormal locations. A small amount of pelvic fluid, normal in most settings, may also help delineate the ovary. When large amounts of fluid (ascites) or blood are present in the pelvis, the ovaries are easily outlined. If all attempts to image the ovary using transvaginal sonography fail, it is possible to attempt transabdominal sonography in a patient with a full bladder. The bladder, filled to capacity, will 'squeeze' the ovaries towards the side walls of the pelvis enabling their detection in many cases.

In the postmenopausal years, the normal atretic ovaries become more difficult to image.

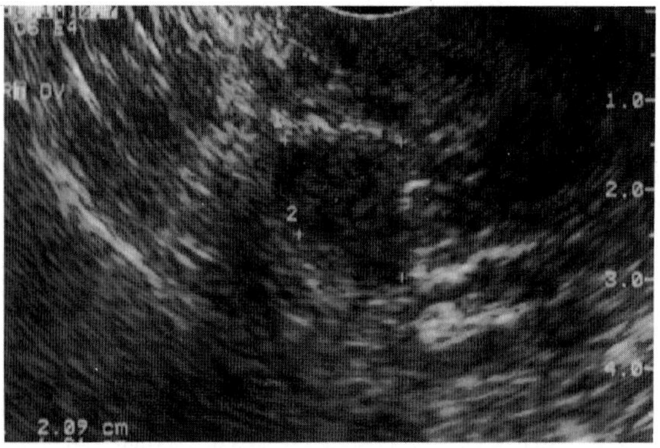

Figure 2 A normal-appearing ovary in a postmenopausal patient; no follicles seen, and relatively smaller and hypoechogenic

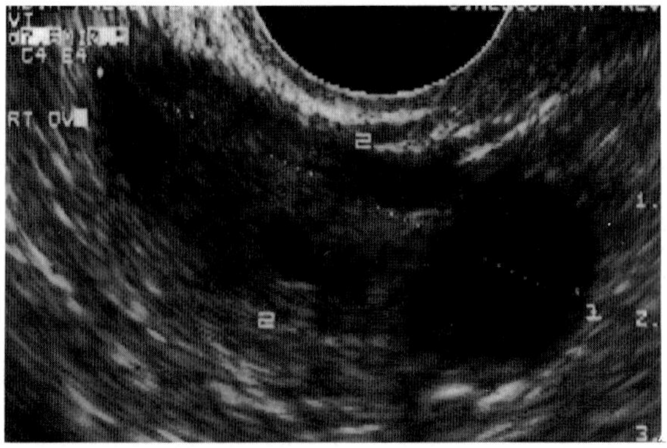

Figure 3 A normal ovary containing a sonolucent dominant follicle

This is due to several factors, including the disappearance of follicles and functional cysts, the smaller size of the ovary itself, and the decreased quantity of pelvic fluid present. The postmenopausal ovaries appear as small, hypoechoic ellipsoid structures located in the above-named locations (Figure 2). In a significant number of patients, the ovaries may not be detected, even after considerable time spent searching for them. There is no consistent view as to whether the inability to visualize a postmenopausal ovary assures a lack of pathology or malignancy. The general consensus seems to favor the view that lack of visualization of postmenopausal ovaries and a negative bimanual examination suggests ovarian atrophy and lack of disease. A study by Rodriguez and colleagues[1] supports this view: 85 of 104 ovaries in postmenopausal women were imaged prior to surgery unrelated to adnexal disease. Of the 19 ovaries that were not seen, all were subsequently found to be atrophic, with no evidence of disease.

The size of the normal ovary changes with the phase of the menstrual cycle and generally decreases with age. The ovary containing the dominant or ovulatory follicle is usually larger. Several studies have attempted to define normal ovarian size[2–6], and the general conclusion is that it should not exceed 2 × 3 × 4 cm. Fleischer and associates[4] examined the ovaries of 30 postmenopausal patients by transvaginal sonography prior to surgery. In this study, at least one ovary was detected 80% of the time, and both ovaries were imaged 60% of the time. The mean size of the normal sonographically-imaged postmenopausal ovary was 2.2 × 1.2 × 1.1 cm. Other authors, including Campbell and co-workers[7], measured ovarian volume rather than size, and found a correlation between estimates of ovarian volume and pathological examination. Differences in ovarian volume may also be secondary to several factors that affect ovarian size, including years since menopause, patient's weight, parity, and hormone replacement regimen.

Functional cysts and polycystic ovaries

A functional ovarian cyst is the most common abnormality found in the ovary, and is always solitary. It is often thin and smooth-walled, with sonolucent fluid within, and exhibits no abnormalities of internal wall structure, such as papillations (Figure 3). It is usually transient in nature and less than 5 cm, although it can persist through several menstrual cycles, and can attain a large size, often reaching 6–7 cm (Figure 4). Large ovarian cysts can be followed by serial ultrasound scans, hormonal suppression, or both. A follow-up scan in 6 weeks is often suggested, if clinically indicated, for large follicular cysts.

The corpus luteum is a functional ovarian cyst that has a myriad of appearances when imaged transvaginally[8]. Once its usual monthly degeneration begins, intrafollicular bleeding may be seen within, with characteristic low-level echoes,

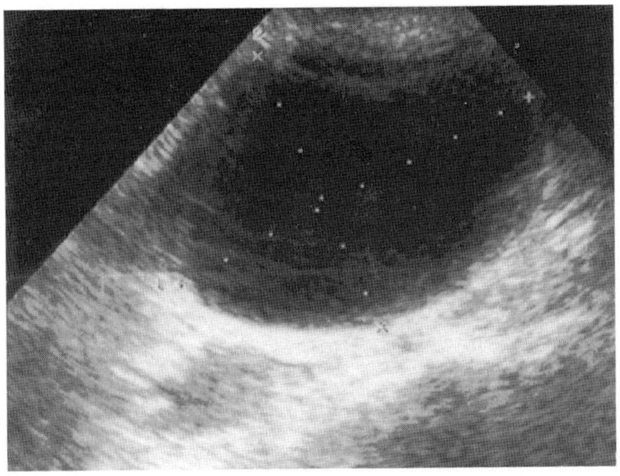

Figure 4 An 8 × 7 cm simple ovarian cyst, appearing completely sonolucent with a thin, smooth wall without internal excrescences

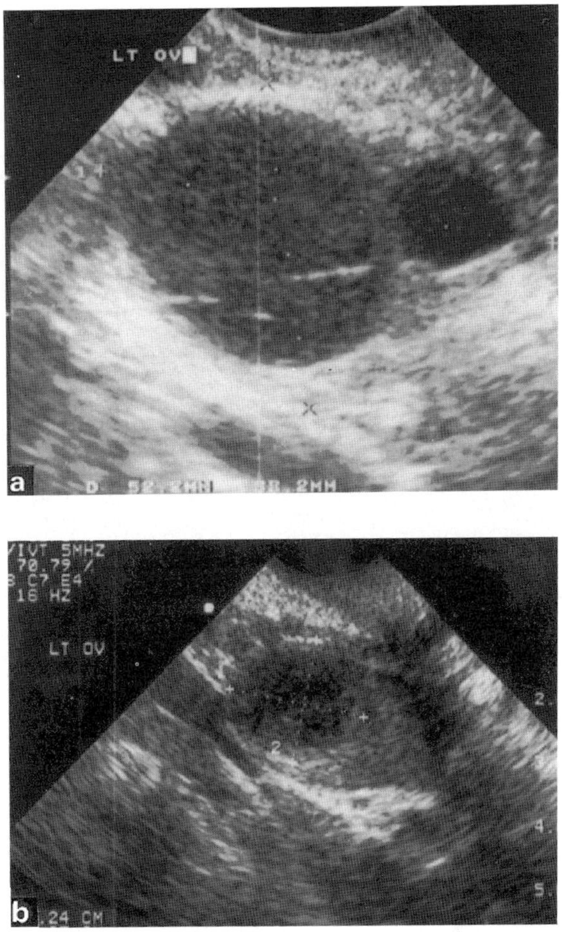

Figure 5 Two corpora lutea, with (a) the typical uniformly low echogenicity; and (b) more varied internal texture

although a multiloculated, irregular and/or complex internal image may be seen (Figures 5,6). Correct diagnosis is correlated with the appropriate time of the menstrual cycle and the presence of surrounding ovarian tissue. The corpus luteum is usually smaller than the persistent follicular cyst in the non-pregnant state, often less than 2 cm. Ruptured corpus luteum cysts are rare and often difficult to diagnose, but the presence of free blood and blood clots in the pelvis and cul-de-sac in a non-pregnant patient raises this suspicion. Color Doppler studies may be used to assist in identification of corpora lutea. The characteristic low impedence to flow caused by the proliferation of new blood vessels may easily be seen.

The polycystic ovary has a characteristic appearance sonographically: it is normal-sized or slightly larger than normal, with multiple, peripherally located, small (immature) follicles[9,10] (Figure 7). This presence of small (less than 8 mm) subcapsular follicles may be the first evidence of the polycystic ovary syndrome (PCOS), or it may confirm an otherwise consistent clinical picture. Among those in whom this typical sonographic picture is noted incidentally, approximately 50% will manifest the classic symptom complex of PCOS, 25% will have an atypical presentation of PCOS, and 25% will be asymptomatic[11].

Ovarian torsion is a difficult diagnosis to make using transvaginal sonography alone, but the recent development of color Doppler flow markedly improves the detection rate by demonstrating absence of flow in the affected ovary. The presence of follicular cysts around a markedly enlarged ovary or the presence of a solid-appearing ovarian mass are sonographic clues when Doppler studies are unavailable, although these characteristic findings are not consistently seen[12].

Benign ovarian masses

Benign ovarian masses are most easily divided into cystic and solid, although several types of ovarian mass contain both components. In general, transvaginal sonography can distinguish cystic from solid masses with a high degree of certainty, and in

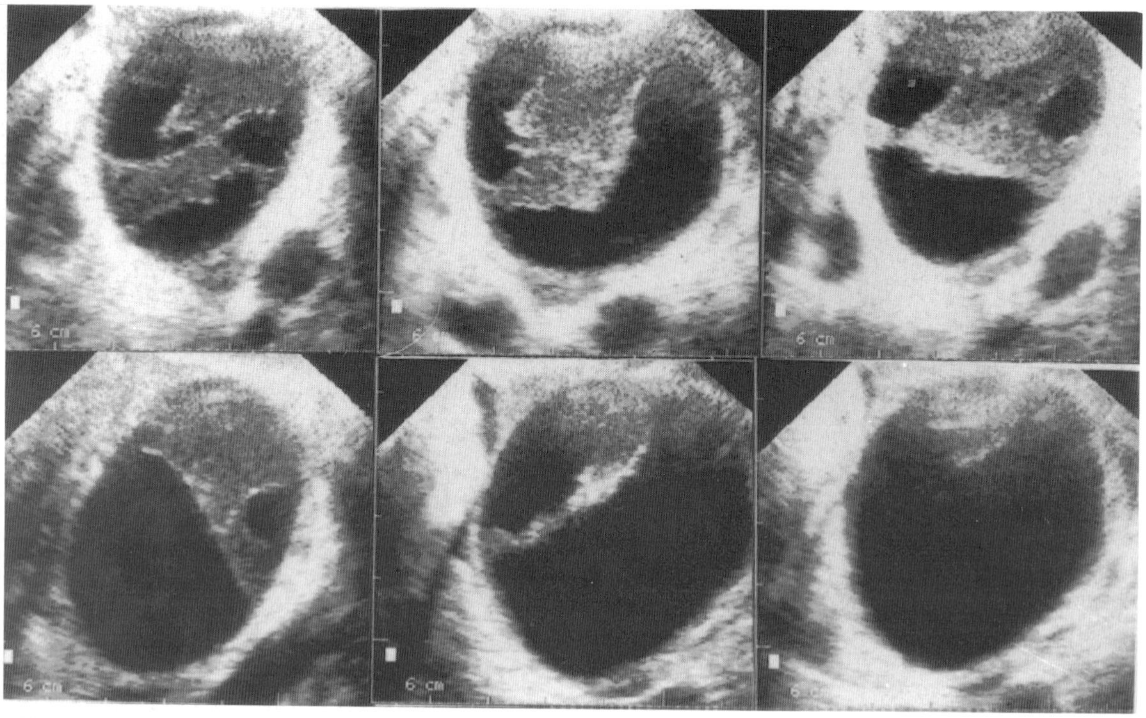

Figure 6 Six different sections of the same corpus luteum, emphasizing the multitudes of shapes and internal appearances created by the retracting clot

addition, may further categorize cystic masses based on the visualization of internal morphological features. This ability to image the internal structure of the ovarian mass is crucial in the differentiation of benign from malignant ovaries. A limited differential diagnosis can often be suggested based on the sonographic appearance of the ovarian mass, and when used in conjunction with consideration of the patient's age, menopausal status, clinical symptoms, and prior surgical history, can often offer a correct diagnosis.

Cystic masses may be further divided into simple and complex, and are not limited to ovarian origin. Paraovarian cysts, peritoneal inclusion cysts, hydrosalpinges, and tubo-ovarian masses may be present in a patient with an abnormal pelvic examination and sonographically normal ovaries.

Sonographic features of simple cystic ovarian masses include a thin, smooth wall, lack of septation within the cystic cavity, and sonolucent (anechoic) fluid within the cavity. These are most often functional ovarian cysts, but may also include non-ovarian etiologies such as paraovarian or paratubal cysts. If the cyst is not follicular and clearly ovarian, the most common diagnoses are cystadenoma, and less often endometrioma or benign cystic teratoma, although the benign teratomas usually demonstrate a more complex and characteristic sonographic picture. Although the studies using transabdominal sonography are inconclusive[13–17], one author, using transvaginal sonography, has found that simple cystic ovarian masses have little or no risk of malignancy, regardless of the cyst size or the patient's age[17].

A cystadenoma is a benign ovarian mass, and can be either mucinous or serous. It often presents in postmenopausal women, but can be found at any time of reproductive life. It has a variable appearance, although serous cystadenomas are often imaged as unilocular and simple, resembling a functional-type cyst (Figure 8), while mucinous cystadenomas often contain septations and more complex sonographic elements (Figure 9). Serous or mucinous tumors of low malignant potential are ovarian masses that contain malignant-type epithelium without evidence of stromal invasion. Sonographically, they may appear more complex

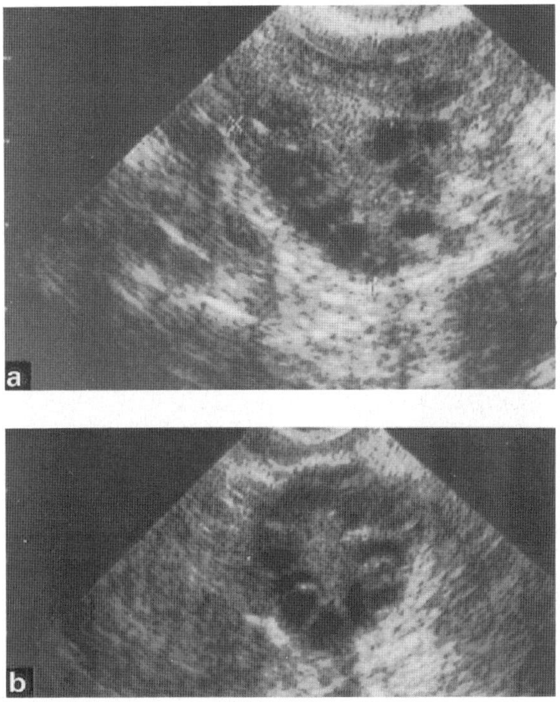

Figure 7 Two views (a and b) of a typical polycystic ovary. The sonolucent follicles crowded beneath the ovarian surface are of approximately equal size, and the central hilar region appears relatively echogenic. These ovaries are typically larger than the normal mean size during the reproductive years

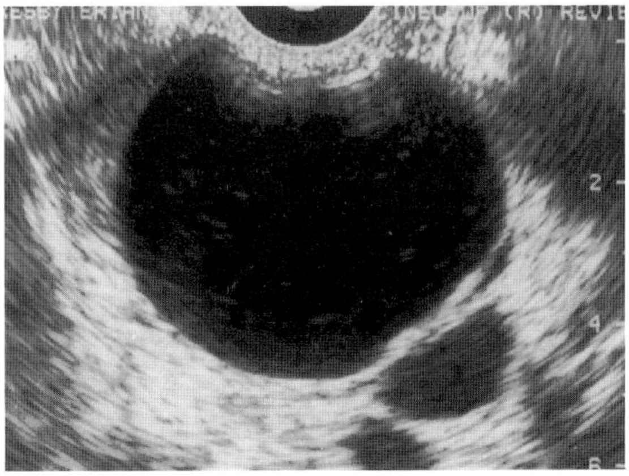

Figure 8 The almost typical appearance of serous cystadenoma. Note the uniform echogenicity, thin, smooth walls, and lack of internal or external protrusions; one or two thin septations can be seen

than their purely benign cystadenoma counterpart, containing thicker septations, solid nodules, and other more ominous-appearing structural

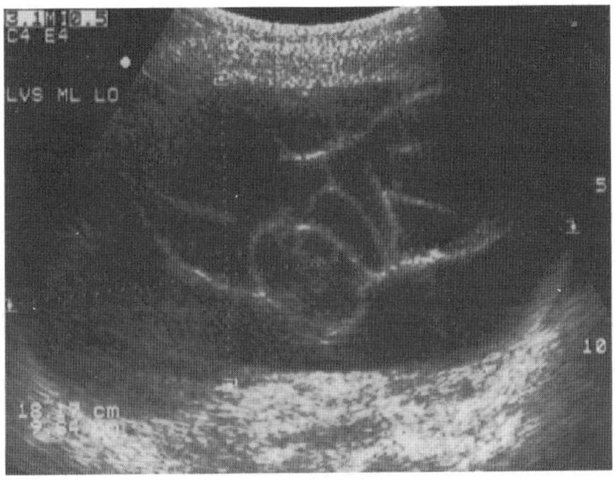

Figure 9 An 18 × 10 cm mucinous cystadenoma, exhibiting a typical multiloculated appearance and low internal echogenicity; these tumors often achieve great size

details (Figure 10). A cystadenofibroma appears as a complex ovarian mass (Figure 11). It may be identified at any time in reproductive life, but is frequently encountered in postmenopausal women. These benign masses have a varied appearance sonographically, often seen as both solid and cystic masses with wall irregularities and areas of calcification. They often appear structurally complex, and may mimic the appearance of tumors of low malignant potential or frank cystadenocarcinoma.

An endometrioma has a typical appearance on ultrasound examination (Figure 12) and these masses are becoming more clinically relevant as the prevalence of endometriosis continues to rise. Endometriosis, the precursor to endometriomata, occurs when functional endometrial tissue grows in abdominal or pelvic sites other than the endometrium itself. This ectopic endometrium functions much as the normally located endometrium does, and responds to cyclical and hormonal changes. With no passage of efflux for this sloughing endometrial tissue, persistent and untreated endometriosis accumulates into cysts of blood and cellular debris, and may cause an intense inflammatory response causing extensive adhesion formation. Small endometriotic implants are unable to be visualized sonographically, but the more advanced, localized form of endometriosis may be seen as a unilocular or multilocular mass containing uniform low-level

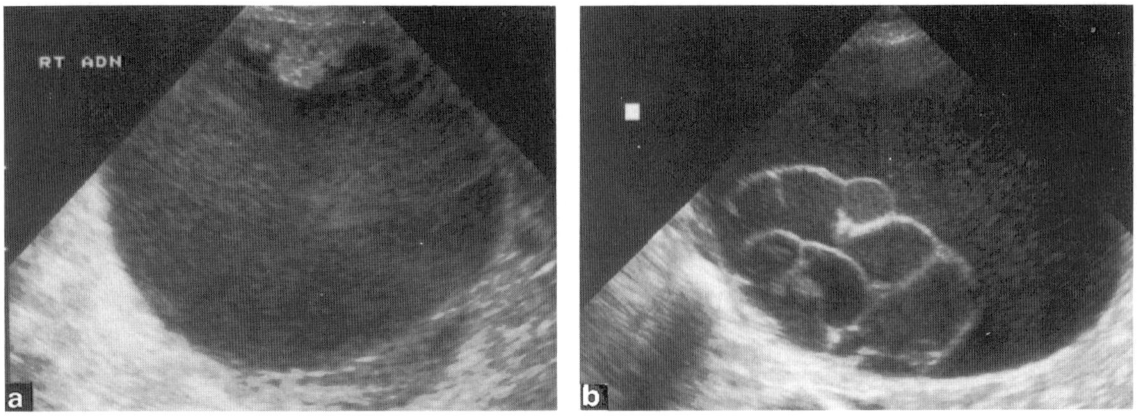

Figure 10 Two tumors of low malignant potential (LMP); (a) serous tumor of LMP showing a complex-appearing inner wall papillation close to the transducer site; (b) mucinous tumor of LMP is large and contains a complex, multiloculated area

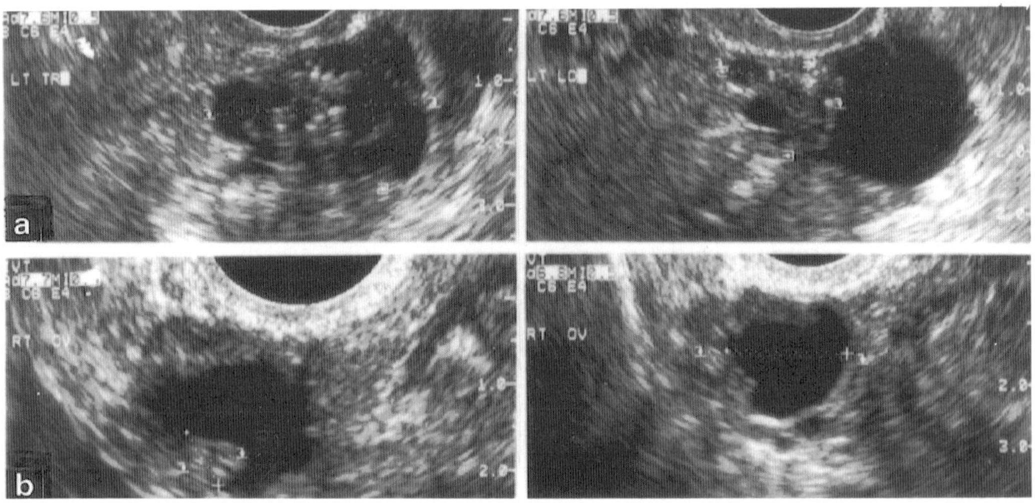

Figure 11 Two cystadenofibromata, (a) on left side; (b) on right side, showing mixed echogenicities, with both solid and cystic areas. These benign tumors can appear complex and be mistaken sonographically for malignancy

echoes within. This classic appearance of an endometrioma is consistently visualized using the higher frequency transvaginal probe, although it may appear solid transabdominally. In a recent study by Kupfer and colleagues in 1992[18], this characteristic homogeneous, hypoechoic 'carpet' of low-level echoes was imaged 82% of the time. An endometrioma may be indistinguishable from a hemorrhagic cyst, although hemorrhagic cysts usually resolve or decrease in size on follow-up scans, while endometriomata usually remain constant and persist on subsequent examinations.

A benign cystic teratoma is the most common benign germ cell ovarian tumor and is derived from all three germ cell layers. They commonly occur during the reproductive years but may also be encountered as a newly palpable ovary on bimanual examination in a postmenopausal woman. They are often asymptomatic, and bilateral approximately 15% of the time. Due to their frequent large size and dense, often solid core, benign teratomas have been known to twist, and less often, to rupture, causing diffuse peritonitis and clinically apparent abdominal pain. Sono-

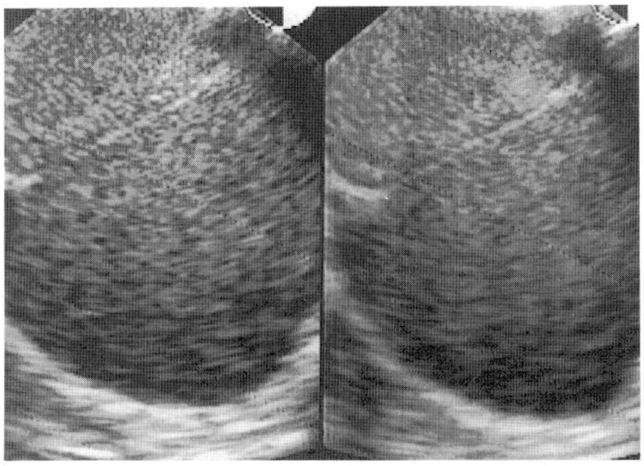

Figure 12 Two sections of an endometrioma, showing typical uniformly low echogenicity, representing the bloody material with which it is filled; this cyst has a thin septation, commonly seen

graphically, a benign cystic teratoma has a variety of appearances[19], ranging from primarily solid to primarily cystic. Often, a characteristic highly echogenic core or 'plug' may be imaged, greatly improving discriminatory ability (Figure 13). This echogenic core usually exhibits a sonographic feature known as shadowing, where the acoustic echoes distal to the core are lost. In the more cystic teratomas, homogeneous fat and sebum deposits may appear sonolucent or low-level echogenic, and teeth may be imaged as highly echogenic nodules within this cystic area. As 10–20% of benign cystic teratomas are bilateral, the contralateral ovary must be carefully imaged for evidence of these characteristic findings, even when normal in size. Any unusual hyperechoic structure imaged within the ovary necessitates a follow-up scan during the early follicular phase of the patient's following menstrual cycle.

Benign solid masses are much less common than benign cystic masses, and are quite difficult to differentiate sonographically from malignant ovarian masses. These primarily consist of fibroma, thecoma, and Brenner tumors although pedunculated myomas often mimic the appearance of a solid ovarian mass. It is almost impossible to distinguish sonographically the fibroma–thecoma from the pedunculated myoma, although the visualization of a fibrous stalk inserting into the uterus improves differentiation. By transvaginal sonography, fibroma and thecoma appear solid and homogeneous, and may exhibit shadowing when calcified (Figure 14). Rarely; these solid tumors appear as a complex mass with mixed echogenicity. Brenner tumors are benign ovarian tumors that often appear as hypoechoic, solid, homogeneous, and well circumscribed. They can grow to a size of 5–8 cm or more, and are rarely bilateral. Any one of these benign solid masses may be part of a complex known as Meigs' syndrome, which contains the triad of benign solid ovarian tumor, ascites, and hydrothorax[20]. The presence of a solid ovarian tumor should instigate a search for evidence of pelvic ascites and pleural fluid.

THE ABNORMAL OVARY

Malignant ovarian masses

Ovarian carcinoma is the leading cause of death from gynecological malignancy, and the fourth leading cause of death from all cancers in women. It accounts for 4% of the cancers by site of incidence, and 5% of the deaths by cancer site[21]. In the United States, every female at birth has a 5–7% risk of developing this deadly disease. The cure rate is dismal, with an overall 5-year survival rate between 30 and 40%, as a result of the late and advanced clinical presentation. Since 1965, and Sunden's pioneering work[22], much progress has been made in evaluating the diagnostic value of sonography in the evaluation of ovaries suspected of malignancy, although no universally accepted criteria are present. Pelvic sonography is more sensitive than pelvic examination in the detection of malignant ovarian tumors[1,23,24], although the combination of transvaginal and transabdominal sonography appears to be superior to either modality alone[4]. While transvaginal sonography delineates finer structural detail within the cyst, transabdominal sonography provides an overview of pelvic anatomy, confirms the presence of ascites or hydronephrosis, and can guide the transvaginal approach.

When an ovarian mass is encountered on transvaginal sonography, the structural details within the mass provide information regarding the possibility of its malignancy. Factors associated with a greater risk of malignancy include a

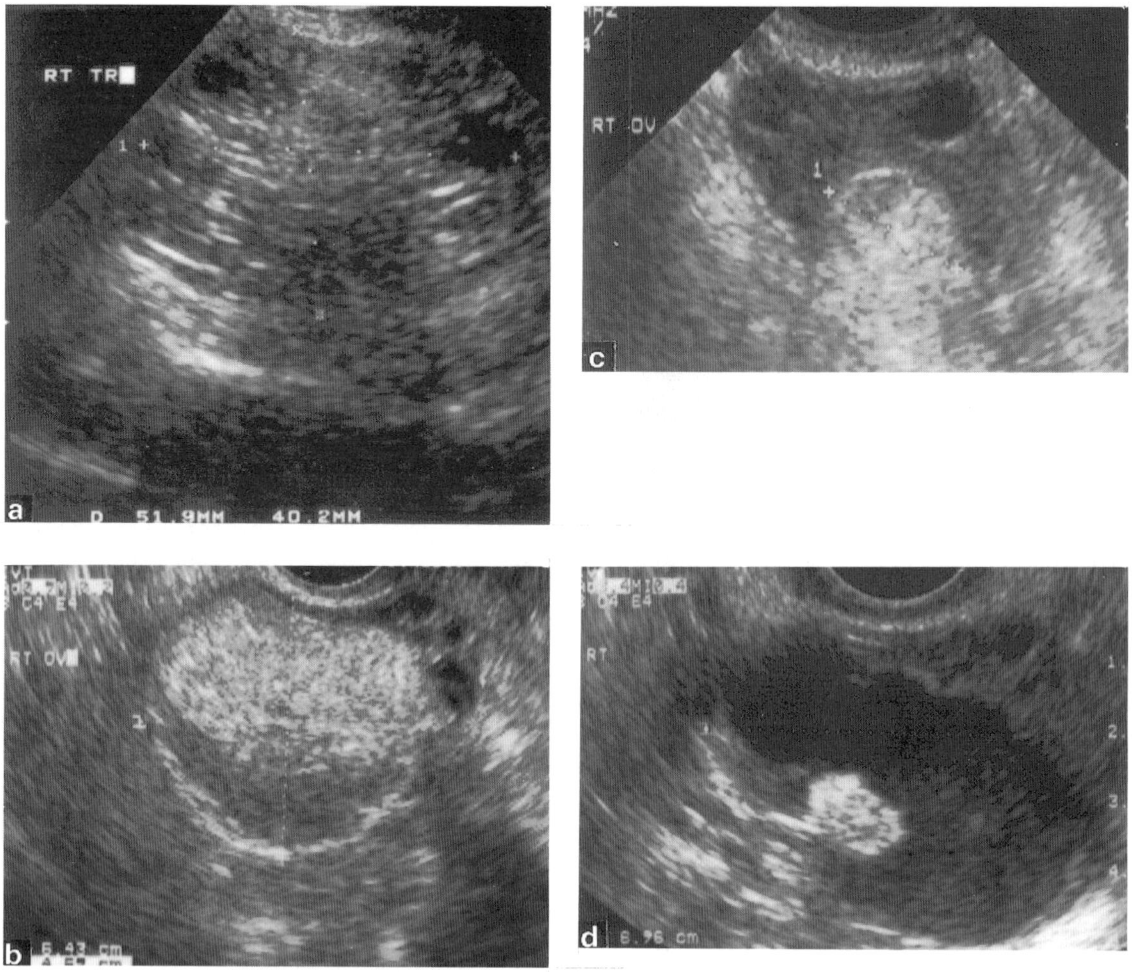

Figure 13 Benign cystic teratoma (BCT), a frequently encountered tumor of the ovary that may exhibit a diversity of morphological characteristics. (a) Tumor showing dispersed, small, bright echoes representing sebaceous material and hair; (b) the larger central hyperechoic structure is the hallmark of the teratoma; (c) an ovary of normal size, containing a small 2 × 2 cm central BCT, seen as the hyperechoic structure in this view; (d) view clearly demonstrating the common echogenic 'core'

size larger than 5 cm[25,26], a complex or solid appearance[4,13,17,27–30], and persistence over time[29]. Size as an independent variable has been questioned, as it is quite common to find benign cysts larger than 5 cm, and malignant masses smaller than 5 cm[13,29].

Epithelial ovarian tumors are the most common ovarian neoplasms, and serous ovarian tumors are the most common malignant epithelial neoplasms. Benign and malignant serous masses make up 25% of all ovarian tumors. The serous cystadenocarcinoma is typically a multiloculated mass containing prominent papillary excrescences and varying degrees of solid echogenic core (Figure 15). Between 30 and 50% are bilateral and approximately 10% are completely solid, without cystic elements.

Mucinous tumors are the second most common epithelial tumor of the ovary, although the vast majority (75%) are benign. Mucinous cystadenocarcinoma often appears as a multiloculated cystic mass that can also exhibit papillary projections or solid components sonographically (Figure 16). Endometrioid carcinoma of the ovary is much less common than serous or mucinous cystadenocarcinoma, representing 15% of all ovarian carcinomas. It typically appears as a cystic mass with solid components, the cystic areas filled with low-level echogenic fluid, probably representing blood.

Sex cord-stromal ovarian tumors are much less common than epithelial ovarian tumors, and may be associated with active hormone secretion. Granulosa cell tumors may secrete estrogen, or less commonly androgens, and may be associated with endometrial hyperplasia or carcinoma.

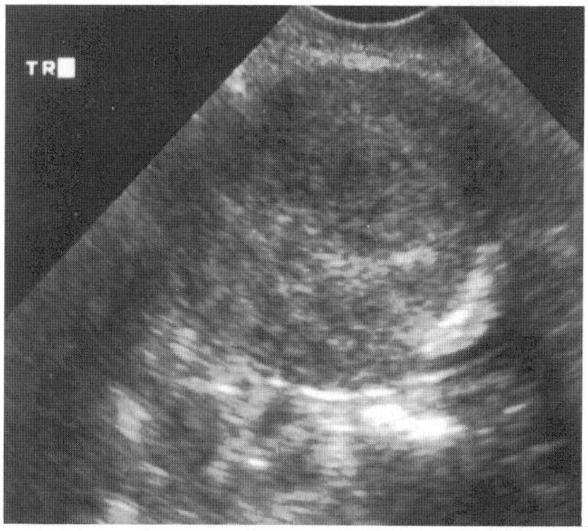

Figure 14 Fibroma thecoma, a uniformly solid tumor exhibiting relatively high overall echogenicity. An area of even higher echogenicity is seen in the lower right aspect of this view, representing an area of calcification

Unlike epithelial ovarian tumors which have a late presentation, granulosa cell tumors often present at Stage 1, have a low malignant potential, and subsequently a lower mortality rate and better prognosis. Sonographically, granulosa cell tumors are most often solid, although they may have areas of cystic degeneration or hemorrhage (Figure 17). Sertoli–Leydig tumors are much less common, may secrete virilizing hormones, and often appear solid sonographically. Diagnosis is often made by the rapid or prepubertal appearance of virilizing characteristics and the presence of an enlarged, solid ovarian mass.

A dysgerminoma is the most common malignant germ cell tumor, although it is rare. It usually appears solid sonographically and may be hyperechoic (Figure 18). An immature teratoma is an unusual variant of the much more common benign cystic teratoma and has a variable appearance by sonography. Metastatic ovarian tumors may include carcinoma of the breast, endometrium, stomach, or colon, or leukemia and lymphoma. A Krukenberg tumor, an ovarian metastasis from a gastric carcinoma, usually appears sonographically as a bilateral, asymmetrically enlarged, solid mass. In general, when compared with primary ovarian carcinoma, ovarian metastasis often appears more hyperechoic and solid[31], although it often has a complex, mixed appearance (Figure 19).

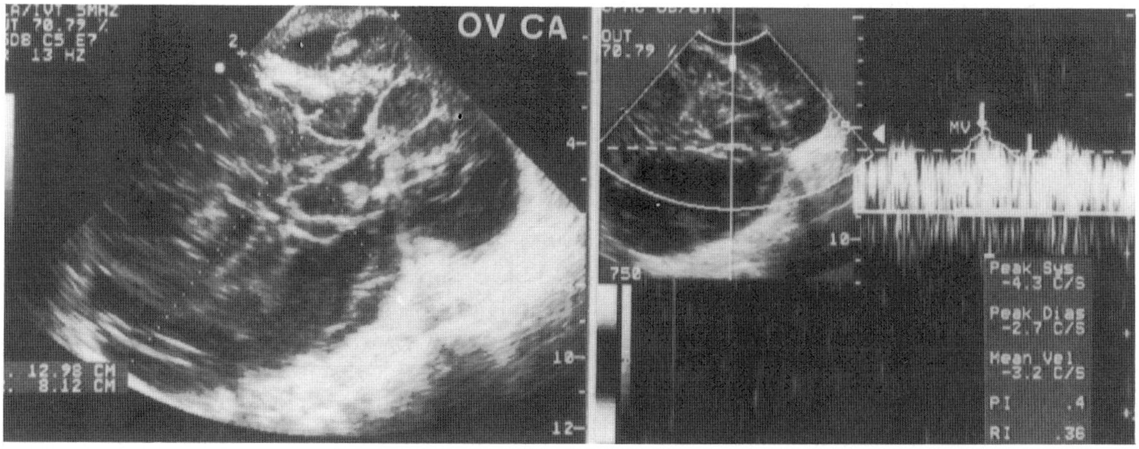

Figure 15 This large and complex ovarian tumor was found to be serous cystadenocarcinoma at surgery. The mass is multiloculated, with mixed echogenicity and thick septations; right side of view displays Doppler flow characteristics for this tumor: high diastolic flow resulting in low pulsatility and resistance indices

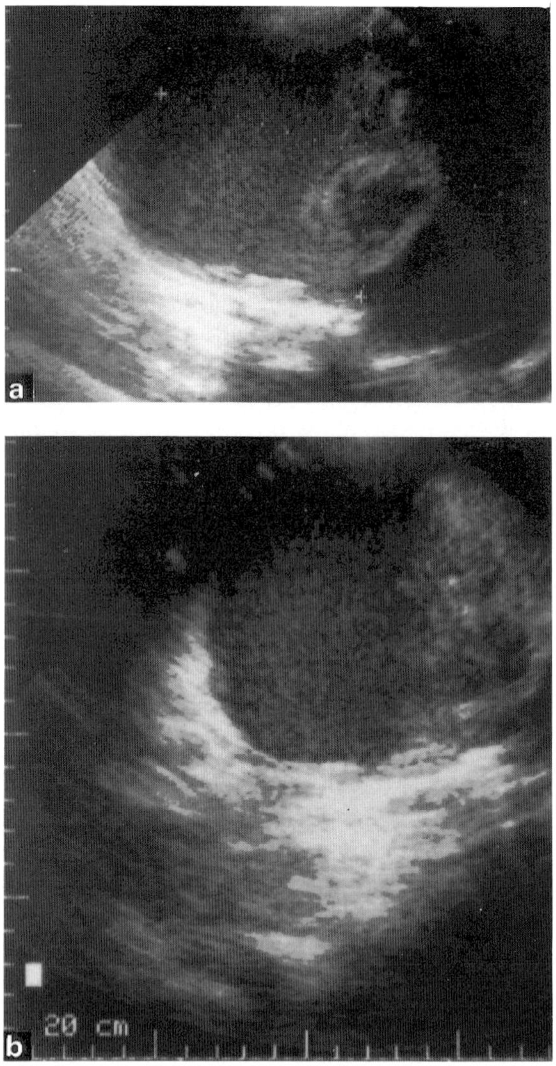

Figure 16 Two examples of tumors found to be mucinous cystadenocarcinoma, showing (a) mixed echogenicity and complex architecture; (b) differences in echogenicity and wall thickness, and irregularities of the inner wall structure

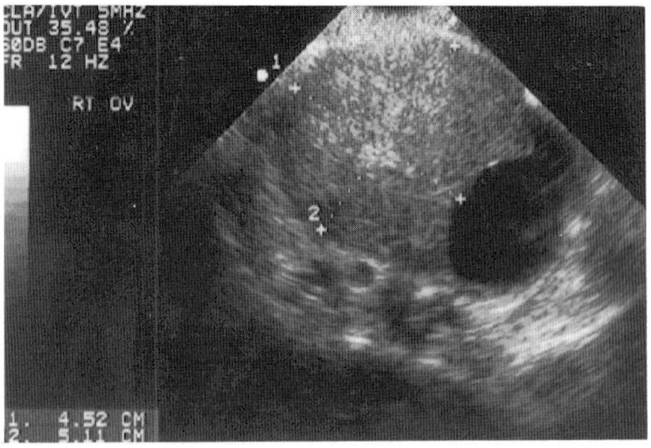

Figure 17 This primarily solid and hyperechoic mass in a postmenopausal woman is a granulosa cell tumor

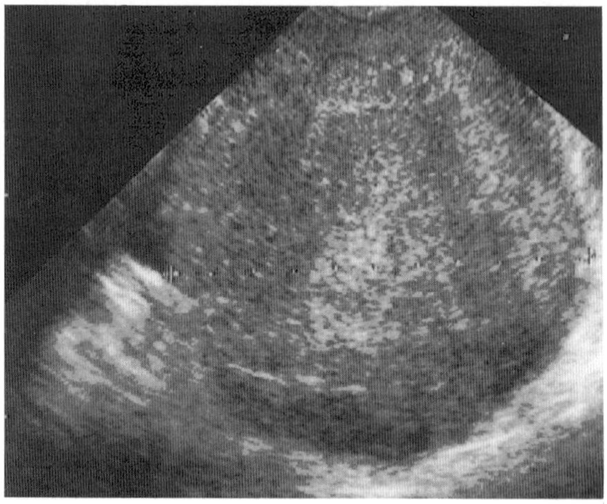

Figure 18 Large dysgerminoma found in a premenopausal patient; solid tumor typically exhibiting very high echogenicity

CRITERIA FOR ULTRASONOGRAPHIC DIAGNOSIS OF OVARIAN LESIONS

The first studies attempting to differentiate benign from malignant ovarian masses utilized transabdominal sonography. In the late 1970s, two studies by Lawson and Albarelli[32] and Deland and colleagues[33] began to characterize ovarian and pelvic masses. Lawson and Albarelli demonstrated an accuracy of 91% in determining the existence, size, location, and consistency of 251 pelvic masses. Deland and colleagues were able to diagnose ovarian cancer in 13 of 14 patients. Campbell and associates[7], in 1980, performed one of the first sophisticated prospective studies using transabdominal sonography in postmenopausal women, although the sensitivity and specificity of this pioneering work was not established. The two most important and oft-quoted studies are those of Andolf and co-workers[34] and Campbell and associates[15]. Both of these studies are based on the premise that diseased ovaries increase in size. Campbell and associates studied over 5000 asymptomatic and self-referred women who underwent three annual screening tests to detect enlarged or grossly abnormal ovaries, and found 97% specificity with only 2.3% false positives. The conclusions to be derived from the studies using transabdominal sonography are that ultrasound screening does detect ovarian cancers missed on bimanual examination; that very large numbers of scans must be performed to detect one ovarian cancer; and that morphological characteristics detected by transabdominal sonography cannot be used to distinguish benign from malignant lesions.

Since the advent of the high-frequency transvaginal probe, structures as small as 1–2 mm may be visualized, revolutionizing our ability to characterize ovarian masses. Although a multitude of sonographic shapes and patterns previously described assist in the differentiation of benign from malignant ovaries, a significant degree of overlap exists. The great accuracy in depicting these structural features transvaginally has prompted several authors to attempt classification of ovarian masses based on the presence or absence of several sonographic components including septae, papillae, loculations, daughter cysts, solid structure and fluid appearance. Bourne and colleagues[35] performed a prospective study to screen for ovarian cancer using a scoring system based on transvaginal sonography in a high-risk group of symptomatic women. The lesions were characterized and scored on texture, presence of loculations, cyst outlines, and degree of echogenicity, with benign lesions scoring low and malignant lesions scoring invariably higher. In another study, the same group explored the possibility of detecting the familial ovarian cancer syndrome as early as possible by transvaginal sonography[36].

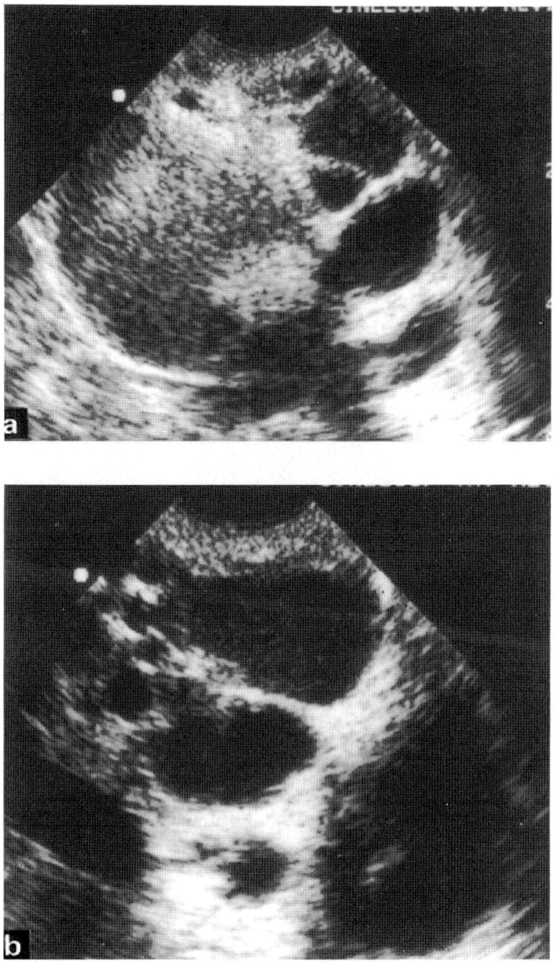

Figure 19 Two of the typical sonographic appearances of metastatic carcinoma of the ovary (a and b), with a multitude of echogenicities and complex structures; small micrometastases will not be sonographically imaged and the ovary may appear normal at transvaginal ultrasonography

Using transvaginal sonography, Granberg and colleagues[17] concluded that a unilocular cyst measuring less than 10 cm in diameter, without papillary formations, had an extremely low chance of being malignant, regardless of the woman's age. In a study performed by van Nagell and co-workers[37], transvaginal sonography was employed to screen for ovarian cancer in 1300 asymptomatic postmenopausal women. Of the 33 women (2.5%) found to have persistent ovarian abnormalities, all 27 who underwent exploratory laparotomy were found to have ovarian tumors, including two primary adenocarcinomas and one metastatic carcinoma.

At Columbia–Presbyterian Medical Center, a scoring system was developed to characterize pelvic and ovarian lesions and compare the transvaginal sonographic images to the histopathological results[27] (Figure 20). The four variables described and scored were: inner wall structure, wall thickness, septations, and echogenicity. The individual values in each category were added to represent the final score for any given lesion; the score was assigned to each ovary or mass, not to

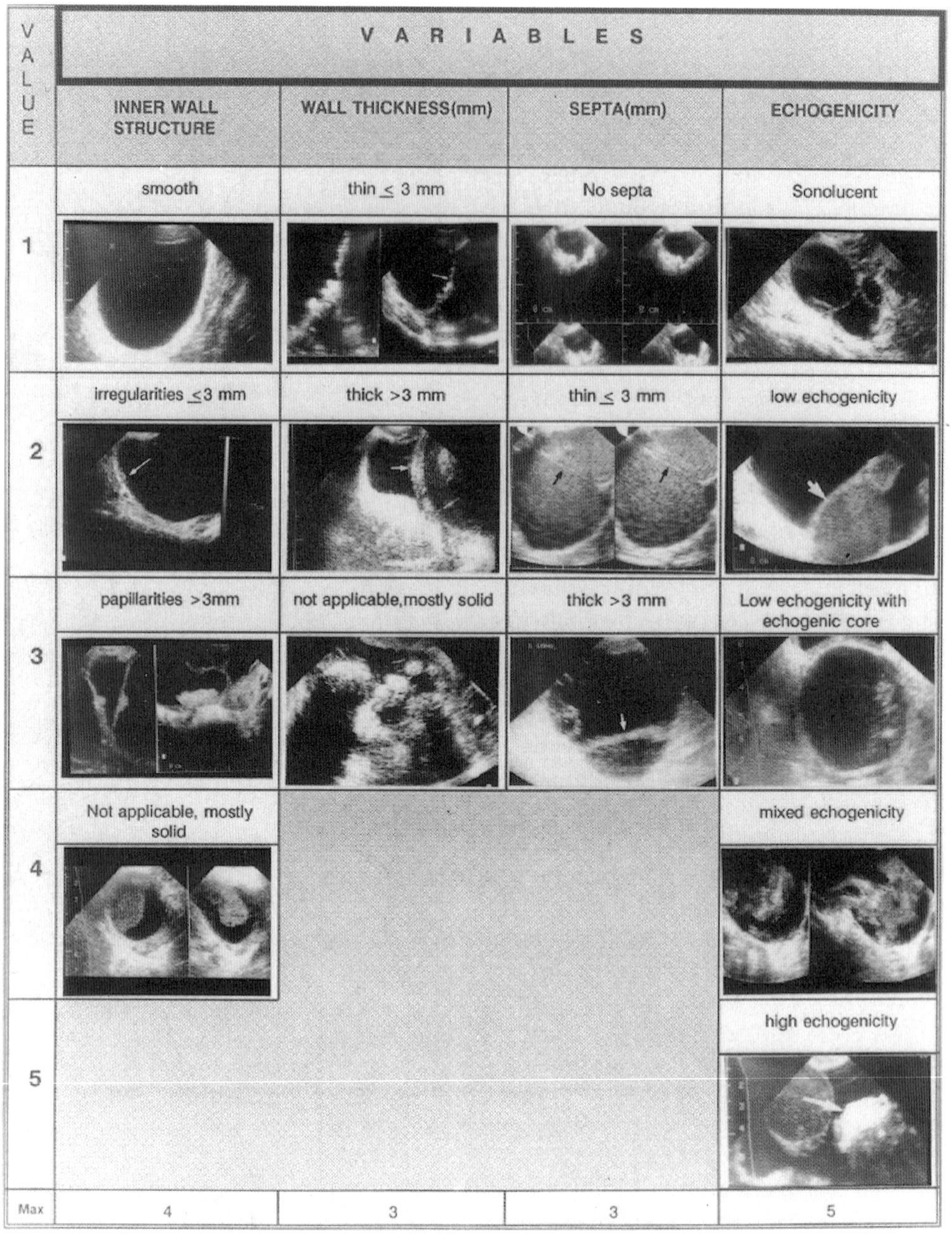

Figure 20 Tabular system for scoring evaluation of abnormal ovaries and extrauterine masses of unclear origin. Reprinted with permission from the American College of Obstetricians and Gynecologists (*Obstet. Gynecol.*, 1991, **78**, 70–6)

each woman. This scoring system was based on previous experience and the general consensus in the literature regarding the most important sonographic features of ovarian malignancy. Increased echogenicity, thick wall or septa, and wall papillarities would raise suspicions of malignancy, and therefore scored higher. The analysis included 143 patients possessing 281 ovaries, and the sensitivity and specificity for each score from 5–13 were obtained. The resulting curve demonstrated that 9 was the score that best distinguished malignant from benign ovaries. Using the score of

9 as the threshold for a positive test resulted in correct identification of all women with malignancy, although these results are less specific than other results reported elsewhere. The choice of a higher threshold would make a scoring system less sensitive and more specific. Several studies have evaluated the sensitivity and specificity of pelvic sonography in the differentiation of benign from malignant ovarian masses, including those by Benacerraf and colleagues[28], Kobayashi[38], Meire and associates[39], Pussel and co-workers[40], Herrmann and colleagues[41], Finkler and associates[42], and Granberg and co-workers[43]. We are at present developing a weighted scoring system using linear regression analysis, in the hopes of less arbitrary point assignments to the mass variables previously described. A fifth variable was added to our new, weighted scoring system: shadowing behind a sound-absorbing structure. This modification allows us to identify correctly the benign cystic teratomas, the source of many of the false-positive results in the previous study.

The latest advance in the characterization of ovarian cysts and masses is represented by the use of color Doppler studies, in conjunction with traditional gray-scale transabdominal and transvaginal sonography. In an attempt to combine gray-scale and color Doppler studies, our group at Columbia–Presbyterian studied 115 ovarian and adnexal masses and correlated them with surgically obtained histopathological findings[44]. The sensitivity and specificity of the previously described scoring system used alone were 94% and 87%, respectively, with a positive predictive value of 60%. By combining the scoring system and the resistance and pulsatility indices (using cut-off points of 0.46 and 0.62, respectively), the sensitivity was 94%, the specificity 99%, and the positive predictive value improved to 94%. These results demonstrate that the combination of morphological and physiological parameters improve differentiation of benign from malignant ovarian masses.

In conclusion, we are confident that transvaginal sonography is an indispensable tool in the evaluation of the ovary. We are also encouraged by the potential to employ this imaging modality in future efforts to screen a larger population for ovarian cancer.

References

1. Rodriguez, H., Platt, L., Medearis, A., *et al.* (1988). The use of transvaginal sonography for evaluation of postmenopausal ovarian size and morphology. *Am. J. Obstet. Gynecol.*, **159**, 810–14
2. Andolf, E., Jorgensen, C., Svelaneius, E., *et al.* (1987). Ultrasound measurement of ovarian volume. *Acta Obstet. Gynecol. Scand.*, **66**, 387–9
3. Cohen, H., Tice, H. and Mandel, F. (1990). Ovarian volumes measured by ultrasound: bigger than we think. *Radiology*, **177**, 189–92
4. Fleischer, A., McKee, M., Gordon, A., *et al.* (1990). Transvaginal sonography of postmenopausal ovaries with pathologic correlation. *J. Ultrasound Med.*, **9**, 637–44
5. Granberg, S. and Wilkland, M. (1988). A comparison between ultrasound and gynecologic exam for detection of enlarged ovaries in a group of women at risk for ovarian cancer. *J. Ultrasound Med.*, **7**, 59–64
6. Goswamy, R., Campbell, S., Royston, J., *et al.* (1988). Ovarian size in postmenopausal women. *Br. J. Obstet. Gynaecol.*, **95**, 795–801
7. Campbell, S., Goswamy, R., Goessens, L., *et al.* (1982). Real time ultrasound for determination of ovarian morphology and volume: a possible early screening test for ovarian cancer? *Lancet*, **1**, 425
8. Yoffe, N., Bronshtein, M. and Brandes, J. (1991). Hemorrhagic ovarian cyst detection by transvaginal sonography: the great imitator. *Gynecol. Endocrinol.*, **5**, 123–9
9. Parisi, L., Tramonti, M., Casciano, S., *et al.* (1982). The role of ultrasound in the study of polycystic ovarian disease. *J. Clin. Ultrasound*, **10**, 167–72
10. Nicolini, U., Ferrazzi, E., Bellotti, M., *et al.* (1985). The contribution of sonographic evaluation of ovarian size in patients with polycystic ovarian disease. *J. Ultrasound Med.*, **4**, 347–51
11. Swanson, M., Sauerbei, E. and Cooperberg, P. (1981) Medical implications of ultrasonically detected polycystic ovaries. *J. Clin. Ultrasound*, **9**, 219–22
12. Graif, M. and Itzchak, Y. (1988). Sonographic evaluation of ovarian torsion in childhood and adolescence. *Am. J. Radiol.*, **50**, 647–9
13. Andolf, E. and Jorgensen, C. (1989). Cystic lesions in elderly women, diagnosed by ultrasound. *Br. J.*

Obstet. Gynaecol., **96**, 1076–9
14. Luxman, D., Bergman, A. and Sagi, J. (1991). The postmenopausal adnexal mass: correlation between ultrasonic and pathologic findings. *Obstet. Gynecol.*, **77**, 726–8
15. Campbell, S., Bhan, V. and Royston, P. (1989). Transabdominal ultrasound screening for early ovarian cancer. *Br. Med. J.*, **299**, 1363–7
16. Maiman, M., Seltzer, V. and Boyce, J. (1991). Laparoscopic excision of ovarian neoplasms subsequently found to be malignant. *Obstet. Gynecol.*, **77**, 563–5
17. Granberg, S., Norstrom, A. and Wilkland, M. (1990). Tumors in the lower pelvis as imaged by vaginal sonography. *Gynecol. Oncol.*, **37**, 224–9
18. Kupfer, M., Schwimer, S. and Lebovic, J. (1992). Transvaginal sonographic appearance of endometriomata: spectrum of findings. *J. Ultrasound Med.*, **11**, 129–33
19. Laing, F., Van Dalsem, V., Marks, W., *et al.* (1981). Dermoid cysts of the ovary: their ultrasonographic appearances. *Obstet. Gynecol.*, **57**, 99–104
20. Meigs, J. and Cass, J. (1937). Fibroma of the ovary with ascites and hydrothorax with a report of 7 cases. *Am. J. Obstet. Gynecol.*, **33**, 249–67
21. Boring, C., Squires, T. and Tong, T. (1993). Cancer statistics, 1993. *Cancer J. Clin.*, **43**, 7–26
22. Sunden, B. (1965). Diagnostic application of ultrasound in genetics. *Gynaekol. Rudsch.*, **2**, 296–359
23. Andolf, E. and Jorgensen, C. (1988). A prospective comparison of clinical ultrasound and operative examination of the female pelvis. *J. Ultrasound Med.*, **7**, 617–20
24. van Nagell, J., Higgins, R., Donaldson, E., *et al.* (1990). Transvaginal sonography as a screening method for ovarian cancer. *Cancer*, **65**, 573–7
25. Sparks, J. and Varner, R. (1991). Ovarian cancer screening. *Obstet. Gynecol.*, **77**, 787–92
26. Rubin, S., Hoskins, W., Hakes, T., *et al.* (1988). Recurrence after negative second look laparotomy for ovarian cancer: analysis of risk factors. *Am. J. Obstet. Gynecol.*, **159**, 1094–8
27. Sassone, A., Timor, I., *et al.* (1991). Transvaginal sonographic characterization of ovarian disease: evaluation of a new scoring system to predict ovarian malignancy. *Obstet. Gynecol.*, **78**, 70–6
28. Benacerraf, B., Finkler, N., Wojciechowski, C., *et al.* (1990). Sonographic accuracy in the diagnosis of ovarian masses. *J. Reprod. Med.*, **35**, 491–5
29. Goldstein, S., Subramanyan, B. and Snyder, J. (1989). The postmenopausal cystic adnexal mass: the potential role of ultrasound in conservative management. *Obstet. Gynecol.*, **73**, 8–10
30. Hurwitz, A., Yagel, S., Zion, I., *et al.* (1988). The management of persistent clear pelvic cysts diagnosed by ultrasonography. *Obstet. Gynecol.*, **72**, 320–2
31. Shimizu, H., Yamasaki, M., Ohama, K., *et al.* (1990). Characteristic ultrasonographic appearance of Krukenberg tumor. *J. Clin. Ultrasound*, **18**, 697–703
32. Lawson, T. and Albarelli, J. (1977). Diagnosis of gynecologic pelvic masses by gray scale ultrasonography: analysis of specificity and accuracy. *Am. J. Roentgenol.*, **128**, 1003–6
33. Deland, M., Field, A., van Nagell, J., *et al.* (1979). Ultrasonography in the diagnosis of tumors of the ovary. *Surg. Gynecol. J. Obstet.*, **18**, 346–48
34. Andolf, E., Svolenius, E. and Astedt, B. (1986). Ultrasonography for early detection of ovarian carcinoma. *Br. J. Obstet. Gynaecol.*, **93**, 1286–9
35. Bourne, T., Campbell, S., Whitehead, M. *et al.* (1990). Transvaginal ultrasound screening for ovarian cancer in a high risk group. Presented at the *Third World Congress on Vaginosonography in Gynecology*, June 14–17, San Antonio, Texas
36. Bourne, T., Campbell, S., Whitehead, M., *et al.* (1991). Ultrasound screening for sporadic and familial early ovarian cancer. *J. Ultrasound Med.*, **10**, 43
37. van Nagell, J., *et al.* (1991). Ovarian cancer screening in asymptomatic postmenopausal women by transvaginal sonography. *Cancer*, **68**, 458–62
38. Kobayashi, M. (1976). Use of diagnostic ultrasound in trophoblastic neoplasms and ovarian tumors. *Cancer*, **38**, 441–52
39. Meire, H., Farrant, P. and Guha, T. (1978). Distinction of benign from malignant ovarian cysts by ultrasound. *Br. J. Obstet. Gynaecol.*, **85**, 893–9
40. Pussel, S., Cosgrove, D., Hinton, J. *et al.* (1980). Carcinoma of the ovary: correlation of ultrasound with second look laparotomy. *Br. J. Obstet. Gynaecol.*, **87**, 1140–4
41. Herrmann, U., Locher, G. and Goldhirsch, A. (1987). Sonographic patterns of ovarian tumors: prediction of malignancy. *Obstet. Gynecol.*, **69**, 777–81
42. Finkler, N., Benacerraf, B., Lavin, P., *et al.* (1988). Comparison of serum CA 125, clinical impression, and ultrasound in the postoperative evaluation of ovarian masses. *Obstet. Gynecol.*, **72**, 659–64
43. Granberg, S., Wilkland, M. and Jannson, I. (1989). Macroscopic characterization of ovarian tumors and the relation to the histologic diagnosis: criteria to be used for ultrasound evaluation. *Gynecol. Oncol.*, **35**, 139–44
44. Timor-Tritsch, I., Lerner, J., Monteagudo, A., *et al.* (1993). Transvaginal sonographic characterization of ovarian masses using color flow directed Doppler measurements and a morphologic scoring system. *Am. J. Obstet. Gynecol.*, **168**, 909–13

Benign and malignant ovarian tumors 9

J. Menczer

The ovary is a complex organ and each one of its cellular components, i.e. germ cells, stromal cells and epithelial (mesenchymal) cells, may give rise to a variety of benign and malignant tumors. In addition, the ovary is also the site of metastasis from malignant tumors in other organ systems.

The most commonly used classification of ovarian tumors is the one recommended by the World Health Organization (WHO) which is based on the histogenesis of the tumor.

This chapter will deal mainly with malignant ovarian neoplasms of epithelial origin and only briefly with benign ovarian tumors and the less common non-epithelial ovarian neoplasms.

BENIGN OVARIAN TUMORS

The majority of ovarian tumors are benign[1]. In addition to the histogenetic classification, benign ovarian tumors may be divided into cystic and solid tumors. One should be aware that cystic tumors may also represent functional ovarian cysts (follicular and luteal cysts) which are not neoplasms in the true sense of the word, but are part of the functional cycle of the ovary, and usually regress spontaneously. Theca luteal cysts are also physiological cysts, associated with multiple pregnancy, hydatidiform mole or ovulation stimulation.

The most common benign cystic neoplasms of the ovary are of epithelial origin (serous and mucinous cystadenomas) or germ cell origin (benign cystic teratomas).

Endometriotic cysts should be mentioned as well. They result from recurrent bleeding into areas of ovarian endometriosis. Pregnancy luteoma is a benign, frequently bilateral tumor which occurs predominantly in Black women and may be associated with maternal and fetal virilism.

The common benign solid ovarian tumors are fibromas, fibrothecomas and Brenner tumors. Fibromas may also contain cystic elements and are then designated as cystadenofibromas. Fibromas were originally described as associated with Meigs' syndrome. This rare syndrome is characterized by the presence of ascites and hydrothorax and it may also be associated with a variety of other ovarian tumors. Brenner tumor is a fibro-epithelial tumor which probably arises from Walthard's cell rests. It is usually unilateral, solid and benign. Occasionally it coexists with mucinous cystadenoma. Bilateral ovarian enlargement may also be caused by polycystic ovaries.

Symptoms

Benign ovarian tumors are frequently asymptomatic. Subjective complaints, mainly discomfort, pain or a sensation of pressure, will usually occur when the tumor is of a large size, or due to the presence of complications such as torsion, rupture, hemorrhage or infection.

Diagnosis

The presence of an adnexal mass is diagnosed because of symptoms or at the time of routine pelvic examination.

The differential diagnosis should also include non-gynecological space-occupying lesions such as a low-lying distended cecum or redundant rectosigmoid, tumor of the lower gastrointestinal tract, diverticulum, appendiceal abscess, desmoid tumor, urachal cyst, peritoneal cyst, pelvic kidney and retroperitoneal tumor. It is beyond the scope of this chapter to detail the process of elimination of non-ovarian pelvic masses. Obtaining a very careful history will be helpful in the elimination of some of these conditions. Additional tests including imaging procedures, laparoscopy and occasionally even laparotomy may be necessary in order to arrive at an accurate diagnosis.

The consistency of adnexal masses may be helpful in the diagnosis. When the adnexal tumor is solid, a pedunculated myoma should be ruled out. Ultrasonography may aid in the differential diagnosis. When the ovaries can be demonstrated separately, the tumor mass is most probably not of ovarian origin. The distinction between masses of ovarian and uterine origin can ultimately be made by laparoscopy. Functional ovarian cysts do not usually exceed a diameter of 5–6 cm and cannot be present in premenarchal or postmenopausal women, or in women of reproductive age who are taking contraceptive pills.

Serous cystadenomas as a group are usually smaller, and more often bilateral and unilocular than mucinous cystadenomas. In spite of these different characteristics, the clinical and ultrasonographic distinction between these cysts is not feasible on an individual basis. Serous cystadenomas may have papillomatous excrescences on the external or internal surface and yet be histologically benign.

Patients with an endometrioma will usually have a history consistent with endometriosis and physical examination will frequently reveal other findings typical of endometriosis.

Polycystic ovaries are found in women with a complex syndrome which includes menstrual irregularity, hirsutism, obesity and anovulatory infertility.

The preoperative diagnosis of benign cystic teratoma (dermoid cyst) can sometimes be made by pelvic X-ray or ultrasonography, especially when calcification, bone elements or teeth are present. Such cysts are occasionally combined with cystadenomas generally of the mucinous type. Benign cystic teratomas very seldom undergo malignant transformation. Nowadays, the more frequent performance of pelvic ultrasonography for a variety of reasons, reveals the presence of previously undetected, small asymptomatic ovarian cysts. Although such cysts are usually benign, they are of concern mainly in postmenopausal women because the possibility of malignancy is difficult to rule out.

Ultrasonographic criteria may be helpful in the differential diagnosis of benign and malignant cysts. Tumor-marker assays (mainly CA 125) may also be of assistance. Ultimately in many instances only surgical excision and histological examination can give a definite diagnosis of the type of adnexal tumor.

Treatment

Since functional ovarian cysts regress spontaneously, expectant management is indicated. Luteal cysts associated with molar pregnancy or ovulation stimulation, also regress spontaneously. Occasionally, such cysts undergo complications such as rupture, bleeding or torsion and may then require surgical intervention. Luteoma of pregnancy invariably regresses postpartum and requires no treatment. The other benign solid and cystic tumors are treated surgically. Actually, any persistant ovarian mass greater than 6–7 cm should be treated surgically. The type of operation will depend on the age of the patient and the desire for fertility preservation. In young women an effort should be made to excise the tumor and preserve the involved ovary. This is possible in most instances. Even when torsion is encountered the involved ovary can be preserved by performing detorsion. In older women the involved ovary can be removed and in peri- and postmenopausal women, bilateral oophorectomy is indicated. The uterus can, in our opinion, be left *in situ* in these cases.

Until recently, surgical intervention, because of presumed benign ovarian tumors, consisted of laparotomy. Nowadays, all the above-mentioned surgical interventions (tumor resection, cystectomy, oophorectomy) can be done by operative laparoscopy. This procedure is supposedly less extensive and is associated with lower morbidity, shorter hospital stay, faster recuperation and improved cosmetic outcome. After excision of the tumor, histological examination by frozen section is advisable. If malignancy is diagnosed, laparotomy and a more extensive procedure is performed for staging and therapeutic purposes.

OVARIAN CANCER OF EPITHELIAL ORIGIN

Among the ovarian malignant neoplasms the most common (90%) are of epithelial origin. In the USA approximately 20 000 new cases are diagnosed yearly and the tumor ranks second in frequency after cancer of the body of the uterus, producing the fourth highest cancer-related mortality rate[2]. The various benign and malignant ovarian neoplasms of epithelial origin are presented in Table 1.

The main problems concerning ovarian cancer of epithelial origin are unknown etiology, unknown natural history, ineffective methods of prevention, screening and early diagnosis, insidious clinical onset and unsatisfactory treatment methods. In spite of great progress in some of these aspects, the management of this neoplasm remains a major challenge in gynecological oncology.

Epidemiology, etiology and risk factors

Ovarian carcinoma is infrequent before the age of 45 years and occurs most frequently in the 6th and 7th decades. The incidence is low in underdeveloped countries and is high in urban areas and industrialized countries with the exception of Japan. While the incidence during the last decades in Western countries has been more or less constant, it has increased in underdeveloped countries[2]. The etiology of the disease is unknown. However, a variety of risk factors have been described[3].

In many, but not all studies, it was found that, as compared to controls, ovarian carcinoma patients belonged to a higher socioeconomic class, were more educated, had earlier onset of menarche and later menopause and were more frequently nulliparous and of single marital status.

An inconsistent association between dietary factors such as fat intake, lactose and copious coffee consumption, has been reported. The consumption of ethanol has been found to be protective. Although the role of perineal exposure to talc has not been definitively established, its use for hygienic purposes should be discouraged.

The possible association between mumps, which is caused by a gonadotropic virus, and ovarian carcinoma is intriguing. We have found[4] that in response to past viral infection, ovarian carcinoma patients appeared to be more likely than controls to have developed subclinical mumps and tended to present with lower persistent mumps complement-fixation antibody titers. This possibly indicates an immunological incompetence that enables the development of ovarian carcinoma while the direct role of the mumps is highly speculative.

Incessant ovulation is a well established risk factor. There is a direct correlation between the number of ovulatory years and the risk for ovarian carcinoma. The relative risk for women with 25 to 29 years of ovulatory activity is 2.1, in contrast to 4.5 in women with more than 40 years of ovulatory activity. Full-term pregnancy and delivery, as well as breast feeding (events during which ovulation does not occur), have a protective effect[3]. Early age at first pregnancy and incomplete pregnancy, may also be protective. It has been postulated that the trauma of ovulation to the ovarian surface epithelium induces its proliferation and promotes the formation of inclusion cysts, which may eventually undergo malignant transformation.

The most potent protective effect is exerted by the intake of oral contraceptive pills[5,6]. The relative risk in users is reduced by about half and the favorable effect persists many years after the use has ceased. No protective effect has been demonstrated for intake of hormonal replacement therapy.

A prominent risk factor is genetic predisposition, as manifested by familial aggregation reported from several countries in different parts of the world[7,8]. Three familial ovarian carcinoma-prone conditions have been recognized[9]:

(1) Site-specific ovarian carcinoma, where familial risk is restricted to ovarian cancer;

(2) Breast/ovarian cancer syndrome, where carcinoma of the breast is associated with ovarian carcinoma; and

(3) Cancer family syndrome, consisting of hereditary non-polyposis colorectal cancer with proximal colonic predominance associated with endometrial and/or ovarian carcinoma.

The hereditary pattern seems consistent with an autosomal dominant gene with incomplete penetrance[9]. Although this risk factor is relevant for

Table 1 World Health Organization histological classification of common epithelial ovarian tumors

(A) *Serous tumors*
- (1) Benign
  - (a) Cystadenoma and papillary cystadenoma
  - (b) Surface papilloma
  - (c) Adenofibroma and cystadenofibroma
- (2) Of borderline malignancy (carcinoma of low malignant potential)
  - (a) Cystadenoma and papillary cystadenoma
  - (b) Surface papilloma
  - (c) Adenofibroma and cystadenofibroma
- (3) Malignant
  - (a) Adenocarcinoma, papillary adenocarcinoma, and papillary cystadenocarcinoma
  - (b) Surface papillary carcinoma
  - (c) Malignant adenofibroma and cystadenofibroma

(B) *Mucinous tumors*
- (1) Benign
  - (a) Cystadenoma
  - (b) Adenofibroma and cystadenofibroma
- (2) Of borderline malignancy (carcinoma of low malignant potential)
  - (a) Cystadenoma
  - (b) Adenofibroma and cystadenofibroma
- (3) Malignant
  - (a) Adenocarcinoma and cystadenocarcinoma
  - (b) Malignant adenofibroma and cystadenofibroma

(C) *Endometrioid tumors*
- (1) Benign
  - (a) Adenoma and cystadenoma
  - (b) Adenofibroma and cystadenofibroma
- (2) Of borderline malignancy (carcinoma of low malignant potential)
  - (a) Adenofibroma and cystadenofibroma
- (3) Malignant
  - (a) Carcinoma
    - (i) Adenocarcinoma
    - (ii) Adenoacanthoma
    - (iii) Malignant adenofibroma
  - (b) Endometrioid stromal sarcomas
  - (c) Mesodermal (Müllerian) mixed tumors, homologous and heterologous

(D) *Clear cell (mesonephroid) tumors*
- (1) Benign: adenofibroma
- (2) Of borderline malignancy (carcinoma of low malignant potential)
- (3) Malignant: carcinoma and adenocarcinoma

(E) *Brenner tumors*
- (1) Benign
- (2) Of borderline malignancy (proliferating)
- (3) Malignant

(F) *Mixed epithelial tumors*
- (1) Benign
- (2) Of borderline malignancy
- (3) Malignant

(G) *Undifferentiated carcinoma*

(H) *Unclassified epithelial tumors*

only a small fraction of ovarian cancer, varyingly estimated to range between 3% and 10%, it is of great importance. The probability that a female member of an ovarian cancer-prone family will develop the tumor is 11–18 times higher than in the general population, and close female relatives may have as much as a 50% chance of developing ovarian cancer[10]. On this basis prophylactic oophorectomy has been advised for all healthy members of ovarian cancer-prone families over the age of 35 who have completed childbearing. It does, however, not confer absolute protection. Widespread intraperitoneal malignancy ('primary peritoneal carcinoma'), histologically undistinguishable from ovarian cancer, has been reported in 1.8% of women after prophylactic oophorectomy[11]. Recently it was reported that the chromosomal region 17q12–23 is associated with a proportion of hereditary ovarian cancers[12]. This will probably allow, in the future, improved identification of women at risk and the performance of prophylactic oophorectomy based on gene-linkage findings.

Receptors for estrogen/progesterone have been demonstrated in ovarian tumors but their role in etiology and progression is undefined. More insight into the etiology of ovarian cancer may be gained by oncogene research. Evidence is already present for high expression of the c-*erb*-B_2 protein, amplification and over-expression of the c-*myc* gene and Ki-*ras* oncogene in a proportion of ovarian cancers[13,14]. High expression of the suppressor gene *p53*[15] and some growth factors have also been reported.

Clinical aspects, diagnosis and screening

The onset of ovarian carcinoma is notoriously insidious. Initially only vague gastrointestinal symptoms are present which are usually not suspected to indicate an ovarian tumor. Abdominal pain and distension due to tumor mass or ascites are the most common symptoms leading to diagnosis. When these symptoms are present the disease has, however, already usually spread beyond the ovaries. Most adnexal masses in premenopausal women represent benign or functional tumors. The presence of an adnexal mass in premenarchal or postmenopausal women has a greater chance of being malignant and should therefore be promptly investigated. Pelvic examination is not reliable for the evaluation of the ovaries, especially in overweight or uncooperative women. The diagnosis of early ovarian cancer by palpation of an asymptomatic ovarian mass thus usually occurs by chance.

Ultrasonographic pelvic examination is a more accurate method of ovarian examination. It enables the identification of clinically unsuspected ovarian masses as well as the accurate determination of their size and volume and their morphology. Benign ovarian cysts are characteristically smaller than 5 cm in diameter, unilateral, unilocular, anechoic and without intracystic papillations. The specificity and predictive value of these criteria are, however, low. Transvaginal ultrasonography provides greater image resolution and may be more sensitive. The recent clinical introduction of color Doppler transvaginal ultrasonography, by which blood-flow resistance or the pulsatility index can be assessed, may improve the ability to distinguish between benign and malignant adnexal masses[16–18]. The role of this technique for screening purposes remains to be evaluated. The various aspects of ultrasonography of adnexal masses are discussed in greater detail in other chapters of this book. Improvement in detection of ovarian cancer in the future may be achieved by conjugation of radiolabelled markers with monoclonal antibodies directed against ovarian cancer-associated antigens[19].

Computed tomography has no advantage over ultrasound in the distinction between benign and malignant masses. It has, however, greatly improved the preoperative determination of the extent of the disease, although tumor nodules smaller than 1.5 cm cannot be visualized[20]. Magnetic resonance imaging (MRI) is probably not more accurate, although its value remains to be determined.

A large number of tumor-associated antigens have been identified in ovarian cancer of epithelial origin[21]. The most useful and most widely clinically employed marker is CA 125. It is demonstrable in approximately 80% of non-mucinous epithelial ovarian cancers. A value greater than 35 U/ml is considered positive. Although 99% of healthy individuals will have less than this value, and 99.7% will have less than 65 U/ml, CA 125 is not specific for ovarian carcinoma. It can be elevated in normal individuals as well as in a great variety of other gynecological and non-gynecological malignancies and benign diseases such as endometrial, cervical, and breast cancer, pregnancy, endometriosis, pelvic inflammatory disease and others. However, CA 125 is of great importance in the follow up of ovarian cancer patients and for monitoring the disease status. Serial determinations of serum CA 125 levels accurately reflect regression and progression of ovarian carcinoma. Falling titers indicate regression of the disease and persistent titers indicate residual disease. A rising CA 125 titer, often preceding clinically demonstrable tumor, is a very reliable indicator of recurrence. The rate of CA 125 decrease in response to therapy is an important prognostic indicator. Thus, patients with a CA 125 level of less than 10 U/ml 1 month after the third postoperative course of chemotherapy have a more favorable outcome than patients with higher CA 125 levels[22].

Attempts are being made to improve the sensitivity and specificity of CA 125 by its use in combination with other tumor markers such as NB/70K, serum lipid-associated sialic acid, CA 19–9 and others. Although the results are diverse, some improvement can probably be achieved by the use of a combination of markers.

Since the 5-year survival rate of patients with tumor confined to the ovaries is better than that of patients with disease that has spread beyond the ovaries, attempts have been made to use several tests for screening and early diagnosis of the disease.

The potential screening efficacy of CA 125 was evaluated by its prospective determination in asymptomatic women who were 40 years or older, or postmenopausal[23]. On the basis of this study, it has been suggested[24] that even with a specificity of 99.5%, only 6–11% of all women with elevated CA 125 levels would actually have ovarian cancer even if the sensitivity was 100%.

In the largest reported screening project by abdominal ultrasonography comprising more than 5000 women, the overall specificity of the procedure was 97.7% and the odds of being affected with ovarian cancer, given a positive result, were 1:67[25]. Screening of 1000 asymptomatic women older than 40 years by vaginal ultrasonography yielded a sensitivity of 100% but a specificity of only 97.8%[26].

The combination of a vaginal examination, CA 125 determination and transabdominal ultrasonography has been evaluated in 4000 postmenopausal volunteers older than 44 years. If a patient had an elevated CA 125 level and an abnormal pelvic or ultrasound examination, the specificity was 100%[27]. The cost-effectiveness of screening for ovarian cancer and its impact on mortality reduction has not been prospectively evaluated. It is generally agreed that no single technique is currently available for effective routine screening. Screening of high risk groups, such as women with a family history or nulliparous women over the age of 45 who have not used oral contraceptives or women with early-onset breast cancer, should be considered.

Histopathology, dissemination and staging

Epithelial ovarian carcinoma arises from the surface epithelium which is composed of a single layer of modified mesothelial cells that cover the ovarian surface. The carcinoma comprises several subtypes histologically, namely: serous, mucinous and endometrioid adenocarcinoma, clear cell carcinoma and borderline tumors. In its malignant form the ovarian surface epithelium may thus have features resembling tubal (serous), endometrial (endometrioid), or endocervical (mucinous) epithelium. The most common subtype is serous cystadenocarcinoma.

Epithelial cysts of borderline malignancy (carcinoma of low malignant potential), which account for up to 10% of ovarian carcinomas, are characterized by cellular stratification, the presence of papillae, increased mitotic activity, cellular atypia and lack of invasion into the stroma. The identification of this histological subset is of great importance since it occurs at a much younger age and offers a much more favorable prognosis.

The histological grade of the tumor is of great

prognostic significance in stage I and II, but in more advanced stages it is not an important variable.

Ovarian cancer is believed to spread from the primary lesion by exfoliation of malignant cells which follow the circulation pattern of peritoneal fluid. These cells attach to peritoneal surfaces and produce dissemination frequently involving the omentum and right hemidiaphragm, but all peritoneal surfaces are at risk. Lymphatic spread to retroperitoneal lymph nodes often occurs, while hematogenic spread is less frequent. Widespread intraperitoneal carcinomatosis consistent with ovarian origin but without ovarian involvement is occasionally encountered. This is considered to indicate that the entire peritoneal mesothelium is at risk for malignant transformation into one of the histological categories typical of ovarian carcinoma.

The natural history of ovarian carcinoma is not well understood. Benign counterparts of the malignant tumors do exist, but their capacity for malignant conversion and the time required for this transformation is not known. Borderline malignancy is an entity by itself. A premalignant state has not been recognized, nor is it known whether all widespread tumors were initially confined to the ovaries and have gradually disseminated and if so, over what time period such progression occurs. It has been suggested that some of the tumors diagnosed as widespread ovarian carcinoma may actually represent a multifocal malignancy which developed synchronously in various areas of epithelium of mesothelial origin. On the other hand, it should be mentioned that recent molecular genetic studies indicate that ovarian carcinoma is a monoclonal disease[28].

Staging of ovarian carcinoma according to the International Federation of Gynecology and Obstetrics (FIGO) is presented in Table 2. It should be performed at the time of exploratory laparotomy. A longitudinal incision adequate for thorough exploration of the pelvic organs and the organs of the lower and upper abdomen is mandatory. Information with regard to the presence of tumor on the surface of the ovaries, the size of the tumor masses, the presence of malignant cells in ascitic fluid or in peritoneal washings, the involvement of the diaphragm, omentum and retroperitoneal lymph nodes, is required for accurate staging. Allocation of a patient to stage IA or IB can only be done by such a comprehensive staging procedure which should also include multiple biopsies from pelvic and abdominal peritoneal areas at risk. The identification of this subset of patients is of great importance since they probably do not require postoperative treatment.

Operative and postoperative treatment

The basis of the therapeutic approach to ovarian carcinoma is surgery. Exploratory laparotomy is performed in order to establish the diagnosis, determine the histological type of the tumor and its grade, and assess the extent of the disease for staging purposes.

The majority (80%) of borderline tumors are confined to the ovaries and treatment consists of hysterectomy and bilateral adnexectomy[29]. In young women who have not yet completed childbearing, more conservative surgery, namely adnexectomy of the involved ovary or even cystectomy, is probably sufficient[30]. The treatment of borderline tumors with lesions also present beyond the ovaries is controversial. While some authors claim that surgical excision alone is sufficient, others recommend the same treatment as for advanced carcinoma[31].

In comprehensively staged IA and IB tumors which are well or moderately differentiated and without adhesions, hysterectomy, adnexectomy and omentectomy may be the definitive treatment[32]. Other stage I patients require additional postoperative treatment. In advanced ovarian carcinoma, comprising the majority (80%) of cases, the aim of surgery is cytoreduction (debulking). There are numerous reports which show that patients with postoperative small residual tumor masses have a more favorable outcome[33,34]. Patients are considered to have had optimal debulking if the diameter of the largest residual tumor mass after the operation is less than 1.5 or 2 cm. The rationale for cytoreduction is manyfold. Chemotherapy molecules diffuse and interact better with small tumors. A smaller tumor may

Table 2 FIGO staging of ovarian cancer

Stage I	Growth limited to the ovaries
Stage Ia	Growth limited to one ovary; no ascites; no tumor on the external surface; capsule intact
Stage Ib	Growth limited to both ovaries; no ascites; no tumor on the external surface; capsule intact
Stage Ic	Tumor either stage Ia or Ib, but with tumor on surface of one or both ovaries, or with capsule ruptured, or with ascites present containing malignant cells, or with positive peritoneal washings
Stage II	Growth involving one or both ovaries with pelvic extension
Stage IIa	Extension and/or metastases to the uterus and/or tubes
Stage IIb	Extension to other pelvic tissues
Stage IIc	Tumor either stage IIa or IIb, but with tumor on surface of one or both ovaries, or with capsule(s) ruptured, or with ascites present containing malignant cells, or with positive peritoneal washings
Stage III	Tumor involving one or both ovaries with peritoneal implants outside the pelvis and/or positive retroperitoneal or inguinal nodes. Superficial liver metastasis equals stage III. Tumor is limited to the true pelvis but with histologically proven malignant extension to small bowel or omentum
Stage IIIa	Tumor grossly limited to the true pelvis with negative nodes but with histologically confirmed microscopic seeding of abdominal peritoneal surfaces
Stage IIIb	Tumor involving one or both ovaries with histologically confirmed implants of abdominal peritoneal surfaces, none exceeding 2 cm in diameter. Nodes are negative
Stage IIIc	Abdominal implants greater than 2 cm in diameter and/or positive retroperitoneal or inguinal nodes
Stage IV	Growth involving one or both ovaries with distant metastases. If pleural effusion is present, there must be positive cytology to allow a case to stage IV. Parenchymal liver metastasis equals stage IV

enhance immunological competence, and requires fewer cycles of treatment, thereby decreasing the likelihood of resistance, and excision of large tumor masses is expected to improve functional and nutritional status.

Hysterectomy, adnexectomy, excision of pelvic masses and omentectomy are the most common operations that achieve cytoreduction and can often be accomplished even in cases with extensive and adherent pelvic tumors by using a retroperitoneal approach. However, in order to achieve optimal cytoreduction, additional surgical procedures, including bowel surgery, urological surgery and a great variety of other operations, often have to be performed[35,36]. The extent of the surgical effort that is worthwhile has never been clearly defined. The morbidity after aggressive cytoreduction may be as high as 67% and mortality has also been reported. In most series, optimal cytoreduction is accomplished in 20–40% of the patients. However, much higher rates are achieved in tertiary referral centers[37].

Primary cytoreductive surgery has gained general acceptance, but its value has never been established by prospective trials and it is not clear whether the better outcome in patients who have undergone optimal debulking is due to an inherent property of the tumor that made optimal resection possible. The concept of debulking is therefore not unchallenged[38]. It has been suggested that residual disease should not exceed 0.5 cm for optimal effect and in one study it was found that only women with no residual macroscopic disease had a significantly better outcome[39]. Interval (delayed) debulking, i.e. a preplanned attempt at debulking after several courses of chemotherapy, yields conflicting results[40,41]. The value of secondary cytoreductive surgery is also uncertain but may be justified in patients with solitary metastases or patients with a long interval between primary surgery and the subsequent appearance of recurrence[42–44].

Postoperative chemotherapy is indicated in most ovarian carcinoma patients. Although a great variety of chemotherapeutic drugs are active in ovarian carcinoma[45], platinum compounds and platinum-based combination chemotherapy are nowadays the most commonly used in the postoperative management of ovarian carcinoma.

A recent overview[46] of randomized clinical trials indicated a survival advantage for platinum-based chemotherapy combination over single non-platinum agents up to 6 years after diagnosis. A comparison of platinum-based combination regimens vs. treatment with platinum alone found a 15% reduction in mortality in the group receiving the combination – a difference of borderline significance.

Initially the standard postoperative chemotherapeutic regimen consisted of cytoxan, adriamycin and cisplatin (CAP). After several trials indicated that this combination is not superior to treatment with cisplatin plus cytoxan (CP), the latter became the standard postoperative treatment. A four-drug combination consisting of hexamethylmelamine in addition to CAP may have some long-term survival advantage over CP in patients with small-volume residual disease.

Carboplatin is a platinum analog with a less toxic effect. It has a decreased incidence of neuro-, oto-, and nephrotoxicity but its myelosuppressive effect, especially thrombocytopenia, is more prominent. Several large studies have indicated that single-agent carboplatin and combinations are equally effective to single-agent cisplatin and cisplatin combination[46,47]. Because of the reduced toxicity, the combination of carboplatin and cytoxan may replace the regimen of CP as initial postoperative treatment. No effective second-line salvage chemotherapy regimens are available for patients who fail initial aggressive postoperative platinum-based chemotherapy. Nevertheless, patients who initially responded to cis- or carboplatin with a long disease-free interval, may respond to second-line treatment with these compounds[48]. A 20% response rate was also obtained in one study by second-line chemotherapy with ifosfamide. Objective responses may also be obtained in less than 10% of patients by second-line treatment with hormones (tamoxifen, megestrol or leuprolide).

Mechanisms of drug resistance are currently being elucidated. Increase in metallothioneins and glutathione[49] and enhanced capacity of DNA repair[50] have been implicated in the resistance to some chemotherapeutic agents, including cisplatin. Inhibition of glutathione synthesis by the synthetic amino acid analog buthionine sulfoximine, reverses drug resistance[51]. Aphidicolin inhibits enzymes important in the DNA repair process thus also reversing drug resistance[52]. Novel therapeutic approaches are also under investigation. Trials using lethal monoclonal conjugates, interferon and other biological response modifiers are in progress.

Taxol is potentially the most active new experimental drug. It is extracted from the bark of the western yew tree (*Taxus brevifolia*) and has a unique mechanism of action. It causes increased polymerization and stabilization of microtubules, thereby disrupting mitosis. Remission in 30–40% of previously platinum-treated advanced ovarian cancer patients has been reported[53–55]. New combinations for the initial chemotherapy (taxol plus cisplatin, taxol plus carboplatin, carboplatin plus cisplatin, carboplatin plus ifosfamide, and others) are also being tested.

Since there is evidence for a direct relationship between dose intensity and survival, trials of dose-intense chemotherapy schedules have been undertaken. Some of these trials incorporate agents which may reduce toxicity. It has been shown that the agents WR2721[56] and ORG-2766 reduce platinum-induced neurotoxicity[57], glutathione may decrease renal toxicity[58], the cytokines G-CSF and GM-CSF reduce neutropenia and growth factors IL-1α and IL-3 may reduce thrombocytopenia. Dose intensification with autologous bone marrow transplantation and peripheral stem cell transplantation are also being investigated[59].

Intraperitoneal chemotherapy is an additional treatment mode. By using this route of administration a pharmacological advantage over the intravenous route is gained. The peak concentration of the drugs administered into the peritoneal cavity is manyfold higher than the peak plasma concentration and the drug comes into direct contact with the tumor. Cisplatin and cisplatin combinations have been used. Because of poor penetration, only patients with small-volume disease are suitable for this treatment. No advantage of initial postoperative intraperitoneal chemotherapy over the intravenous administration has so far been demonstrated. The role of intraperitoneal cisplatin chemotherapy as second-line treatment remains to be determined, although a high response rate has been reported in patients with small-volume disease, with an initial response to intravenous cisplatin[60–62].

Abdominopelvic irradiation is also a postoperative treatment modality in ovarian cancer. It has been shown to be effective in patients with small-volume residual disease, especially when the tumor is not undifferentiated[63]. As second-line treatment, abdominopelvic irradiation has little curative effect in patients with macroscopic disease[64]. Single fraction irradiation is an effective modality for palliation of pain and bleeding. The use of intraperitoneal radioactive agents, mainly ^{32}P, are undergoing clinical trials in patients with small-volume disease.

About half of the patients who finish postoperative chemotherapy achieve complete clinical remission, i.e. they have no clinical, radiological and marker evidence of disease. The optimal treatment of these patients has hitherto not been determined. At second-look laparotomy, approximately half of these patients will have residual macroscopic or microscopic disease. No effective salvage therapy is available for those with residual disease. A large proportion of those with a pathologically confirmed complete response (negative second-look laparotomy) will eventually suffer recurrence, and secondary debulking at the time of second-look laparotomy is of doubtful value. Therefore, second-look laparotomy does not affect survival and is no longer considered to be a routine procedure in the management of ovarian carcinoma[65]. Additional treatment thus seems justified in all patients who are clinically in complete remission. We have shown that intraperitoneal cisplatin chemotherapy with systemic thiosulfate kidney protection in patients with a clinical complete response gives more favorable results than abdominopelvic irradiation or no treatment[66,67]. Other potential treatments in this group include systemic ifosfamide or hexamethylmelamine, intraperitoneal ^{32}P or interferon.

Prognosis and survival

Well-established unfavorable prognostic factors include advanced stage, grade and age, low performance status, suboptimal cytoreduction, large tumor masses at the time of initial operation and large volume of ascites. In contrast to grade, histological type is generally believed to have little effect on prognosis, with the exception of clear cell carcinoma which is considered to have a poor prognosis.

Newly recognized prognostic factors may assist in defining subsets of patients for whom more aggressive treatment is warranted. The presence of aneuploidy and a high S fraction determined by flow cytometric analysis, the inability to form colonies in a clonogenic assay and the amplification–overexpression of the Her-2*neu* oncogene, unfavorably affect survival[68–71]. The introduction of morphometry which allows automated quantitative microscopic image-analysis of morphological features, such as mitotic index, epithelial cell volume and nuclear area, allows a more objective evaluation of histological criteria that correlates well with prognosis[72].

The prognosis of ovarian cancer of epithelial origin is unfavorable and the overall 5-year survival rate for these patients is 37%. The 5-year survival rate for comprehensively staged patients with stage I disease is 80–90%, for stage II disease 60–80% and for patients with stage III and IV disease 15–20% and 5%, respectively. The longest survival of patients with advanced ovarian carcinoma is observed in those with a negative second-look laparotomy. The 5-year survival rate of stage I borderline tumors (95%) and of more advanced borderline tumors (75%) is superior to that of patients with invasive carcinoma. Late recurrences are, however, observed.

GERM CELL TUMORS

The malignant variants of germ cell tumors account for about 3% of ovarian cancers. Dysger-

Table 3 World Health Organization histological classification of ovarian germ cell tumors

(A) *Dysgerminoma*
(B) *Endodermal sinus tumor*
(C) *Embryonal carcinoma*
(D) *Polyembryoma*
(E) *Choriocarcinoma*
(F) *Teratomas*
  (1) Immature
  (2) Mature
    (a) Solid
    (b) Cystic
      (i) Dermoid cyst (mature cystic teratoma)
      (ii) Dermoid cyst with malignant transformation
  (3) Monodermal and highly specialized
    (a) Struma ovarii
    (b) Carcinoid
    (c) Struma ovarii and carcinoid
    (d) Others
(G) *Mixed forms*

minoma accounts for about 50% of germ cell tumors, endodermal sinus tumor and immature teratoma for about 20% each, and embryonal carcinoma, choriocarcinoma and mixed tumors comprise the remaining 10%.

The prognosis of patients with these tumors has improved considerably since the introduction of cisplatin combination chemotherapy. Not only is long-term survival achieved, but fertility is preserved as well. This is considered as one of the achievements in gynecological oncology. The germ cell tumors are listed in Table 3.

Dysgerminoma

Dysgerminoma is the most common germ cell tumor. It is a solid tumor composed of cells which resemble embryonal primordial germ cells. The stroma is infiltrated with lymphocytes. Bilaterality may occur in 10 to 20% of the cases. Extensive histological sampling of the tumor is mandatory in order to determine that no other germ cell elements are present and that the tumor represents a pure dysgerminoma. A grossly normal-appearing contralateral ovary may harbor tumor foci. Dysgerminomas may be associated with pregnancy in up to 20% of cases[73], probably due to the young age of patients.

Endodermal sinus (yolk sac) tumor

This tumor is unilateral in most cases. Histologically, various patterns (reticular, endodermal sinus, glandular, hepatoid) are discernible. Hyaline bodies which stain with periodic acid–Schiff are often present. Schiller–Duval bodies consisting of tumor cell-lined papillae containing a central vessel are also often seen in the reticular tumors. The tumors are almost always composed of cells that contain α-fetoprotein.

Immature teratoma

These tumors may be solid or cystic and are also usually unilateral. They contain cells derived from all three germ layers (ectoderm, mesoderm and endoderm) and are graded from I to III according to the amount of immature tissue present. Neural tissue is the most commonly found immature element.

Embryonal and choriocarcinoma

Pure forms of these tumors are extremely rare. They may secrete human chorionic gonadotropin (hCG) and cause sexual precocity or irregular uterine bleeding. Many choriocarcinomas occur in children.

An extremely rare and highly malignant germ cell tumor is polyembryoma, which is composed of numerous embryoid bodies resembling normal embryos.

Mixed germ cell tumors

These tumors may contain any mixture of germ cell elements, but the most common is a combination of endoderm sinus tumor and dysgerminoma. If dysgerminoma elements are present, the contralateral ovary may be involved in 10% of cases. The exact determination of the different components that these tumors contain is considered to be important for therapeutic and prognostic purposes.

Clinical aspects

These tumors occur mainly in girls and young women. The most common symptom is abdominal pain. Other symptoms include abdominal distension, fever and, rarely, isosexual precocious puberty or irregular bleeding due to hCG secretion (mainly by choriocarcinoma, embryonal carcinoma and mixed tumors). Acute pain may also occur, due to rupture, bleeding or torsion.

Endodermal sinus tumors, almost without exception, produce α-fetoprotein, which may also be produced by immature teratomas, mixed germ cell tumors and embryonal carcinoma. α-Fetoprotein and hCG are therefore important markers used in the preoperative diagnosis and follow up of patients with these tumors. Additional markers that may be elevated are lactic dehydrogenase, CA 125 and neuron-specific enolase[74–76].

Physical examination will usually reveal a unilateral pelvic mass 5–15 cm in diameter, but much larger masses have been reported. Ascites may also be present.

The tumors spread on the peritoneal surfaces or by lymphatic dissemination. Surgical staging is performed as for malignant tumors of epithelial origin. It should consist of cytological sampling of peritoneal fluid or washings, meticulous inspection of all abdominal and pelvic peritoneal surfaces, and sampling of pelvic and para-aortic lymph nodes. When no gross lesions are seen, random biopsies should be obtained. If the tumor is macroscopically confined to one ovary, biopsy of the contralateral ovary should be considered mainly in the case of dysgerminoma, because of its greater tendency for bilaterality.

Treatment and survival

The primary treatment of malignant germ cell tumors is surgical. Most of the patients are young and since bilaterality is infrequent in most tumors and preservation of fertility is important, unilateral adnexectomy is adequate. When a disseminated tumor is encountered, the principles of cytoreduction may also apply to these malignant tumors[77]. It should, however, be kept in mind that malignant germ cell tumors are chemosensitive, and very aggressive resection should be avoided.

The most effective postoperative chemotherapy regimens in patients with advanced disease are cisplatin-based combinations, namely vinblastine, cisplatin and bleomycin (VPB) or bleomycin, etoposide (VP16) and cisplatin (BEP)[77–79]. Although dysgerminoma, similarly to testicular seminoma, is a highly radiosensitive tumor, postoperative treatment, when indicated, should nowadays consist of cisplatin-based chemotherapy as in other germ cell tumors.

There is some evidence that adjuvant BEP chemotherapy may be effective in completely resected, advanced-stage malignant germ cell tumors as well as in advanced-grade stage I immature teratoma, stage I endodermal sinus tumor and mixed germ cell tumors[80]. Normal pregnancy can occur after combination chemotherapy of patients with malignant germ cell tumors[77,81,82].

Second-look laparotomy is probably not indicated in these tumors. Persistent and recurrent tumors also respond to second-line chemotherapy such as cisplatin, vinblastin and ifosfamide[83]. Therapeutic trials with dose intensification, with autologous bone marrow rescue, or phase II drugs, are currently under investigation[84]. With new chemotherapy regimens, survival rates higher than 95% can be achieved. Almost all appropriately staged patients with stage I disease, and a considerable percentage of patients with advanced disease, survive.

GONADAL STROMAL (SEX CORD) TUMORS

These tumors comprise about 6% of ovarian neoplasms and about 2% of ovarian cancers. Their histogenesis is not clear and they may originate either from celomic epithelium or from subcelomic mesenchymal cells of the gonadal ridge. The gonadal stromal tumors are listed in Table 4. The vast majority of functioning, i.e. hormone-producing, tumors belong to this group. Each functioning tumor is able to produce multiple steroids at the same time and the clinical manifestations depend on the predominant steroid produced.

Granulosa cell tumor

This is a relatively rare tumor which may occur at any age, but 45% are diagnosed in postmenopausal women and only 5% before puberty. Granulosa cell tumors are solid and fleshy or occasionally

Table 4 World Health Organization histological classification of ovarian sex cord stromal tumors, other tumors, tumor-like conditions, and lipid (lipoid) cell tumors

Sex cord stromal tumors
(A) Granulosa–stromal tumors
  (1) Granulosa cell tumor
  (2) Tumors in the thecoma–fibroma group
    (a) Thecoma
    (b) Fibroma
    (c) Unclassified
(B) Androblastomas: Sertoli–Leydig cell tumors
  (1) Well differentiated
    (a) Tubular androblastoma: Sertoli cell tumor (tubular adenoma of Pick)
    (b) Tubular androblastoma with lipid storage: Sertoli cell tumor with lipid storage (folliculome lipidique of Lecene)
    (c) Sertoli–Leydig cell tumor (tubular adenoma with Leydig cells)
    (d) Leydig cell tumor: hilus cell tumor
  (2) Of intermediate differentiation
  (3) Poorly differentiated (sarcomatoid)
  (4) With heterologous elements
(C) Gynandroblastoma
(D) Unclassified

Gonadoblastoma
(A) Pure
(B) Mixed with dysgerminoma or other form of germ cell tumor

Soft tissue tumors not specific to the ovary
Secondary (metastatic) tumors
Tumor-like conditions
(A) Pregnancy luteoma
(B) Hyperplasia of ovarian stroma and hyperthecosis
(C) Massive edema
(D) Solitary follicle cyst and corpus luteum cyst
(E) Multiple follicle cysts (polycystic ovaries)
(F) Multiple luteinized follicle cysts and/or corpora lutea
(G) Endometriosis
(H) Surface-epithelial inclusion cysts (germinal inclusion cysts)
(I) Simple cysts
(J) Inflammatory lesions
(K) Paraovarian cysts

cystic. They are rarely (3%) bilateral. Cystic granulosa cell tumors occur in children and are usually unilateral and benign. Several histological patterns have been described and include micro- and macroglandular, tubular, sarcomatoid and other patterns. An admixture of patterns is often present. The cells are usually pale and grooved. The typical Call–Exner bodies, i.e. granulosa cells around clear spaces, are characteristic of the microfollicular pattern.

Most granulosa cell tumors also contain theca cells – hence the term granulosa–theca cell tumors. The theca cells are a benign component of the tumor and do not metastasize.

Juvenile granulosa cell tumors are encountered mainly in children and their histological pattern may be lobular, macrofollicular or a solid admixture of granulosa and theca cells. The cells are usually darker than in the adult type and contain no grooves. Although numerous mitotic figures and marked atypia are often present, these tumors metastasize only rarely (15%).

Although granulosa cell tumors may produce a variety of steroids, most of them produce estrogens. This may cause isosexual precocious puberty in premenarchal girls, irregular bleeding in women of reproductive age or postmenopausal bleeding which may be associated with endometrial hyperplasia or carcinoma[85]. Other symptoms are those of a pelvic mass.

The histological features of the tumors are not considered reliable prognostic indicators. Characteristics indicating malignant potential are age over 40, large diameter (≥ 15 cm), bilaterality, rupture, increased mitotic activity, atypia and vascular or capsular invasion[86,87].

In girls and young women, when the tumor is confined to one ovary, excision of the involved adnexa is adequate. Reproductive function can thus be preserved in these patients.

In older women, the standard treatment is hysterectomy and bilateral adnexectomy. No difference in survival has been observed between stage I patients treated by surgery alone and those treated by surgery and adjunctive postoperative radiotherapy[88].

Advanced or recurrent disease is usually treated by postoperative radiotherapy or chemotherapy but the relative merits of these treatment modalities cannot be assessed. No advantage of any drug or drug combination has yet been demonstrated.

Sertoli tumors

A Sertoli tumor is usually a unilateral, solid tumor which may occur at any age but is diagnosed mainly in young women. Several histological patterns have been described. Most tumors contain cells with intracytoplasmic lipid. When the lipid accumulation is substantial, the tumor has been called 'folliculome lipique'. A variant of a complex Sertoli tumor (sex cord tumor with annular tubules) may be associated with the Peutz–Jeghers syndrome.

Most of the tumors are functioning and are mainly virilizing, but may also produce estrogens and progesterones. Clinical manifestations depend on the predominant hormone produced. Rarely, Cushing's syndrome is caused.

These tumors recur or metastasize only rarely. Unilateral adnexectomy is adequate treatment when the tumor is confined to one ovary and when conservation of fertility is a consideration. Otherwise, hysterectomy and bilateral adnexectomy is standard treatment.

Sertoli–Leydig tumors

These very rare tumors occur in young women of reproductive age. Histologically, they present as an admixture of Sertoli, Leydig and undifferentiated gonadal stromal cells. Heterologous elements (cartilage, muscle, etc.) may also be present[89].

Characteristically they produce androgens and gradually produce virilization manifested by oligomenorrhea followed by amenorrhea, breast atrophy, acne, hirsutism, clitoral enlargement and deepening of the voice.

Bilaterality and extraovarian spread is rare and therefore unilateral adnexectomy is usually adequate treatment. Removal of the tumor is usually associated with return of regular menstrual cycles within several weeks, but hirsutism may persist longer and clitoral enlargement and voice changes may not regress. Stage I and differentiation at diagnosis are not dependable prognostic indicators. Therefore, when fertility is not an issue, hysterectomy and bilateral adnexectomy are indicated[90,91].

When the disease has spread beyond the ovaries, combination chemotherapy such as cisplatin, adriamycin and cyclophosphamide or bleomycin, etoposide and cisplatin has been used[92].

Lipid cell tumors

These are extremely rare tumors which may produce androgens, but also a variety of other steroids. Typically, the tumor is virilizing. Histologically, it contains Leydig (hilar) cells resembling adrenal cortical cells.

These tumors are usually unilateral and generally benign. They are treated by adnexectomy in young women when confined to one ovary. In older women, or advanced stages, hysterectomy and bilateral adnexectomy are indicated.

SECONDARY OVARIAN TUMORS

The ovary is a frequent site for metastases from other organs, and approximately 10% of ovarian tumors are not primarily ovarian in origin[93,94]. Ovarian involvement is often bilateral. Metastatic ovarian tumors may arise in other gynecological neoplasms or from tumors in other organ systems. The most common gynecological tumor metastasizing to the ovary is endometrial carcinoma. When the endometrioid histological pattern is encountered, it is often difficult to establish whether the tumor is metastatic or a second primary. The most common metastatic tumors from other organ systems are metastases from breast tumors and the gastrointestinal tract, mainly the colon. The term Krukenberg tumor should be reserved for tumors that contain abundant signet-ring cells. The origin of almost all such tumors is in the stomach, although other sites of origin (mainly breast and small intestine) have also been reported. The diagnosis of tumors metastatic to the ovary may precede detection of the primary neoplasm. The survival of patients with secondary ovarian tumors is very poor.

References

1. Beck, R. P. and Latour, J. P. A. (1960). Review of 1019 benign ovarian neoplasms. *Obstet. Gynecol.*, **16**, 479–82
2. Muir, C. S., Waterhouse, J., Mack, T., Powell, J. and Whelan, S. (1987). *Cancer Incidence in Five Continents*, vol. V, Publ. 88. (Lyon: IARC Science Publishers)
3. Parazzini, F., Franceschi, S., La Vecchia, C. and Faroli, M. (1991). The epidemiology of ovarian cancer. *Gynecol. Oncol.*, **43**, 9–23
4. Menczer, J., Modan, M., Ranon, L. and Golan, A. (1979). Possible role of mumps virus in the etiology of ovarian cancer. *Cancer*, **43**, 1375–8
5. Cramer, D. W., Hutchison, G. B., Welch, W. R., Scully, R. E. and Knapp, R. C. (1982). Factors affecting the association of oral contraceptives and ovarian cancer. *N. Engl. J. Med.*, **307**, 1047–51
6. The Cancer and Steroid Hormone Study of the Centers for Disease Control and the National Institute of Child Health and Human Development (1987). The reduction in risk of ovarian cancer associated with oral-contraceptive use. *N. Engl. J. Med.*, **316**, 650–5
7. Piver, M. S., Mettlin, C. J., Tsukada, Y., Nasco, P., Greenwald, P. and McPhee, M. F. (1984). Familial ovarian cancer registry. *Obstet. Gynecol.*, **64**, 195–9
8. Menczer, J. and Ben-Baruch, G. (1991). Familial ovarian cancer in Israeli Jewish women. *Obstet. Gynecol.*, **77**, 276–7
9. Lynch, H. T., Bewtra, C. and Lynch, J. F. (1986). Familial ovarian carcinoma. Clinical nuances. *Am. J. Med.*, **81**, 1073–6
10. Piver, M. S. (1990). *The Gilda Radner Familial Ovarian Cancer Registry Newsletter*, Roswell Park Memorial Hospital, Buffalo
11. Piver, M. S., Jishi, M. F., Tsukada, Y. and Natarajan, N. (1993). Primary peritoneal carcinoma after oophorectomy in women with a family history of ovarian cancer. *Cancer*, **71**, 2751–5
12. Narod, S. A., Feunteun, J., Lynch, H. T., Watson, P., Conway, T., Lynch, J. and Lenoir, G. M. (1991). Familial breast–ovarian cancer locus on chromosome 17q12-q23. *Lancet*, **338**, 82–3
13. Zhou, D. J., Gonzales-Cadavid, N., Ahuja, J., Battifora, H., Moore, G. E. and Cline, M. J. (1988). A unique pattern of proto-oncogene abnormalities in ovarian adeno-carcinomas. *Cancer*, **62**, 1573–6
14. Yasue, H., Takeda, A. and Ishibashi, M. (1987). Amplification of the c-*myc* gene and the elevation of its transcripts in human ovarian tumor lines. *Cell Struct. Func.*, **12**, 121–4
15. Marks, J. R., Davidoff, A. M., Kerns, B. J., Humphrey, P. A., Pence, J. C., Dodge, R. K., Clarke-Pearson, D. L., Iglehart, J. D., Bast, R. C. Jr and Berchuck, A. (1991). Overexpression and mutation of p53 in epithelial ovarian cancer. *Cancer Res.*, **51**, 2979–84
16. Bourne, T. H. (1991). Transvaginal color Doppler in gynecology. *Ultrasound Obstet. Gynecol.*, **1**, 359–73
17. Kurjak, A., Zalud, I. and Alfirevic, Z. (1991). Evaluation of adnexal masses with transvaginal color ultrasound. *J. Ultrasound Med.*, **101**, 295–7
18. Weiner, Z., Thaler, I., Beck, D., Rottem, S., Deutsch, M. and Brandes, J. M. (1992). Differentiating malignant from benign ovarian tumors with transvaginal color flow imaging. *Obstet. Gynecol.*, **79**, 159–62
19. Averete, H. E. and Donato, D. M. (1990). Ovarian carcinoma: advances in diagnosis, staging and treatment. *Cancer*, **65**, 703–8
20. Stehman, F. B., Calkins, A. R., Wass, J. L., Smirz, L. R., Sutton, G. P. and Ehrlich, C. E. (1988). A comparison of findings at second-look laparotomy with pre-operative computed tomography in patients with ovarian carcinoma. *Gynecol. Oncol.*, **29**, 37–42
21. Montag, W. (1990). Tumor markers in gynecologic oncology. *Obstet. Gynecol. Surv.*, **45**, 94–105
22. Mogensen, O. (1992). Prognostic value of CA 125 in advanced ovarian cancer. *Gynecol. Oncol.*, **44**, 207–12

23. Einhorn, N., Sjovall, K. and Schoenfeld, G. (1990). Prospective evaluation of CA 125 levels in a normal population. *Am. Soc. Clin. Oncol.*, **9**, 157
24. Creasman, W. T. and DiSaia, P. J. (1991). Screening in ovarian cancer. *Am. J. Obstet. Gynecol.*, **165**, 7–10
25. Campbell, S., Bhan, V., Royston, P., Whitehead, M. I. and Collins, W. P. (1989). Trans-abdominal ultrasound screening for early ovarian cancer. *Br. Med. J.*, **299**, 1363–7
26. Van Nagell, J. R., Higgins, R. V., Donaldson, E. S., Gallion, H. H., Powell, D. E., Pavlik, E. J., Woods, C. H. and Thompson, E. A. (1990). Transvaginal sonography as a screening method for ovarian cancer. A report of the first 1000 cases screened. *Cancer*, **65**, 573–7
27. Jacobs, I. J. and Oram, D. A. (1989). Potential screening tests for ovarian cancer. In Sharp, F., Mason, W. P. and Leake, R. E. (eds.) *Ovarian Cancer*, pp. 197–205. (London: Chapman and Hall Medical)
28. Tsao, S. W., Mok, C. H., Knapp, R. C., Oike, K., Muto, M. G., Welch, W. R., Goodman, H. M., Sheets, E. E., Berkowitz, R. S. and Lau, C. C. (1993). Molecular genetic evidence of a unifocal origin for human serous ovarian carcinomas. *Gynecol. Oncol.*, **48**, 5–10
29. Chambers, J. T. (1989). Borderline ovarian tumors: a review of treatment. *Yale J. Biol. Med.*, **62**, 351–65
30. Lim-Tan, S. K., Cajigas, H. E. and Scully, R. E. (1988). Ovarian cystectomy for serous borderline tumors: a follow-up study of 35 cases. *Obstet. Gynecol.*, **72**, 775–81
31. Gershenson, D. M. and Silva, E. F. (1990). Serous ovarian tumors of low malignant potential with peritoneal implants. *Cancer*, **65**, 578–85
32. Young, R. C., Walton, L. A., Ellenberg, S. S., Homesley, H. D., Wilbanks, G. D., Decker, D. G., Miller, A., Park, R. and Major, F. Jr (1990). Adjuvant therapy in stage I and II epithelial ovarian cancer. Results of two prospective randomized trials. *N. Engl. J. Med.*, **322**, 1021–7
33. Griffiths, C. T., Parker, L. M. and Fuller, A. F. (1979). Role of cytoreductive surgical treatment in the management of advanced ovarian cancer. *Cancer Treat. Rep.*, **63**, 235–40
34. Hainsworth, J. D., Grosh, W. W. and Burnett, L. S., Jones, H. W. 3rd, Wolff, S. N. and Greco, F. A. (1988). Advanced ovarian cancer. Long term results of treatment with intensive cisplatin based chemotherapy of brief duration. *Ann. Intern. Med.*, **102**, 165–70
35. Wharton, J. T., Edwards, C. L. and Rutledge, F. N. (1984). Long term survival after chemotherapy for advanced epithelial ovarian carcinoma. *Am. J. Obstet. Gynecol.*, **148**, 997–1005
36. Piver, M. S. and Baker, T. (1986). The potential for optimal (≥2) cytoreductive surgery in advanced carcinoma at a tertiary medical center. A prospective study. *Gynecol. Oncol.*, **24**, 1–8
37. Heintz, A. P., Hacker, N. F., Berek, J. S., Rose, T. P., Munoz, A. K. and Lagasse, L. D. (1986). Cytoreductive surgery in ovarian carcinoma. Feasibility and morbidity. *Obstet. Gynecol.*, **67**, 783–8
38. Menczer, J. (1992). Cytoreductive surgery in the treatment of advanced ovarian carcinoma. Some controversial aspects. *Eur. J. Gynecol. Oncol.*, **13**, 320–2
39. Schwartz, P. E., Chambers, J. T., Kohorn, E. I., Chambers, S. K., Weitzman, H., Voynick, I. M., MacLusky, N. and Naftolin, F. (1989). Tamoxifen in combination with cytotoxic chemotherapy in advanced epithelial ovarian cancer. A prospective randomized trial. *Cancer*, **63**, 1074–8
40. Wils, J., Blijham, G., Naus, A., Belder, C., Bron, H., Ceelan, T., Eekhout, A., von Erp, J. and Geelan, P. (1986). Primary or delayed debulking surgery and chemotherapy consisting of cisplatin, doxorubicin and cyclophosphamide in Stage III–IV epithelial ovarian carcinoma. *J. Clin. Oncol.*, **4**, 1068–73
41. Gershenson, D. M., Wharton, J. K. T., Copeland, L. J., Stringer, C. A., Edwards, C. L., Kavanagh, J. J. and Freedman, R. S. (1989). Treatment of advanced epithelial ovarian cancer with cisplatin and cisplatin and cyclophosphamide. *Gynecol. Oncol.*, **32**, 336–41
42. Vogl, S. E., Seltzer, V., Calanog, A., Moukhtar, M., Camacho, F., Kaplan, B. H. and Greenwald, E. (1984). 'Second-effort' surgical resection for bulky ovarian cancer. *Cancer*, **54**, 2220–5
43. Morris, M., Gershenson, D. M. and Wharton, J. T. (1989). Secondary cytoreductive surgery in epithelial ovarian cancer. Non-responders to first-line therapy. *Gynecol. Oncol.*, **33**, 1–5
44. Jacob, J. H., Gershenson, D. M., Morris, M., Copeland, L. J., Burke, T. W. and Wharton, J. T. (1984). Neoadjuvant chemotherapy and interval debulking for advanced epithelial ovarian cancer. *Gynecol. Oncol.*, **42**, 146–50
45. Ozols, R. F. and Young, R. C. (1984). Chemotherapy of ovarian cancer. *Semin. Oncol.*, **11**, 251–63
46. Advanced Ovarian Cancer Trialists group (1991). Chemotherapy in advanced ovarian cancer: an overview of randomized clinical trials. *Br. Med. J.*, **303**, 884–93
47. Alberts, D. S., Green, S., Hannigan, E. V., O'Toole, R., Stock-Novack, D., Anderson, P., Surwit, E. A., Malvlya, V. K., Nahhas, W. A. and Jolles, C. J. (1992). Improved therapeutic index of carboplatin plus cyclophosphamide versus cisplatin plus cyclophosphamide. Final report by the Southwest Oncology Group of a phase III randomized trial in stages III (suboptimal) and IV ovarian cancer. *J. Clin. Oncol.*, **10**, 706–17

48. Markman, M. and Hoskins, W. (1992). Responses to salvage chemotherapy in ovarian cancer: a critical need for precise definitions of the treated population. *J. Clin. Oncol.*, **10**, 513–14
49. Perez, R. P., Hamilton, T. C. and Ozols, R. F. (1990). Resistance to alkylating agents and cisplatin: insights from ovarian carcinomal model systems. *Pharmacol. Ther.*, **48**, 19–27
50. Parker, R. J., Eastman, A., Bostick-Bruton, F. and Reed, E. (1991). Acquired cisplatin resistance in human ovarian cancer cells is associated with enhanced repair of cisplatin–DNA lesions and reduced drug accumulation. *J. Clin. Invest.*, **87**, 772–7
51. Louie, K. G., Hamilton, T. C., Winker, M. A., Behrens, B. C., Tsuruo, T., Klecker, R. W. Jr, McKoy, W. M., Grotzinger, K. R., Myers, C. E. and Young, R. C. (1986). Augmentation of adriamycin accumulation and metabolism in adriamycin sensitive and resistant human ovarian cancer cell lines. *Biochem. Pharm.*, **35**, 467–72
52. Katz, E. J., Andrews, P. A. and Howell, S. B. (1990). The effect of DNA polymerase inhibitors on the cytotoxicity of cisplatin in human ovarian carcinoma cells. *Cancer Commun.*, **2**, 159–64
53. McGuire, W. P., Rowinsky, E. K., Rosenshein, N. B., Grumbine, F. C., Ettinger, D. S., Armstrong, D. K. and Donehower, R. C. (1989). Taxol, a unique antineoplastic agent with significant activity in advanced ovarian epithelial neoplasms. *Ann. Intern. Med.*, **111**, 273–9
54. Einzig, A. I., Wiernik, P. H., Sasloff, J., Garl, S., Runowicz, C., O'Hanlan, K. A. and Goldenberg, G. (1990). Phase II study of taxol in patients with advanced ovarian cancer. *Proceedings of the American Association of Cancer Research*, **31**, 187
55. Thigpen, T., Blessing, J. and Ball, H. (1990). Phase II trial of Taxol as second-line therapy for ovarian carcinoma (Abstr.). *Proc. Am. Soc. Clin. Oncol.*, **9**, 156
56. Kemp, G. M., Glover, D. J. and Schein, P. S. (1990). The role of WR-2721 in the reduction of combined cisplatin and cyclophosphamide toxicity (Abstr.). *Proc. Am. Soc. Clin. Oncol.*, **9**, 67
57. Van der Hoop, R. G., Vecht, C. J., Van der Burg, M. E., Elderson, A., Boogerd, M., Heimans, J. J., Vries, E. P., van Houwelingen, J. C., Jennekens, F. G. and Gispen, W. H. (1990). Prevention of cisplatin neurotoxicity with an ACTH (4–9) analogue in patients with ovarian cancer. *N. Engl. J. Med.*, **322**, 89–94
58. Di-Re, F., Bohm, S., Oriana, S., Spatt, G. B. and Zunino, F. (1990). Efficacy and safety of high dose cisplatin and cyclophosphamide with glutathione protection in the treatment of bulky advanced epithelial ovarian cancer. *Cancer Pharm.*, **25**, 355–60
59. Shpall, E. J., Clarke-Pearson, D., Soper, J. T., Berchuk, A., Jones, R. B., Bast, R. C. Jr, Ross, M., Lidor, Y., Vanacek, K. and Tyler, T. (1990). High-dose alkylating agent chemotherapy with autologous bone marrow support in patients with stage III/IV epithelial ovarian cancer. *Gynecol. Oncol.*, **38**, 386–91
60. Howell, S. B. (1988). Intraperitoneal chemotherapy for ovarian cancer. *J. Clin. Oncol.*, **6**, 1673–5
61. Markman, M. (1989). Intraperitoneal cisplatin chemotherapy in the management of ovarian carcinoma. *Semin. Oncol.*, **16**, 79–82
62. Markman, M., Reichman, B., Hakes, T., Jones, W., Lewis, J. L. Jr, Rubin, S., Almadrones, L. and Hoskins, W. (1991). Responses to second line cisplatin-based intraperitoneal therapy in ovarian cancer. Influence of a prior response to intravenous cisplatin. *J. Clin. Oncol.*, **9**, 1801–5
63. Dembo, A. J. (1985). Abdominopelvic radiotherapy in ovarian cancer. A 10 year experience. *Cancer*, **55**, 2285–90
64. Menczer, J., Ben-Baruch, G., Modan, M. and Brenner, H. (1986). Abdominopelvic irradiation for stage II–IV ovarian carcinoma patients with limited or no residual disease at second-look laparotomy after completion of cisplatinum based combination chemotherapy. *Gynecol. Oncol.*, **24**, 149–54
65. Friedman, J. B. and Weiss, N. S. (1990). Sounding board, second thoughts about second look laparotomy in advanced ovarian cancer. *N. Engl. J. Med.*, **322**, 1079–81
66. Menczer, J., Ben-Baruch, G., Modan, M. and Brenner H. (1989). Intraperitoneal cisplatin chemotherapy vs. abdominopelvic irradiation in ovarian carcinoma after second-look laparotomy. *Cancer*, **63**, 1509–13
67. Menczer, J., Ben-Baruch, G., Rizel, S. and Brenner, H. (1992). Intraperitoneal chemotherapy vs. no treatment in ovarian carcinoma patients who are in complete clinical remission. *Cancer*, **70**, 1956–9
68. Friedlander, M. L., Taylor, I. W., Russell, P., Musgrove, E. A., Hedley, H. and Tattersall, M. H. (1983). Ploidy as a prognostic factor in ovarian cancer. *Int. Gynecol. Pathol.*, **2**, 55–63
69. Friedlander, M. L., Headly, D. H., Taylor, I., Russell, P., Coates, A. S. and Tattersall, M. H. (1984). Influence of cellular DNA content on survival in advanced ovarian cancer. *Cancer Res.*, **44**, 397–400
70. Dittrich, C., Dittrich, E., Sevelda, P., Hudec, M., Salzer, H., Grunt, T. and Eliason, J. (1991). Clonogenic growth *in vitro*. An independent biologic prognostic factor in ovarian carcinoma. *J. Clin. Oncol.*, **9**, 381–8
71. Slamon, D. J., Godolphin, W., Jones, L. A., Holt, J. A., Wong, S. G., Keith, D. E., Levin, W. J., Stuart, S. G., Udova, J. and Ullrich, A. (1989). Studies of the Her-2*neu* proto-oncogene in human breast and ovarian cancer, *Science*, **244**, 707–12
72. Baak, J. P., Schipper, N. W., Wisse-Brekelmans, E.

C., Ceelen, T., Bosman, F. T., van Geuns, H. and Wils, J. (1988). The prognostic value of morphometrical features and cellular DNA content in cisplatin treated late ovarian cancer patients. *Br. J. Cancer*, **57**, 503–8
73. Krepart, G., Smith, J. P., Rutledge, F. and Delclos, L. (1978). The treatment for dysgerminoma of the ovary. *Cancer*, **41**, 986–90
74. Awais, G. M. (1983). Dysgerminoma and serum lactic dehydrogenase levels. *Obstet. Gynecol.*, **61**, 99–101
75. Bahari, C. M., Lurio, M., Schoenfeld, A. and Joel-Cohen, S. J. (1980). Ovarian teratoma with peritoneal gliomatosis and elevated serum alpha-fetoprotein. *Am. J. Clin. Pathol.*, **73**, 603–7
76. Kuzmits, R., Schernthaner, G. and Krisch, K. (1987). Serum neuron-specific enolase, a marker for response to therapy in seminoma. *Cancer*, **60**, 1017–21
77. Williams, S. D., Blessing, J. A., Moore, D. H., Homesley, H. D. and Adcock, L. (1989). Cisplatin, vinblastine and bleomycin in advanced and recurrent ovarian germ cell tumors. *Ann. Intern. Med.*, **111**, 22–7
78. Gershenson, D. M., Wharton, J. T., Kline, R. C., Larson, D. M., Kavanagh, J. J. and Rutledge, F. N. (1986). Chemotherapeutic complete remission in patients with metastatic ovarian dysgerminoma. *Cancer*, **58**, 2594–9
79. Williams, S. D., Birch, R., Einhorn, L. H., Irwin, L., Greco, F. A. and Loehrer, P. J. (1987). Disseminated germ cell tumors, chemotherapy with cisplatin plus bleomycin plus either vinblastine or etoposide. *N. Engl. J. Med.*, **316**, 1435–40
80. Williams, S. D., Blessing, J. A. and Slaytor, R. (1989). Ovarian germ cell tumors. Adjuvant trials of the gynecologic oncology group (Abstr.). *Proc. Am. Soc. Clin. Oncol.*, **8**, 150
81. Loehrer, P. J. Sr, Lauer, R., Roth, B. J., Williams, S. D., Kalasinski, L. A. and Einhorn, L. H. (1988). Salvage therapy with VP-16 or vinblastine plus ifosfamide plus cisplatin in recurrent germ cell cancer. *Ann. Intern. Med.*, **109**, 540–6
82. Schwartz, P. E. (1984). Combination chemotherapy in the management of ovarian germ cell malignancies. *Obstet. Gynecol.*, **64**, 564–72
83. Sessa, C., Bonazzi, C., Landoni, F., Pecorelli, S., Sartori, E. and Mangioni, C. (1987). Cisplatin, vinblastine and bleomycin combination chemotherapy in endodermal sinus tumor of the ovary. *Obstet. Gynecol.*, **70**, 220–4
84. Gershenson, D. M. (1993). Update on malignant ovarian germ cell tumors. *Cancer*, **71** (Suppl. 4) 1581–90
85. Evans, A. T., Gaffey, T. A., Malkasian, G. D. and Annegers, J. F. (1980). Clinicopathologic review of 118 granulosa and 82 theca cell tumors. *Obstet. Gynecol.*, **55**, 231–8
86. Bjorkholm, E. and Silfversward, C. (1981). Prognostic factors in granulosa-cell tumors. *Gynecol. Oncol.*, **11**, 261–74
87. Fox, H., Agrawal, K. and Langley, F. A. (1975). A clinicopathologic study of 92 cases of granulosa cell tumor of the ovary with special reference to the factors influencing prognosis. *Cancer*, **35**, 231–41
88. Stenwig, J. T., Hazekamp, J. T. and Beecham, J. B. (1979). Granulosa cell tumors of the ovary. A clinicopathological study of 118 cases with long-term follow-up. *Gynecol. Oncol.*, **7**, 136–52
89. Prat, J., Young, R. H. and Scully, R. E. (1982). Ovarian Sertoli–Leydig cell tumors with heterologous elements. II Cartilage and skeletal muscle. A clinicopathologic analysis of twelve cases. *Cancer*, **50**, 2465–75
90. Zaloudek, C. and Norris, H. J. (1984). Sertoli–Leydig tumors of the ovary. A clinicopathological study of 64 intermediate and poorly differentiated neoplasms. *Am. J. Surg. Pathol.*, **8**, 409–18
91. Young, R. H. and Scully, R. E. (1985). Ovarian Sertoli–Leydig cell tumors. A clinicopathological analysis of 207 cases. *Am. J. Surg. Pathol.*, **9**, 543–69
92. Gershenson, D. M., Copeland, L. J., Kavanagh, J. J., Stringer, C. A., Saul, P. B. and Wharton, J. T. (1987). Treatment of metastatic stromal tumors of the ovary with cisplatin, doxorubicin and cyclophosphamide. *Obstet. Gynecol.*, **70**, 765–9
93. Petru, E., Pickel, H., Heydarfadai, M., Lahousen, M., Haas, J., Schaider, H. and Tamussino, K. (1992). Nongenital cancers metastatic to the ovary. *Gynecol. Oncol.*, **44**, 83–6
94. Young, R. H. and Scully, R. E. (1991). Metastatic tumors in the ovary. A problem-orientated approach and review of the recent literature. *Semin. Diagn. Pathol.*, **8**, 250–76

Ovarian tumors in pregnancy

10

I. R. McFadyen and D. W. Pilling

Most swellings of the ovary discovered during pregnancy are asymptomatic and benign. Malignant neoplasms are rare. Routine clinical or ultrasound examination reveals the majority of ovarian tumors, but a sizeable minority presents with symptoms which may be severe. They may be discovered at any stage of pregnancy or early in the puerperium. Not only is the mother affected, the fetus is at risk from consequences of their treatment or from their hormonal effects.

The majority of ovarian tumors found in pregnancy are corpora lutea, particularly in the first trimester[1,2]. They are found in 7–9% of pregnancies examined by ultrasound in the first 10 weeks but decrease thereafter; by 16–20 weeks they are present in only 0.3%[1]. Rarely more than 5 cm in diameter, these are unilocular and are almost always unilateral. Maximum diameter is achieved before 12 weeks and then the cyst regresses slowly over the next few weeks. Most other ovarian masses discovered in pregnancy were present at conception. The majority are benign dermoid cysts, which account for 22–40% of ovarian neoplasms[3–5]. This would be expected, since germ cell tumors peak during teenage years, whereas other types of neoplasms increase with age until the age of 45–50[6]. The next most common tumors are benign cystadenomata (10–15%), with others in decreasing frequency. Overall, 88% of ovarian tumors in pregnancy are physiological[2] and less than 1% are malignant[7–9].

The prevalence of ovarian tumors in pregnancy has been reported in three ways: those found on routine ultrasound examination of unselected populations, those found on routine clinical examination and those which required laparotomy during pregnancy. Laparotomy for an ovarian tumor is necessary once in 950 pregnancies[10,11] and routine scanning reveals an ovarian mass once in every 190–350 pregnancies[7,8]. Clinical examination of patients whose pregnancies were being terminated revealed a prevalence of one in 600 pregnancies, in both the first and second trimesters[9]. Clinically detectable tumors of 6 cm diameter or more have been found once per 274–815 pregnancies[3,12]. Unilocular cysts which are 5 cm or less in diameter almost invariably disappear spontaneously as pregnancy progresses[7]. Even those with a diameter of up to 10 cm may resolve but larger tumors rarely do so[7,8]. The true prevalence thus depends on the size of the tumor which can be detected by the method used and the stage of pregnancy in which the examination is made.

Corpora lutea are rarely bilateral, but these do occur[1]. Other tumors are more commonly bilateral and a few of these are malignant[1,10]. If, however, the theca lutein cysts which accompany 25% of hydatidiform moles are bilateral, the patient is more likely to develop trophoblastic disease[13]. Polycystic ovaries are bilateral. They are associated with an increased risk of spontaneous abortion because of the high basal levels of luteinizing hormone found in this condition[14]. The ultrasonic appearance is multiple cysts 2–8 mm in diameter peripherally in the ovary or scattered throughout the increased stroma of the organ[15]. Frequently, women with this condition require pharmacological assistance with conception. This may produce hyperstimulation of the ovaries with multiple large cysts and free fluid in the abdomen[16], but this may also occur spontaneously[17].

Malignant ovarian tumors are not common in pregnancy. Among those found on routine clinical or ultrasound examination, about 1% are malignant[7–9]. While more of those presenting with symptoms show malignancy, the reported incidence is not over 2–6%[3,10,11,18]. The ultrasound appearances suggesting malignancy are multilocular cysts (particularly if the septa are thick), solid areas in the tumor, invasion of the capsule, fixation, free fluid in the abdomen and growth on repeated examination. Uterine fibroids also, however, may grow rapidly during pregnancy. The ovarian tumors may be either unilateral or bilateral. The appearances suggestive of malignancy may also be seen in mucinous cystadenomata, teratomata, endometriomata, struma ovarii or infarcted benign tumors[1,19]. Color Doppler helps to identify malignant ovarian masses with certainty by demonstrating angiogenesis within the tumor[20,21].

Both benign and malignant tumors may produce hormones which affect the fetus. This is not common but virilization of girls has been described[22]. Primary Krukenberg tumors are the most common of these functioning tumors. Rarely do they affect the mother, but one mother was reported to develop a spotty complexion and severe hirsutism during the pregnancy[23]. More common than hormonal problems for the fetus are the effects of treatment. Chemotherapy or therapeutic irradiation early in pregnancy are likely to be teratogenic; they may lead to spontaneous abortion but do not always do so. Removal of a luteal cyst may also remove its hormonal support for the pregnancy, but this is not likely to increase the risk of abortion if the operation is later than 7 weeks[12,24,25]. Even clearance of the pelvis of all gynecological organs except the uterus is compatible with a continuing pregnancy. The trauma of laparotomy early in pregnancy is, however, likely to increase fetal loss[26]. This does not occur so frequently with operations in the second trimester but any surgery during pregnancy is associated with increased rates of premature delivery and intrauterine growth retardation[27].

PRESENTATION

Most ovarian tumors are incidental findings on routine clinical or ultrasound examination during pregnancy. If they lie beside the uterus they may appear to be part of it and produce an irregular shape. If they lie below it they can raise the level of the fundus so that the pregnancy appears to be large for dates or to have involution that is delayed in the puerperium. Late in pregnancy, they can produce an unstable lie or prevent the presenting part from engaging. Very occasionally, they are not discovered until labor is obstructed by their presence in the pelvis. While a retroverted gravid uterus or one with fibroids may produce acute retention of urine in pregnancy, it is almost unknown for an ovarian tumor in the pelvis to interfere with bladder emptying, although it may be associated with increased frequency.

A minority of ovarian tumors present symptomatically, usually with pain. This may be acute or chronic, continuous or intermittent. The precipitating cause most frequently is torsion of the cyst on its stalk or acute hemorrhage into its substance. Hemorrhage into the corpus luteum occurs about once in 300 pregnancies[28]. Like volvulus of the intestine, spontaneous torsion of the ovary is not uncommon early in the puerperium[2,4,18]. Acute pain is usually felt in the lower abdomen and may be continuous or intermittent. It may be severe, but it can be mild. Vomiting frequently accompanies severe acute episodes. Acute and chronic pain may both be felt in the loin radiating into the iliac fossa and into the thigh, exactly mimicking ureteric pain.

Rupture may occur with trauma at any time, raising the suspicion of malignancy, but is most common at delivery. Benign dermoids are the most common tumors to rupture; their contents are irritants and produce chemical peritonitis with pain and shock. Hemorrhage and torsion can also produce pain and shock. Ovarian tumors are high on the list of causes of an acute abdomen in pregnancy. Infection almost always occurs in the puerperium[10]. Although an occasional ovarian carcinoma presents by secondary spread, almost all ovarian tumors, benign or malignant, are discovered in the first 20 weeks of pregnancy by abdominal or vaginal examination or by ultrasound scan. If the mother books late, these examinations may be omitted, or occasionally a tumor develops after 20 weeks. At any stage in pregnancy from conception to the puerperium, ovarian tumors may produce significant symptoms.

DIFFERENTIAL DIAGNOSIS

The signs and symptoms produced by ovarian tumors in pregnancy may be mimicked by or closely resemble those produced by other pathologies. They must be differentiated not only from other causes of these signs and symptoms in pregnancy, but also from similar signs and symptoms which are accompanied by amenorrhea which is not due to pregnancy. Asymptomatic ovarian tumors may also be difficult to differentiate from other masses.

Early in pregnancy ectopic pregnancies are sometimes difficult to differentiate from bleeding into ovarian cysts or other problems due to ovarian cysts. A tubal pregnancy may present as an acute abdomen but this usually has been preceded by episodes of lower abdominal colic and backache. An ovarian ectopic pregnancy may, however, present as sudden collapse. In each case the period of amenorrhea may not be prolonged; indeed, menstruation may not have been missed. When the mother has collapsed, the differential diagnosis usually is unnecessary, since a laparotomy is obviously required and the diagnosis is made then. Intermittent lower abdominal pain due to tubal contractions to expel the pregnancy may be difficult to differentiate from intermittent torsion of an ovarian cyst. Clinical examination sometimes helps, particularly if the cyst is large. Cervical excitation tenderness frequently is present with an ectopic pregnancy but is uncommon with an ovarian tumor. If there has been 2–3 months of amenorrhea, the mass in the Fallopian tube may resemble an ovarian tumor, particularly in those cases in which there are few other symptoms. Frequently, however, it is necessary to proceed to an ultrasound examination or laparoscopy before the diagnosis can be clarified.

All amenorrhea in women of childbearing age is due to a pregnancy until proved otherwise, but it may also be caused by hormone-producing tumors, acute illness and psychiatric disturbance. A hormone-producing ovarian tumor with amenorrhea may have exactly the same signs and symptoms as those tumors which accompany pregnancy. The acute illness which is most likely to be confused with an ovarian tumor occurring in pregnancy is pelvic inflammatory disease. An acute episode of this (particularly if superimposed on chronic lesions in the pelvis) may produce amenorrhea, lower abdominal pain which may be constant or intermittent, abdominal signs which cannot be differentiated from an ovarian tumor, and signs on bimanual examination which also cannot be differentiated from an ovarian tumor, particularly if there is a large pyosalpinx or hydrosalpinx. Cervical excitation pain is common in pelvic inflammatory disease. Other acute illnesses usually are not difficult to differentiate from ovarian tumors unless there is another unrelated pelvic mass present. Psychogenic amenorrhea may be accompanied by abdominal pain and other symptoms which are related to the psychic upset. This frequently also is accompanied by cervical excitation pain. Since these women frequently are tense and over-anxious, there is tenderness and guarding of the abdomen. The diagnosis is not straightforward, particularly if there are incidental and irrelevant pelvic masses such as a loaded colon.

At any stage in pregnancy or early in the puerperium, the symptoms and signs produced by appendicitis, urinary tract problems, fibroids, orthopedic problems or abruptio placentae may resemble those of an ovarian tumor. It is, therefore, important to make an accurate diagnosis, because the treatment of each of these is different from that for an ovarian tumor.

Appendicitis is frequently difficult to diagnose at any stage in pregnancy. This is particularly true of late pregnancy when there may be no pyrexia or localizing sign, or when the misleading elevation occurs of the site of the appendix to high in the abdomen where it is pushed by the pregnant uterus. Early in pregnancy, intermittent abdominal pain and other gastrointestinal upset may be accompanied by pyrexia and make the diagnosis fairly straightforward. This is not always true, the signs being masked by pregnancy. A retrocecal appendix is always difficult to diagnose even in the non-pregnant subject; a rectal examination may give the only clue.

The urinary tract may produce symptoms from infection, from ureteric stones and from acute retention of urine. Bacteriuria is one of the most common problems to occur in pregnancy. In most populations it is present in 3–8% of all pregnant women. In half of these it is not accompanied by any symptoms, and in half of those with suggestive signs or symptoms, there is no infection. The diagnosis is not so easy as is frequently thought. It cannot be made from a midstream specimen of urine. Midstream specimens of urine in pregnancy and in the puerperium have a false-positive rate of 15–50%[29,30]. Even repeated midstream specimens do not reduce this rate much, because women who contaminate their specimens tend to contaminate recurrently. A catheter specimen of urine or a suprapubic aspiration specimen is essential for accurate diagnosis. Mixed growth may indicate true infection and bacterial counts of less than 10^5/ml may indicate infection if the specimen has been too short a time in the bladder, if the organisms are fastidious or if the mother is in diuresis. Counts greater than 10^5/ml may be due to contamination or to specimens spending too long in getting to the laboratory. The only sign which is of reasonable value is hematuria, but this may also be produced by ureteric stone. A ureteric stone can also produce symptoms very suggestive of a twisting ovarian cyst. Acute retention of urine may well produce acute or subacute lower abdominal discomfort with a cystic swelling rising out of the pelvis. It may be a consequence of a retroverted gravid uterus or of a fibroid impacted in the pelvis. All of these require precision in diagnosis. Many women with intermittent torsion of an ovarian cyst have had a number of courses of antibiotics for 'urinary' symptoms before the final and true diagnosis is made.

Compression of nerves emerging from the spinal canal, injury to the spine (old or new) or other injuries may produce symptoms very similar to those of an ovarian cyst. Rectus sheath hematoma may have a clear history of injury but not necessarily so. Round ligament pain may occasionally be so acute as to mimic an acute abdomen, but when intermittent may mimic an ovarian cyst. Shingles and other lesions of the nervous system may produce acute and severe pain.

Necrobiosis in a uterine fibroid frequently is difficult to differentiate from the pain and abdominal signs produced by an ovarian mass. Lesions in the upper abdomen, such as cholecystitis, or outside the abdomen, may produce symptoms and signs resembling those produced by an ovarian mass. They also may occur at any time in pregnancy or the early puerperium.

In the puerperium, torsion, infection, infarction, rupture or hemorrhage into an ovarian tumor may produce symptoms and signs similar to those produced by after-pains, intestinal complications, acute retention of urine or musculoskeletal problems following delivery. Since the abdomen is considerably less full than during pregnancy, cysts are more easily discovered and the diagnosis is simplified.

METHODS OF DIAGNOSIS

A complete and accurate history and a full clinical examination frequently strongly suggest the cause of symptoms. It is surprising, however, how large an ovarian cyst can be and yet escape clinical detection if it is soft and deformable, if it lies behind the uterus or if the mother is obese.

The nature of the patient's replies to questions and her attitude to her attendants and to examination may point to a psychosocial basis for her complaints. Cervical excitation pain can be due to anxiety and tension as well as to ectopic pregnancy or pelvic inflammatory disease, but tense women may have either of these, so usually this sign indicates the need for further investigation. Examination of the inguinal region may show a hernia, or rectal examination may reveal a pelvic appendix, a pelvic tumor or secondary deposits in the pouch of Douglas. Either of these examinations may be forgotten and the diagnosis missed or delayed. Rarely forgotten is the temperature, but pyrexia requires interpretation. It may be due to infection, but can also be caused by hematoma or deep venous thrombosis, and the temperature may not be raised even if severe pelvic or peritoneal infection is present.

Hematological investigations also may be misleading. The erythrocyte sedimentation rate is raised early in normal pregnancy and may be normal in pelvic inflammatory disease. The white cell count rises in normal pregnancy and may reach 20×10^9/l[31]. A single value is not very informative but sequential specimens may be valuable if they show a rising white cell count. There may be a leukocytosis in pelvic inflammatory disease but frequently there is not. While a single white cell count is potentially misleading, diagnostic information may be obtained from a sequence of specimens, particularly if differential counts are reported. Non-infective lesions such as

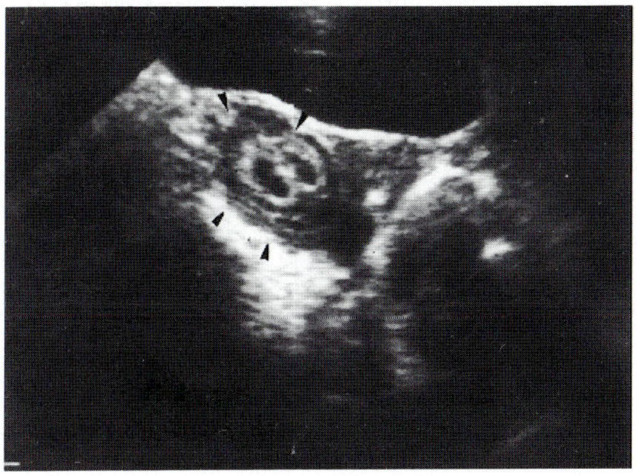

Figure 1 Transabdominal ultrasound scan, transverse section, showing uterus and right adnexal ectopic pregnancy (arrowed)

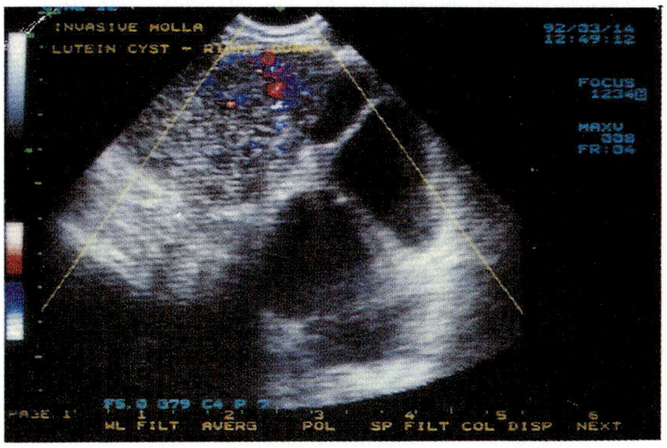

Figure 2 Transvaginal color flow Doppler scan showing molar pregnancy with increased flow within it, and three adjacent corpus luteal cysts (Courtesy of Professor A. Kurjak and Dr R. Matijevic)

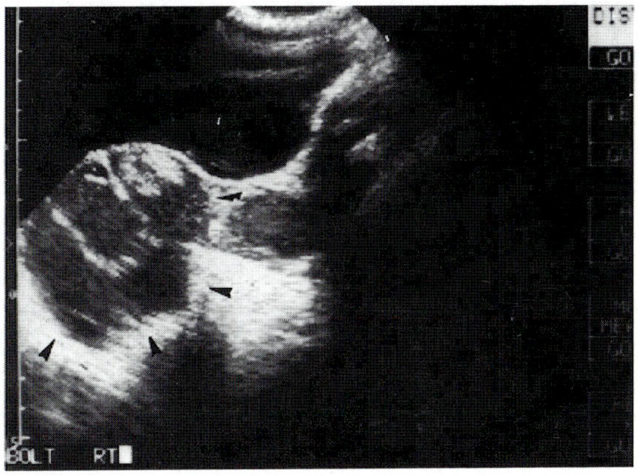

Figure 3 Transabdominal ultrasound scan, transverse section, showing multiloculated endometriotic cyst (arrowed). Note the cyst content is of higher echogenicity than the bladder

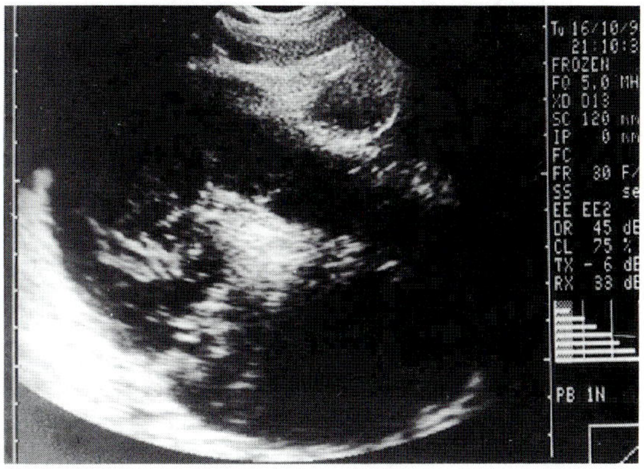

Figure 4 Transabdominal ultrasound scan of adnexal mass containing high-level echoes. This is a dermoid cyst of the ovary

torsion of a cyst are also sometimes accompanied by a leukocytosis.

Urinary pregnancy tests, too, may be very informative, but they also can have false-negative results. If the specimen is not the first passed in the morning, the human chorionic gonadotropin may be too diluted to produce a positive result. Bacteriuria and other abnormal constituents in the urine may interfere with the test and produce errors. For confidence in the result, the test should be carried out in a laboratory. To accept a result from the patient assumes that a dependable kit was used with the correct technique – not always a valid assumption.

Clinical history and examination with standard laboratory tests may suggest a diagnosis with enough confidence for definitive management to be started. If this is not the case, ultrasound examination is necessary to determine whether or not a tumor is present, or to clarify the nature of a tumor. A number of masses may resemble ovarian tumors[32]. A full bladder, the retroverted gravid uterus or a double uterus, uterine fibroids (particularly if they are pedunculated) or a hematocele in the pouch of Douglas may all be mistaken for an ovarian lesion.

If ultrasound confirms the presence of a pelvic lesion, or if it is not sufficiently informative, or if

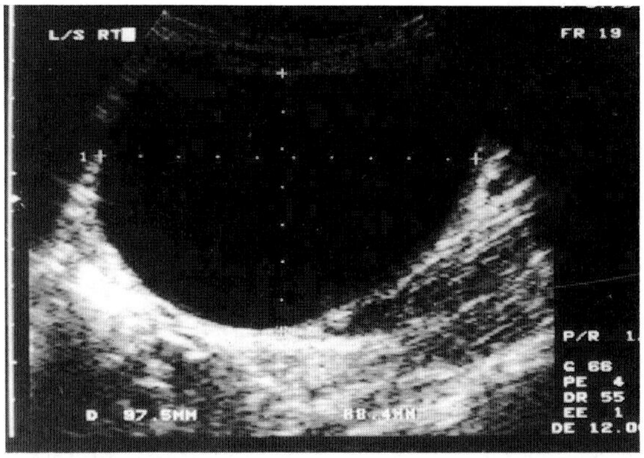

Figure 5 Transabdominal ultrasound scan, longitudinal section, of 10 cm × 9 cm thin-walled, unilocular, simple follicular cyst

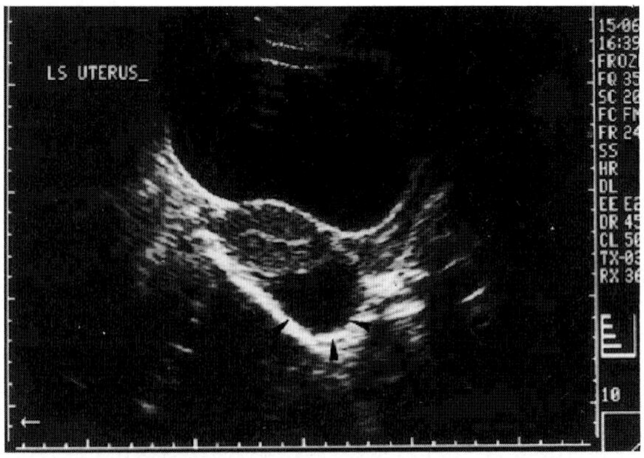

Figure 7 Transabdominal ultrasound scan, transverse section, of small simple follicular cyst behind the uterus (arrowed)

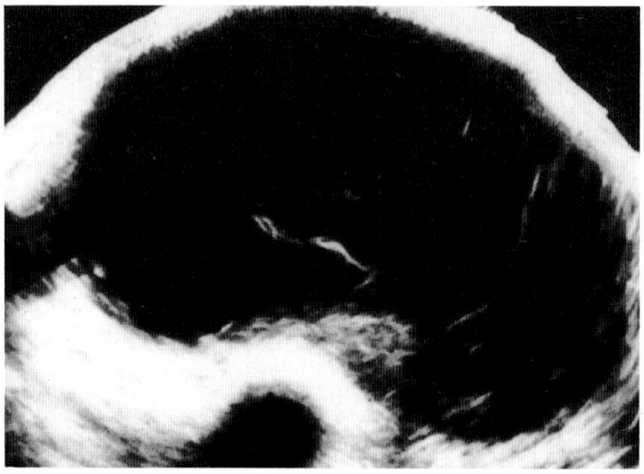

Figure 6 Transabdominal ultrasound scan, transverse section, of massive cyst containing multiple internal septa. This is a serous cystadenoma

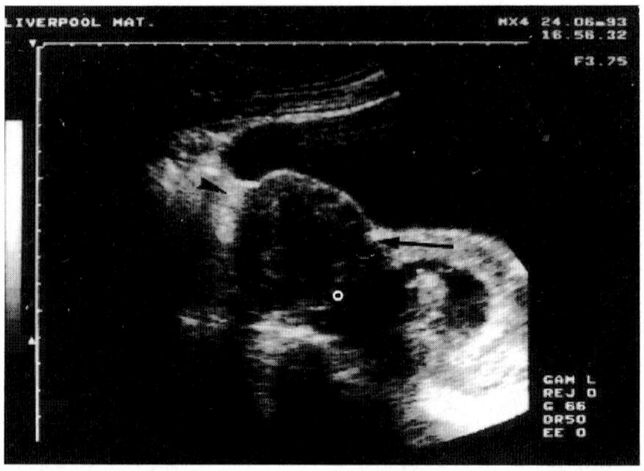

Figure 8 Transabdominal ultrasound scan, longitudinal section, of pregnant uterus containing 5 cm diameter fibroid (arrowed). Note diminished echoes from centre of lesion due to red degeneration in the fibroid. Early necrobiosis can, however, be present without alteration in the ultrasonic appearance of the fibroid

the clinical condition requires it, laparoscopy or laparotomy is the next step.

TREATMENT

Interventions are best left until the midtrimester, unless the condition is acute and requires immediate treatment. This not only reduces the risks for the fetus but also allows time for spontaneous resolution of benign cysts, or to observe any increase in size. If a cyst 10 cm in diameter does decrease in size, or if there is possible malignancy, laparotomy is necessary. Other tumors may be aspirated under ultrasound guidance[33,34]. Not only is this effective treatment safe but it allows cytological examination of the fluid. A single tap is usually sufficient, but repeat aspiration is unlikely to disturb the pregnancy. The technique is most appropriate for single unilocular cysts, 5–10 cm in diameter. Larger unilocular cysts may be aspirated, but not multilocular cysts (particularly if they contain solid areas), endometriomata, or teratomata, if blood or pus is suggested by the clinical condition or if a second pelvic mass is present.

If aspiration of a cyst is not appropriate or is not possible, laparotomy is required for all cysts of 10 cm or more in diameter, since they are unlikely to resolve spontaneously and can produce severe symptoms. In the past, 6 cm cysts were considered

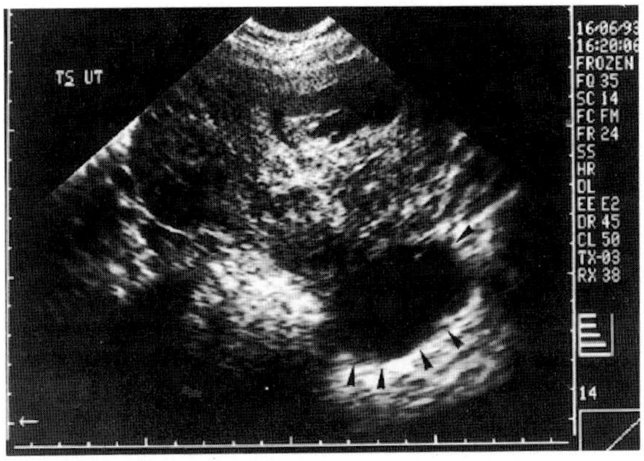

Figure 9 Transabdominal ultrasound scan, transverse section, showing a pregnant uterus containing a small fibroid. Note the corpus luteum cyst (arrowed) behind the uterus

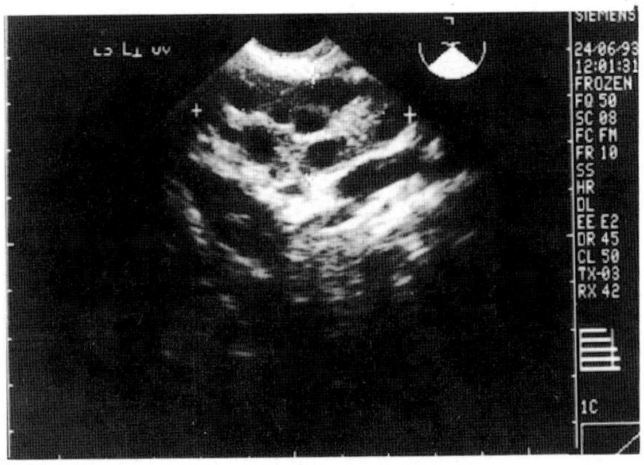

Figure 11 Transvaginal scan showing enlarged ovary with increased stroma and multiple cysts, in a case of polycystic ovary disease

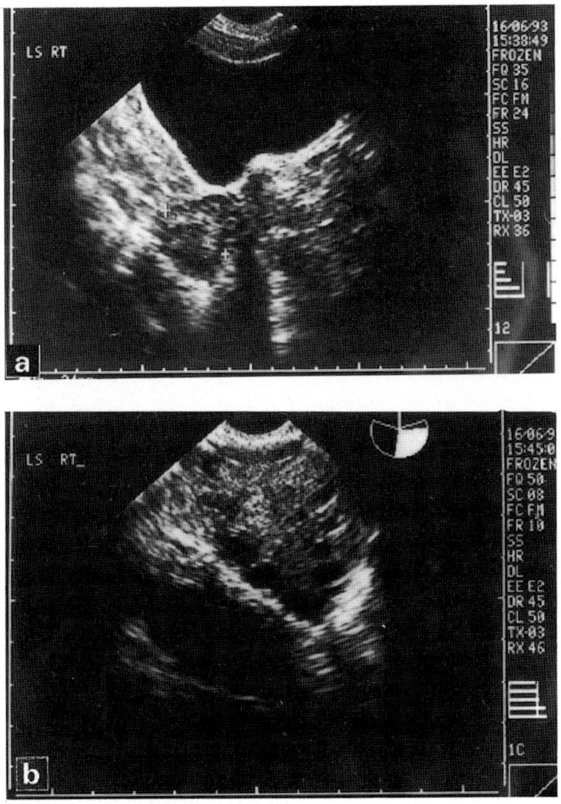

Figure 10 Enlarged right ovary with increased stroma and multiple cysts around the periphery, in a case of polycystic ovary disease. (a) Transabdominal scan, transverse section – increased stroma marked by + +; (b) transvaginal scan, with clearer demonstration of cysts

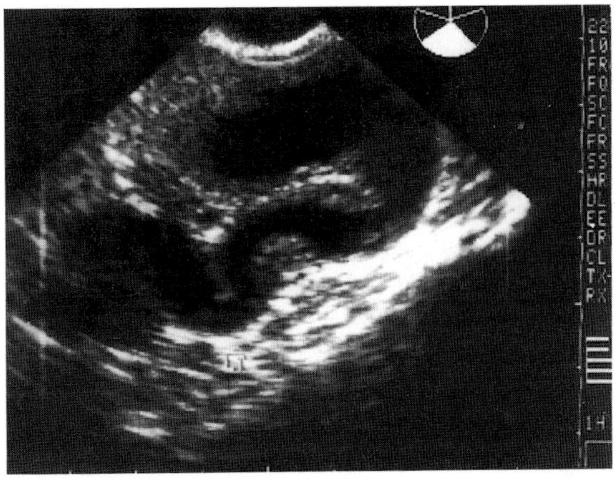

Figure 12 Transvaginal ultrasound scan showing uterus with serpiginous structure, a hydrosalpinx, arising from it

to require laparotomy. With ultrasound surveillance it is now reasonable to aspirate these unless they are symptomatic or there is a suspicion of malignancy. If surgery is necessary, the operation to be performed depends on the lesion present. Ovarian cystectomy with conservation of as much ovarian tissue as possible is the most common procedure. Where the cyst has undergone torsion (even three times) on the pedicle it is possible to unwind the torsion, excise ruptured or necrotic areas, ensure that the circulation returns, replace the cyst in the abdomen and expect the pregnancy to continue uneventfully[16].

Malignant cysts are likely to be suspected

before the laparotomy. This provides an opportunity to discuss treatment options with the parents. Chemotherapy may harm or kill the fetus but it might be considered as an adjuvant to surgery. Total surgical clearance of the pelvis makes cure more likely, but not guaranteed. Leaving the uterus preserves the fetus but prolonging the pregnancy delays the start of any additional therapy. The couple's decision frequently depends on the stage in pregnancy at which the diagnosis is made. The later the malignancy is discovered the more likely are they to wish to produce a viable fetus.

A tumor found late in pregnancy presents problems only in the timing of intervention. Symptomatic tumors can be dealt with by laparotomy provided they are accessible. If they are asymptomatic and an elective section is indicated for another reason, then they may be operated on at the time of Cesarean section. If they are present in the pelvis they may be an indication for Cesarean section. Spontaneous or forceps delivery past a large ovarian tumor is not advisable.

ULTRASOUND AND OVARIAN TUMORS IN PREGNANCY

Ultrasound has shown that ovarian tumors are more common than was discovered by clinical examination. It has confirmed that the majority are physiological and regress spontaneously, particularly those less than 5 cm in diameter, but even larger cysts may disappear. By allowing precision in diagnosis of malignancy and other problems, ultrasound has rationalized treatment so that the most appropriate methods can be used to minimize risks for both fetus and mother. Aspiration of cysts under ultrasound guidance has simplified and increased the safety of management during pregnancy. Screening by scanning has meant that few women go into labor with a large adnexal tumor in the pelvis. In the diagnosis of masses in pregnancy it may demonstrate double pathology: an ovarian cyst may coincide with a tubal pregnancy or abruptio placentae. By demonstrating the presence of an ovarian tumor it stimulates critical assessment of 'urinary' and other symptoms. In every way it has improved care of mother and fetus.

References

1. Lavery, J. P., Koontz, W. L., Layman, L., Shaw, L. and Gumpel, U. (1986). Sonographic evaluation of the adnexa during early pregnancy. *Surg. Gynecol. Obstet.*, **163**, 319–23
2. Tchabo, J.-G., Stay, E. J. and Limaye, N. S. (1987). Ovarian tumors in pregnancy. A community hospital's five year experience. *Int. Surg.*, **72**, 227–9
3. Tawa, K. (1964). Ovarian tumors in pregnancy. *Am. J. Obstet. Gynecol.*, **90**, 511–16
4. Peterson, W. F., Prevost, E. C., Edmunds, F. T., Hundley, J. M. and Morris, F. K. (1955). Benign cystic teratomas of the ovary. A clinico-statistical study of 1007 cases with a review of the literature. *Am. J. Obstet. Gynecol.*, **70**, 368–82
5. Koonings, P. P., Campbell, K., Mishell, D. R. and Grimes, D. A. (1989). Relative frequency of primary ovarian neoplasms: a 10-year review. *Obstet. Gynecol.*, **74**, 921–6
6. Ewertz, M. and Kjaer, S. K. (1988). Ovarian cancer incidence and mortality in Denmark, 1943–1982. *Int. J. Cancer*, **42**, 690–6
7. Thornton, J. G. and Wells, M. (1987). Ovarian cysts in pregnancy: does ultrasound make traditional management inappropriate? *Obstet. Gynecol.*, **69**, 717–21
8. Hogston, P. and Lilford, R. J. (1986). Ultrasound study of ovarian cysts in pregnancy: prevalence and significance. *Br. J. Obstet. Gynaecol.*, **93**, 625–8
9. Ballard, C. A. (1984). Ovarian tumors associated with pregnancy termination patients. *Am. J. Obstet. Gynecol.*, **149**, 384–7
10. Buttery, B. W., Beischer, N. A., Fortune, D. W. and Macafee, C. A. J. (1973). Ovarian tumours in pregnancy. *Med. J. Aust.*, **1**, 345–9
11. White, K. C. (1973). Ovarian tumors in pregnancy. *Am. J. Obstet. Gynecol.*, **116**, 544–8
12. Grimes, W. H., Bartholomew, R. A., Colvin, E. D., Fish, J. S. and Lester, W. M. (1954). Ovarian cyst complicating pregnancy. *Am. J. Obstet. Gynecol.*, **68**, 594–603
13. Montz, F. J., Schlaerth, J. B. and Morrow, C. P. (1988). The natural history of theca lutein cysts. *Obstet. Gynecol.*, **72**, 247–51

14. Homburg, R., Armar, N. A., Eshel, A., Adams, J. and Jacobs, H. S. (1988). Influence of luteinising hormone concentrations on ovulation, conception, and early pregnancy loss in polycystic ovary syndrome. *Br. Med. J.*, **297**, 1024–6
15. Adams, J., Polsen, D. W. and Franks, S. (1986). Prevalence of polycystic ovaries in women with anovulation and idiopathic hirsutism. *Br. Med. J.*, **293**, 355–9
16. Bider, D., Ben-Rafael, Z., Goldenberg, M., Shalev, J. and Mashiach, S. (1989). Pregnancy outcome after unwinding of twisted ischaemic–haemorrhagic adnexa. *Br. J. Obstet. Gynaecol.*, **96**, 428–30
17. Zalel, Y., Katz, Z., Caspi, B., Ben-Hur, H., Dgani, R. and Insler, V. (1992). Spontaneous ovarian hyperstimulation syndrome concomitant with spontaneous pregnancy in a woman with polycystic ovary disease. *Am. J. Obstet. Gynecol.*, **167**, 122–4
18. Hess, L. W., Peaceman, A., O'Brien, W. F., Winkel, C. A., Cruikshank, D. P. and Morrison, J. C. (1988). Adnexal mass occurring with intrauterine pregnancy: report of fifty-four patients requiring laparotomy for definitive management. *Am. J. Obstet. Gynecol.*, **158**, 1029–34
19. Meire, H. B., Farrant, P. and Guha, T. (1978). Distinction of benign from malignant ovarian cysts by ultrasound. *Br. J. Obstet. Gynaecol.*, **85**, 893–9
20. Kurjak, A., Zalud, I., Jurkovic, D., Alferivic, Z. and Miljan, M. (1989). Transvaginal colour Doppler for the assessment of the pelvic circulation. *Acta Obstet. Gynecol. Scand.*, **68**, 131–5
21. Bourne, T., Campbell, S., Steer, C., Whitehead, M. I. and Collins, W. P. (1989). Transvaginal colour flow imaging: a possible new screening technique for ovarian cancer. *Br. Med. J.*, **299**, 1367–70
22. Haymond, M. W. and Weldon, V. (1973). Female pseudohermaphroditism secondary to a maternal virilizing tumour. *J. Pediat.*, **82**, 682–6
23. Bell, R. J. M. (1977). Female virilisation due to maternal Krukenberg tumour. *Lancet*, **1**, 1162–3
24. Csapo, A. I., Pulkinen, M. O., Ruttner, B., Savage, J. P. and West, W. G. (1972). The significance of corpus luteum in pregnancy maintenance. 1 Preliminary studies. *Am. J. Obstet. Gynecol.*, **112**, 1061–7
25. McFadyen, I. R. (1985). Missed abortion, and later spontaneous abortion, in pregnancies clinically normal at 7–12 wk. *Eur. J. Obstet. Gynecol. Reprod. Biol.*, **20**, 381–4
26. Saunders, P. and Milton, P. J. D. (1973). Laparotomy during pregnancy: an assessment of diagnostic accuracy and fetal wastage. *Br. Med. J.*, **3**, 165–7
27. Mazze, R. I. and Kallen, B. (1989). Reproductive outcome after anesthesia and operation during pregnancy: a registry study of 5405 cases. *Am. J. Obstet. Gynecol.*, **161**, 1178–85
28. Hallet, J. G., Steele, C. H. and Snyder, M. (1984). Ruptured corpus luteum with hemoperitoneum: a study of 173 surgical cases. *Am. J. Obstet. Gynecol.*, **149**, 5–9
29. Norden, E. W. and Kass, E. H. (1968). Bacteriuria of pregnancy – a critical appraisal. *Annu. Rev. Med.*, **19**, 431–70
30. McFadyen, I. R., Eykyn, S. J., Gardner, N. H. N., Vanier, T. M., Bennet, A. E., Mayo, M. E. and Lloyd-Davies, R. W. (1973). Bacteriuria in pregnancy. *J. Obstet. Gynaecol. Br. Cwlth.*, **80**, 385–405
31. Cruikshank, J. M. (1970). The effects of parity on the leucocyte count in pregnant and non-pregnant women. *Br. J. Haematol.*, **18**, 531–7
32. Donald, I. (1979). *Practical Obstetric Problems*, 7th edn., p. 279. (London: Lloyd–Luke)
33. Rodin, A., Coltart, T. M. and Chapman, M. G. (1989). Needle aspiration of simple cysts in pregnancy. *Br. J. Obstet. Gynaecol.*, **96**, 994–6
34. De Crespigny, L. C., Robinson, H. P., Davoren, R. A. M. and Fortune, D. W. (1985). Ultrasound-guided puncture for gynecological and pelvic lesions. *Aust. N.Z. J. Obstet. Gynaecol.*, **25**, 227–9

Endometriosis and the ovary

11

I. Brosens and P. Puttemans

The ovaries and the posterior leaf of the broad ligaments are the most frequent locations for endometriosis and adhesions, and for some reason the left side is more frequently affected than the right side[1]. The actual prevalence of endometriosis in the general population is estimated to be 10% which indicates that ovarian endometriosis is a frequent phenomenon. In this chapter the pathogenesis, pathophysiology, diagnosis and therapeutic aspects of ovarian endometriosis will be discussed.

PATHOGENESIS

The first published report of an endometrial cyst of the ovary, by W. W. Russel in 1899[2], gave a detailed description of the ovary 'enveloped in adhesions to the posterior face of the broad ligament' and 'the presence of areas which were an exact prototype of the uterine glands and interglandular connective tissue'. Despite the remarkably accurate description, it took more than two decades before the relationship between the hemorrhagic cyst and the endometrium-like tissue was established[3]. Cullen[3] postulated that the uterine mucosa on the surface of the ovarian cyst was due to an extension of uterine adenomyoma. Sampson[4] observed in the ovary that during menstruation the ectopic mucosa showed the same features of desquamation and bleeding as the uterine mucosa. Following Sampson's theory on the histogenesis of endometriosis, several authors held the view that heterotopic endometrial tissue eats its way into the ovary or invades the follicle or corpus luteum following ovulation. In both theories the endometrial cyst develops like other neoplastic cysts in the medulla of the ovary. Sampson[4] noted that 'structures, like uterine glands are usually most numerous near the site of perforation'. This characteristic association with the presence of adhesions was, however, not explained by the previous theories. The scarified area was regarded as the site of perforation (Figure 1). In 1957 the role of adhesions and scarification in the formation of the endometrial cyst of the ovary was clarified by Hughesdon[5]. His work based on step serial sections of the ovaries containing an endometrioma showed that 'even in the most advanced lesions the ectopic endometrium never in fact leaves the surface: it remains on, and is never in, the ovary' (Figure 2). In fact, in more than 90% of cases, the ovarian cortex is identifiable and forms a pseudocystic wall. The ovarian cortex is invaginated and the so-called site of perforation is the place of invagination and the site of original endometrial implantation with adhesion formation.

PATHOPHYSIOLOGY

The term 'chocolate cyst' is frequently used to describe the endometrial cyst of the ovary but it is misleading, as a similar content can be found in hemorrhagic functional cysts and even in some neoplastic tumors.

The gross features of the ovarian endometrioma are well known to the gynecological surgeon and it has been suggested that they suffice for diagnosis. Although this may be true in many cases, there are several reasons not to rely only on the outside characteristics.

The gross features include the location of the cyst on the frontal side of the ovary in opposition to the posterior leaf of the broad ligament, the presence of adhesions between the ovary and the broad ligament, the fibrotic retracted scar and the pigmented or hemorrhagic lesions suggestive of superficial endometriosis on the cortex and peritoneum. The enlargement of the ovary tends not to produce a general expansion (as is the case in most intraovarian cysts) but is eccentrially located on the medial side. Frequently lysis of the adhesions between the ovary and the parametrium results in

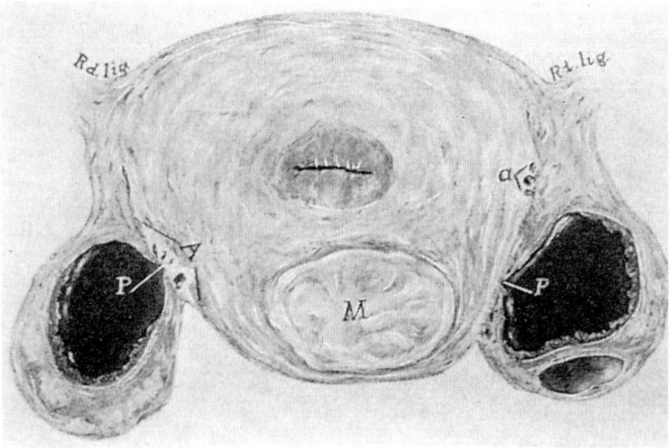

Figure 1 Sampson's drawing of the uterus and ovaries showing the ovaries adherent to the posterior surface of the uterus[4]. The site of perforation (P) (according to the author) represents in fact the invagination of the cortex

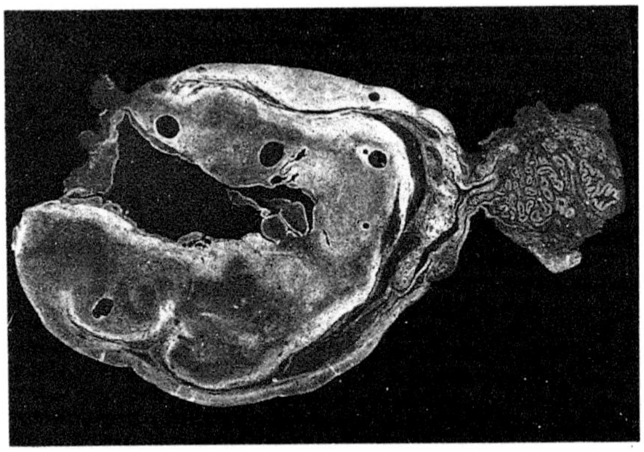

Figure 2 Hughesdon's drawing of a section through the ovary with an endometrioma which demonstrates that the wall of the endometrioma is invaginated ovarian cortex and that the cystic structure is sealed by adhesions at the site of invagination[5]

spilling of the contents and opening of the cyst at the site of the scar.

In the microscopic diagnosis of ovarian endometrioma a wide variation of pictures may occur. The criterion of diagnosis is the presence of endometrial tissue, preferably both glands and stroma. Cases are seen in which the endometrium is so typical, both histologically and functionally, that it cannot be distinguished from eutopic endometrium. On the other hand, no specific pathological diagnosis can be definitively made in about one third of typical endometrial cysts and only the diagnosis of 'compatible with endometriosis' is made[6].

Careful histological studies using step serial sections have demonstrated that in the vast majority of ovarian endometriomas the wall is formed by the inverted ovarian cortex[5]. The frontal surface in proximity to the hilus of the ovary is the most frequent site where the invagination occurs. Using the technique of ovarian cystoscopy[7], the site of retraction and invagination can be identified. The ovarian cortex can in the early stages still be recognized by its pearl-white appearance. Endometrial implants are seen as red, vascularized or hemorrhagic islands at the site of retraction and are scattered over the ovarian cortex. On histological examination the implant frequently has a mucosa-like appearance. Nieminen[8] was the first to observe the difference in hormonal response between free superficial and enclosed implants. The free mucosa-type lesion can undergo secretory changes during the luteal phase of the cycle and vascular necrosis and shedding at the time of menstruation. In many respects the ovarian endometrioma can be compared with a hematometra, an entrapment of blood secondary to obstruction by adhesions.

The pathogenesis of ovarian endometriomas is apparently induced by a sequence of events – the presence of superficial endometriotic implants high in the ovarian fossa (one of the predilection sites), the activity of which causes the ovary to adhere to the side wall of the pelvis, posterior leaf of the broad ligament or sacrouterine ligament. Once tightly fixed, the entrapment of blood induces a progressive invagination of the ovarian cortex following the path of least resistance (Figure 3). The further distension of the endometrioma, sometimes reaching impressive dimensions, can be attributed not only to the shedding of the mucosa-like outgrowths on the surface of the inverted cortex, but also to the chronic irritation of hemorrhoid-like venules seen at cystoscopy around the retracted hilus of the ovary and the secondary involvement of hemorrhagic functional cysts such as hemorrhagic corpora lutea developing on the inverted cortex. This explains the characteristics of most endometriomas, such as the site of implant and adhesions, the retracted scar on the ovarian cortex, the spilling of the contents at dissection and the frequent combination, particularly in large cysts, with hemorrhagic func-

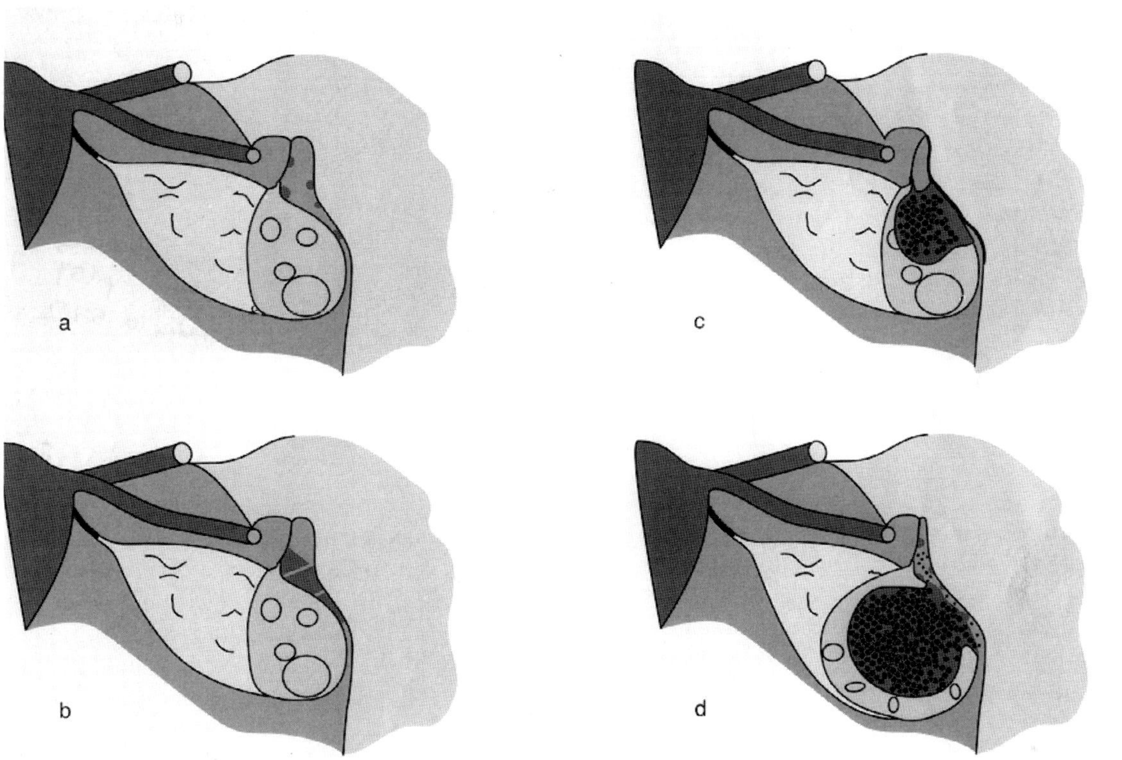

Figure 3 Formation of the endometrial cyst: (a) superficial hemorrhagic lesion in the fossa ovarica; (b) adhesion formation between ovary and peritoneum enclosing the implant; (c) inversion of the ovarian cortex and pseudocyst formation; (d) distension of the pseudocyst

tional cysts[9]. Progressive distension of the cyst and fibrosis of the wall obscure the original structure and result in a dark, fibrotic, pigmented and poorly vascularized surface.

The terminology of deep endometriosis for the ovarian endometrioma is misleading for two reasons. First, the pathogenesis of the endometriomas is in most cases related to superficial and superficially spreading endometriosis and subsequent adhesion formation and second, the mucosal type of implant responds to ovarian steroids much as does eutopic superficial endometrium.

DIAGNOSIS

It needs no argument to understand that the clinical and biochemical assessment of any ovarian mass is of limited diagnostic value due to a low specificity and sensitivity. Vaginal ultrasound has a high sensitivity to detect and measure an ovarian cyst, but its specificity remains low. Ultrasound may be useful, however, to monitor the size of a known cyst in response to therapy or to evaluate its recurrence. Due to the non-specificity, there will continue to be difficulty differentiating, for example, between an endometrioma and a hemorrhagic lutein cyst[10]. Direct visual inspection through a laparoscope of the cyst itself and the pelvic environment will in most cases provide more clues as to the type of ovarian cyst that is present. The indirect signs are especially suggestive of an ovarian endometrioma. These include the localization, the adhesions, the retraction of the ovarian capsule, the presence of ovarian and/or peritoneal endometriotic implants and the chocolate content that is usually freed at the time of ovarian manipulation. These indirect signs, however, are frequently absent when adhesions following previous surgery are present or do not exclude the combination with lutein cysts[11]. Laparoscopic inspection can also fail to diagnose the endometrioma, particularly if the full surfaces of the ovary and especially the frontal and lateral surfaces are not inspected. Puncture and aspiration have been recommended to improve the detection and staging of an ovarian endometrioma[12]. However, the chocolate content can be misleading as it is found in other conditions such as the hemorrhagic lutein cyst and even in some neoplastic cysts[13]. Recommendations to biopsy endometriomas are made mainly to exclude malignancy or detect epithelial atypia in ovarian tumors; however, histopathological examination fails to reveal endometriosis in up to one third of typical ovarian endometriomas. This has led some authors to suggest that ovarian biopsies would seem dispensable for a correct laparoscopic diagnosis of the disease[14]. The clinical problem is, however, the selection of the appropriate site for biopsy. At random biopsies, especially in cases of a large endometrioma, inadequate material is frequently provided for histopathological diagnosis.

The concept of the non-invasive imaging approach to diagnosis is further explored by magnetic resonance imaging (MRI)[15,16]. In the investigation of women with adnexal masses the sensitivity, specificity and predictive accuracy of MRI for the identification of endometriosis were 90%, 98% and 96%, respectively. The appearance of endometriosis in MRI is not pathognomonic but the diffuse pelvic lesions are more readily reflected by MRI than by ultrasonography. The use of MRI may be particularly indicated when the ovarian cyst is obscured by adhesions such as in the postoperative recurrent cyst or in the follow-up once the diagnosis has been made.

Ovarian cystoscopy

To obtain more visual and histological information on this subject, the technique of ovarian cystoscopy, based on the same principle of double optic laparoscopy as the rigid salpingoscopy, was developed[7]. Using minimal invasive surgery (a 3–4 mm opening in the ovarian capsule), the goal was to examine the cyst *in situ* before surgery and to detect and biopsy the endometrial implants under direct vision. The basic principle of endoscopy is to achieve proper distension with an appropriate medium for full visual inspection. The cyst is inspected and the site of entry to the cyst is selected. The hemorrhagic cyst is then punctured and flushed abundantly with sterile saline at body temperature until the fluid becomes clear. Flushing of the cyst is performed with a pressurized suction-irrigator through a 5 mm suprapubic trocar. A sample of the cyst fluid is kept for cytological evaluation. The second endoscope is a 2.8 mm and 6° telescope located in a 13.5 operating sheath with a 5 Fr groove that allows passage of an infusion and small instruments such as a biopsy forceps or a laser fiber (manufactured by Karl Storz GmbH & Co, Tuttlingen, Germany) to be introduced through the operating channel of the laparoscope. Alternatively, the second endoscope is a 4 mm 30° rigid Hamou II hysteroscope (manufactured by Karl Storz GmbH & Co, Tuttlingen, Germany) and is introduced through one of the suprapubic trocars. The larger size of this optic gives an excellent view. After introduction into the cyst through the small puncture hole, a saline infusion is allowed to run freely to distend the cyst so the wall can be inspected in detail (Figure 4). Small biopsies are taken under direct vision for histopathological study.

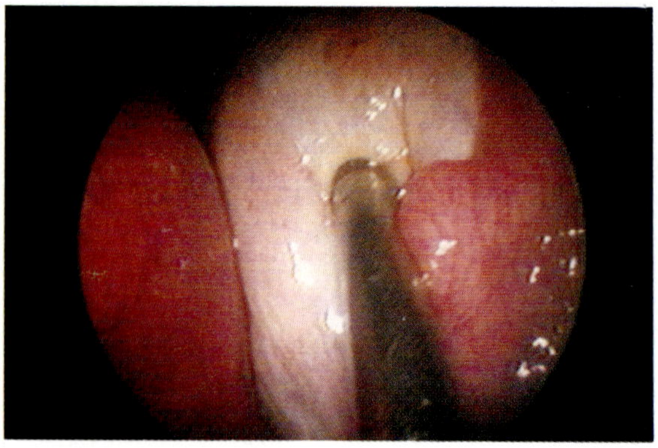

Figure 4 The second optic is introduced in the cyst through a 5 mm puncture hole after aspiration of the contents and abundant flushing

Functional cysts are characterized by a smooth and undulating surface overlying a fine, retinal network of blood vessels (follicular cyst) (Figure 5) or by the presence of areas with a uniform luteinization (lutein cyst) (Figure 6).

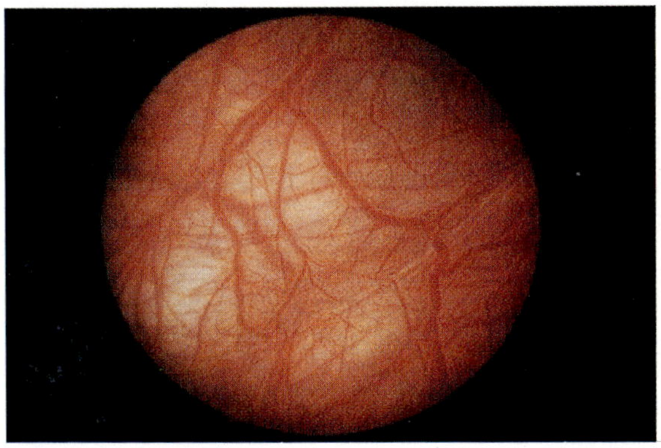

Figure 5 Ovarian cystoscopy showing the smooth surface and retinal network of the vascularization in a follicular cyst

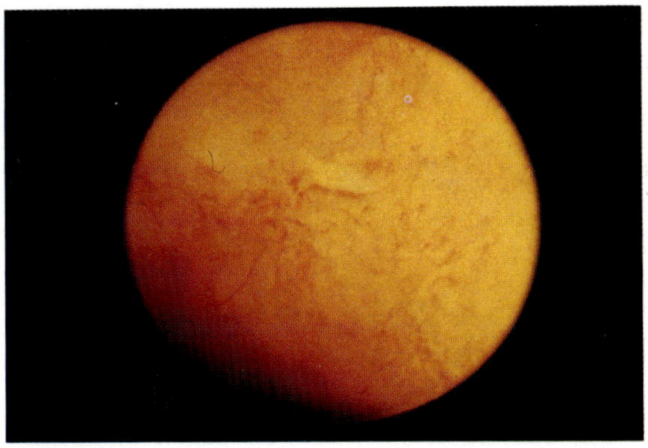

Figure 6 Ovarian cystoscopy showing uniform luteinization in a hemorrhagic lutein cyst

The wall of the true ovarian endometrioma presents different appearances. Vascularization is most prominent at the site of invagination or in proximity to the ovarian hilus, where vessels protrude on the surface as small hemorrhoids. Retraction of the wall is also frequently found in this area (Figure 7). The wall has no uniform lining but presents a pearl-white, dark brown or black surface with an irregular network of vascularization and areas with easily detachable mucosa-like tissue (Figure 8). With the technique of double optic ovarioscopy the wall of the ovary can be inspected in detail and biopsies can be obtained from the representative areas (Figure 9). On biopsy the pearl-white surface is usually confirmed as ovarian capsule/cortex, the dark brown or black non-vascularized areas as pigmented fibroreactive tissue and the vascularized hemorrhagic areas as luteinization or endometrial tissue. The mucosa-like tissue, easily detachable from the white inner surface, can present the full characteristics of superficial endometrium[17] (Figure 6).

The free superficial implants, in contrast to enclosed implants, have been shown to respond during the menstrual cycle in a similar way to eutopic superficial endometrium, including menstrual bleeding[8]. It is likely that these free implants are the cause of bleeding and endometrioma formation. There is no evidence that active and progessive implants of endometriomas are invading the ovarian tissue itself. On the contrary, the endometrial implants seem to extend like explants

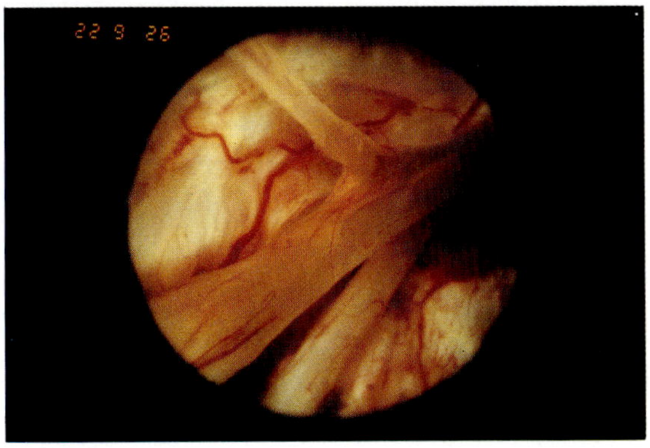

Figure 7 Ovarian cystoscopy of a large endometrioma demonstrating the site of inversion and a hemorrhagic active endometrial implant. The implant and inversion are located in proximity to the hilus of the ovary

over the surface and are easily detachable. In the evolution of endometriomas two stages can be distinguished. In the non-fibrotic (red) stage, the ovarian cortex is still identifiable by its pearl-white appearance and shows extensive vascularization and patches of well vascularized implants. In the fibrotic (brown–black) stage the wall is thickened by dark pigmented fibrotic tissue. Hemorrhagic and vascularized areas are prominent in some areas, particularly at the hilus of the ovary (Figure 7).

THERAPEUTIC ASPECTS

Even with the recent and ongoing achievements in operative endoscopy, the surgical management of the ovarian endometrioma remains a contro-

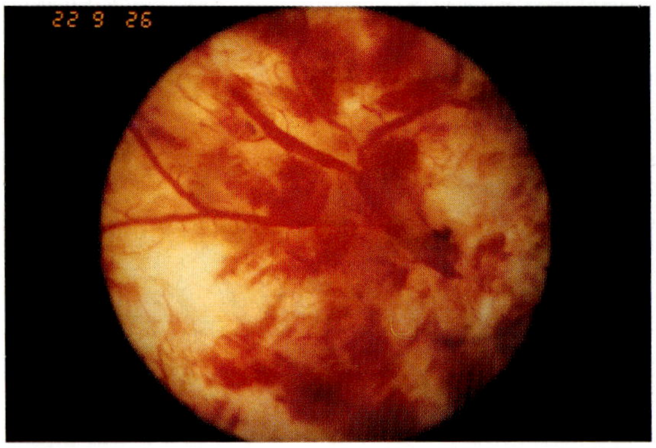

Figure 8 Ovarian cystoscopy of a large endometrioma. The inverted ovarian cortex is covered by an irregular but extensive network of vascularization and islands of mucosa-type endometrial implants

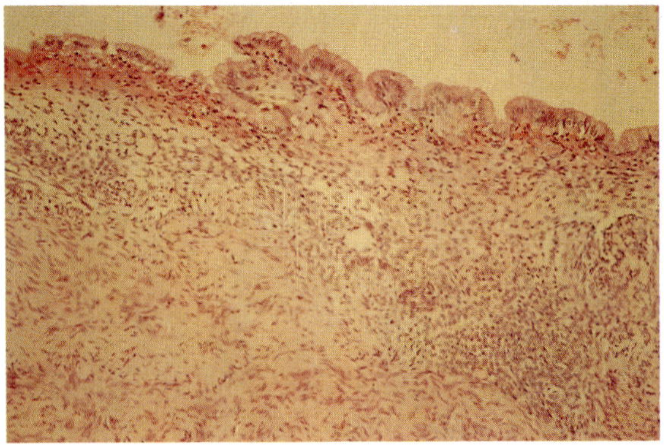

Figure 9 Histological picture of a mucosa-type endometrial implant proliferating on the (inverted) ovarian cortex

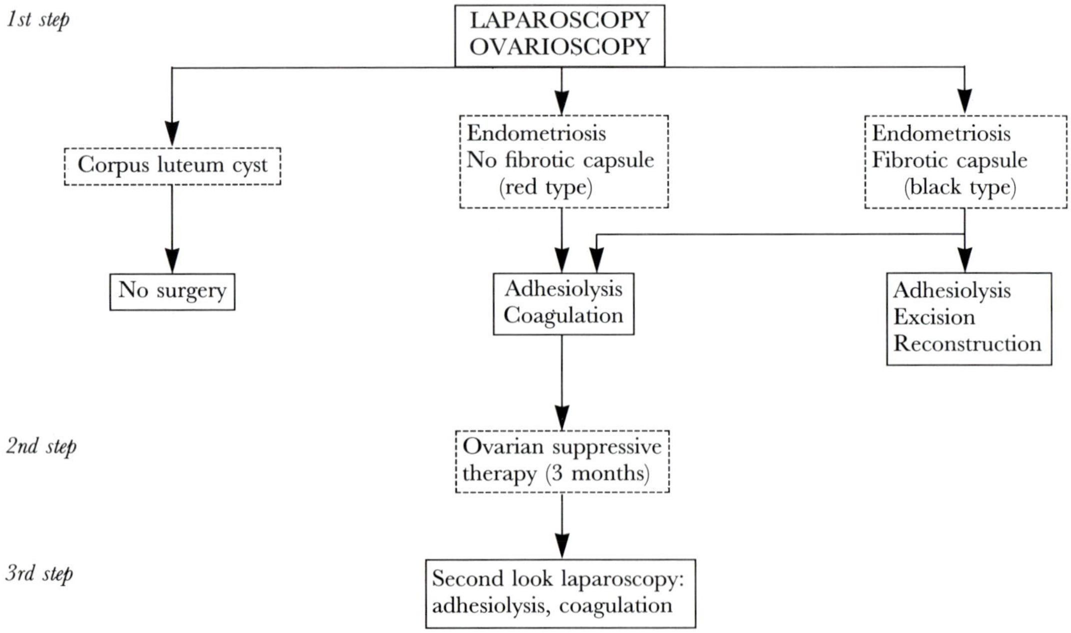

Figure 10 Three-step technique for laparoscopic treatment of large ovarian endometrial cyst

versial issue – in the first place because clinicians are still faced with a problem of correct diagnosis, both in the sense of missing this pathology and of treating a lutein cyst for an endometrioma; in the second place because it is now a well-established fact that surgical damage to the ovarian capsule for whatever purpose is likely to increase the risk of postoperative periovarian adhesive disease and to induce a vicious circle of recurrent dysfunctional cyst formation and repeated surgery.

The pathogenetic mechanism has important therapeutic implications. The well known resistance of endometriomas to any type of medical therapy is likely not to be due to the non-responsiveness of the endometrial implant but to the occlusion of the inverted cortex by adhesions with entrapped old blood similar to a hematometra. The surgical approach should be concentrated on ovariolysis and the identification and destruction of the superficial endometriotic implants, which frequently are located high in the ovarian fossa. In the non-fibrotic red endometrioma, excision or removal of the normal, yet inverted ovarian cortex will initiate the vicious circle of: (1) the postoperative *de novo* formation of dense adhesions as seen after wedge resections; (2) the recurrence of functional cysts; and (3) eventually, repeated surgery. In cases of large endometriomas the combination of the initial ovariolysis, followed by 3-month therapy with gonadotropin-releasing hormone reduces the cystic structures significantly and concentrates the endometriotic implants, which can be more easily destroyed during a second-look procedure[18]. In the older fibrotic endometrioma, it becomes more difficult to ensure complete destruction of all endometriotic areas, buried as they are in thick layers of pigmented fibrotic scar tissue. A complete resection of the cyst pseudowall itself is recommended (Figure 10).

In conclusion, the technique of double optic ovarioscopy is proposed as a useful tool to explore hemorrhagic cysts of the ovary suspected to be endometriosis. Dysfunctional ovarian cysts can be identified, the site of biopsy for histological examination can be selected and the activity and stage of fibrosis of the endometrioma can be assessed. Moreover, the diagnostic tool can guide the endoscopist towards the most appropriate (equivalent to the most conservative) approach of minimal invasive surgery.

References

1. Jenkins, S., Olive, D. L. and Haney, A. F. (1986). Endometriosis: pathogenic implications of the anatomic distribution. *Obstet. Gynecol.*, **67**, 335–8
2. Russel, W. W. (1899). Aberrant portions of the Müllerian duct found in an ovary. *Johns Hopkins Hosp. Bull.*, **10**, 8–10
3. Cullen, T. S. (1920). The distribution of adenomyoma containing uterine mucosa. *Arch. Surg.*, **1**, 215–83
4. Sampson, J. A. (1921). Perforating hemorrhagic (chocolate) cysts of the ovary. *Arch. Surg.*, **3**, 245–323
5. Hughesdon, P. E. (1957). The structure of endometrial cysts of the ovary. *J. Obstet. Gynaecol. Br. Cwlth.*, **44**, 481–7
6. Novak, E. and Woodruff, J. (1974). *Novak's Gynecologic and Obstetric Pathology*, p. 456. (Philadelphia: W. B. Saunders Co)
7. Brosens, I. A. and Puttemans, P. J. (1989). Double-optic laparoscopy. Salpingoscopy, ovarian cystoscopy and endo-ovarian surgery with the argon laser. *Baillière's Clin. Obstet. Gynaecol.*, **3**, 595–608
8. Nieminen, U. (1962). Studies on the vascular pattern of ectopic endometrium with special reference to cyclic changes. *Acta Obstet. Gynecol. Scand.*, **41** (Suppl. 3), 1–81
9. Nezhat, F., Nezhat, C., Allan, C. J., Metzger, D. A. and Sears, D. L. (1992). Clinical and histologic classification of endometriomas: implications for a mechanism of pathogenesis. *J. Reprod. Med.*, **37**, 771–6
10. Athey, P. A. and Diment, D. D. (1989). The spectrum of sonographic findings in endometriomas. *J. Ultrasound Med.*, **8**, 487–91
11. Brosens, I. A., Boeckx, W. and Page, G. (1988). Microsurgery of ovarian endometriosis. *Hum. Reprod.*, **3**, 365–6
12. Candiani, G. B., Vercellini, P. and Fedele, L. (1990). Laparoscopic ovarian puncture for correct staging of endometriosis. *Fertil. Steril.*, **53**, 994–7
13. Martin, D. C. and Berry, J. D. (1990). Histology of chocolate cysts. *J. Gynecol. Surg.*, **6**, 43–6
14. Vercellini, P., Vendola, N., Bocciolone, L., Rognoni, M. T., Carinelli, S. G. and Candiani, G. B. (1991). Reliability of the visual diagnosis of ovarian endometriosis. *Fertil. Steril.*, **56**, 1198–200
15. Arrive, L., Hricak, H. and Martin, M. C. (1989). Pelvic endometriosis: MR imaging. *Radiology*, **171**, 687–92
16. Togashi, K., Nishimura, K., Kimura, I., Tsuda, Y., Yamashita, K., Shibata, T., Nakano, Y., Konishi, J., Konishi, I. and Mori, T. (1991).

Endometrial cysts: diagnosis with MR imaging. *Radiology*, **180**, 73–8

17. Brosens, I. A. (1993). Classification of endometriosis revisited. *Lancet*, **341**, 630
18. Donnez, J., Nisolle, M., Clerckx, F., Gillerot, S., Bourgorjon, D., Wayemberg, M. and Casanas-Roux, F. (1990). The ovarian endometrial cyst: the combined (hormonal and surgical) therapy. In Brosens, I., Jacobs, H. S. and Runnebaum, B. (eds.) *LHRH-Analogues in Gynaecology*, pp. 165–75. (Carnforth, UK: Parthenon Publishing)

Clinical and ultrasound dimensions of infections of the ovary and Fallopian tube

12

M. Toth and F. A. Chervenak

Infections of the ovary and Fallopian tube are of great importance to women's health in that they are a leading cause of infertility, pelvic pain, and ectopic pregnancy. This chapter will review the pathogenesis, epidemiology, prevention, symptoms, and the clinical and ultrasound appearance of acute and chronic pelvic inflammatory disease (PID). The role of color Doppler ultrasound will be emphasized. Hysterosalpingosonography as an important diagnostic tool will be discussed.

Infection of the ovaries usually occurs as a part of an ascending upper genital tract infection process, which also involves the cervix, the uterus, and the Fallopian tubes. Infection of the upper genital tract is generally called PID. PID is the most common sexually transmitted disease of women, and it can cause permanent damage to the upper reproductive tract. This can lead to infertility, ectopic pregnancy and chronic pelvic pain[1,2]. It is estimated that in the United States 10–15% of women of reproductive age have had at least one episode of PID and, each year, about 1 000 000 new cases occur. Annually, nearly 300 000 women are hospitalized for this disease and over 2.5 million outpatient visits to doctors result from PID.

About 30% of infertility and 50% of ectopic pregnancies are caused by PID. In 1988, 200 000 women were hospitalized with this diagnosis; of these, 29 000 required hysterectomy. Nearly 40 000 ectopic pregnancies each year are attributed to pelvic infections. Only about two-thirds of all women can again become pregnant after an ectopic pregnancy[1–4].

There is new evidence suggesting that pregnancies following PID have a higher incidence of adverse outcome. This is most likely due to an increased number of spontaneous abortions in patients with a history of pelvic infection[3]. Moreover, there is a decreased success rate after embryo transfer in women undergoing *in vitro* fertilization after PID[5]. There are two possible explanations for these phenomena: bacteria could create a host response that results in an immunologically hostile environment for the embryo in the uterine cavity, or deep-seated intracellular bacteria (e.g. *Chlamydia trachomatis*) or resistant bacterial particles may survive antibiotic treatment and stimulate an immune response that may be directed against the developing fetus.

The first hypothesis is supported by the finding of elevated anti-*Chlamydia* IgA antibody levels in the cervical secretion of women undergoing *in vitro* fertilization after suffering permanent tubal damage[5]. The finding of *Chlamydia* DNA particles on *in situ* hybridization in the tubal tissue of culture-negative women with infectious tubal damage supports the second hypothesis[6].

PID results in more morbidity than necessary for the following reasons. In most cases the disease is identified too late, women are not hospitalized as often as they should be, they frequently receive inadequate or inappropriate antibiotic treatment, and, in addition, the male sex partner (the most likely source of the infection) is often not identified and treated. PID is thought of by many specialists as 'the most neglected disease in the United States today'[1,4].

PATHOGENESIS

A wide variety of bacteria have been isolated from the cervices, uteri, and tubes of women with PID. This polymicrobial infection usually ascends. The most common anaerobic bacteria in PID are *Bacteroides* species and peptostreptococci. Some bacteria (e.g. mycoplasmas and mycobacteria) reach the pelvis via the bloodstream or by direct extension from another abdominal organ (e.g. during diverticulitis or appendicitis).

Chlamydia trachomatis and *Neisseria gonorrhoea* are the most frequently identified sexually transmitted pathogens. Two-thirds of women infected by *Neisseria* will also be positive for *Chlamydia*[7]. These two organisms inflict damage to the tubes by different mechanisms. *In vitro* experiments have shown that *Neisseria* elicits a more rapid and a more serious tubal scarring than does *Chlamydia*[8]. This is due to the direct effect of the bacterium and its toxins on the ciliated epithelial cells. The reverse is true *in vivo*. *Neisseria* produces very characteristic symptoms with rapid onset of discomfort, for which the patient should seek immediate medical attention. Women with chlamydial infections are the most likely candidates for extensive and irreversible tubal damage that develops over a long period of time and progresses slowly. The symptoms are subtle or may be entirely absent. Present in 60–70% of these cases, *Chlamydia* has evolved as the most serious and most common pathogen of PID. A complicated immunological process is thought to be responsible for the scar tissue formation in women infected by this bacterium[9]. *Chlamydia* has learned to adapt, to its advantage, to the shortcomings of the human immune system. It synthesizes a 57 kDa protein that is a member of the family of the 60 kDa heat shock proteins. These substances are present in many bacteria and also in several eukaryotic organisms, including man. Chlamydial heat shock proteins are capable of sensitizing human T lymphocytes. Because the human and chlamydial heat shock proteins are about 50% homologous, lymphocytes that were sensitized by *Chlamydia* can also respond to human heat shock proteins which are released by the host cells under environmental stress. The end result is a delayed autoimmune hypersensitivity reaction that continues to cause progressive damage even after the elimination of *Chlamydia*[10]. In laboratory experiments, Morrison and colleagues[10] recently demonstrated the continued production of heat shock protein by *Chlamydia* after the bacterium was exposed to high concentrations of antibiotics and interferon. This treatment stopped the synthesis of all other proteins by the bacterium. The experiment suggests that non-replicating bacterial particles that remain in the tissue after antibiotic treatment are still capable of maintaining their antigen status[10]. These DNA particles may be able to stimulate the immune system through continued synthesis of heat shock proteins. Campbell and Patton[6] successfully identified chlamydial DNA particles and antigens in the tissues of women with chronic salpingitis by using immunoperoxidase and *in situ* hybridization techniques. Only early recognition and very aggressive treatment will prevent this bacterium from activating the host immune system and triggering an autoimmune process that is no longer responsive to antibiotic treatment.

EPIDEMIOLOGY AND PREVENTION

PID is the most serious complication of sexually transmitted disease. It occurs very seldom in sexually inactive or pregnant women. Sexually active adolescents with multiple partners are at the greatest risk[1]. Large epidemiological studies have shown that the disease is the most common in behavioral settings where the male sex partner is promiscuous and the female is monogamous[11]. This indicates that PID and sexually transmitted diseases in general have a male-to-female vector, i.e. that more men are infecting women than vice versa.

There is a parallel between the bacterial flora of the cervix of women with PID and the seminal bacteria of their sexual partners. Using the polymerase chain reaction (PCR) technique in six couples in which the women had chlamydial PID, Witkin and Toth identified the bacterium in the semen of all the male partners[12].

The mechanism of ascending chlamydial infection has been extensively studied. Between 8% and 12% of the population is thought to be infected by this bacterium. In most cases, *Chlamydia* is present in a silent or so-called carriage flora, but it may also be associated with lower genital tract infections, such as bartholinitis, cervicitis, and acute urethral syndrome in the female, and in prostatitis and urethritis in the male.

Variables directly associated with the risk of transmission or progression of the disease are

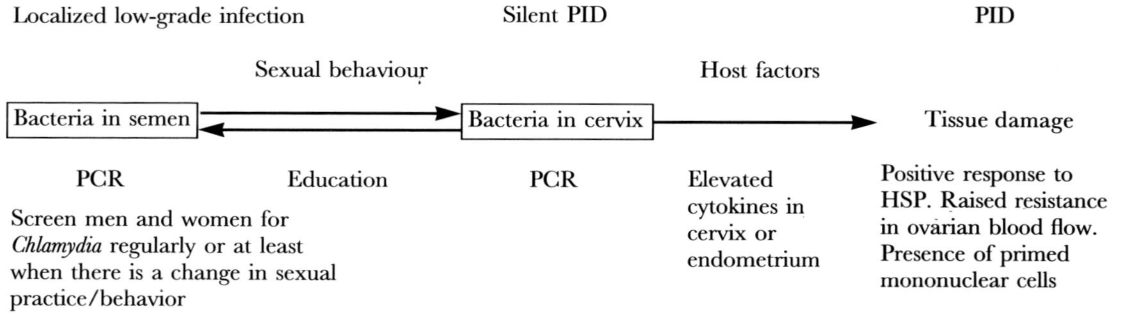

Figure 1 Mechanism of pelvic inflammatory disease (PID). Sexually transmitted bacteria cause localized, low-grade infection of the lower genital tract. Depending on bacterial virulence, bacteria number, and host response to the invading micro-organisms, the infection progresses through silent PID into clinically manifest PID. HSP, heat shock protein; PCR, polymerase chain reaction

called 'risk factors' and those that have an effect mediated through another variable are termed 'risk markers'. Demographic and social risk factors and risk markers include age, race, socio-economic status, marital status, and either rural or urban residence[1,11].

The role of sexual behavior in the development of PID is well documented. Multiple sexual partners, young age at first sexual intercourse, high frequency of sexual intercourse, and high rate of acquiring new sexual partners within the 30 days prior to developing PID appear to be the most important risk factors. Vaginal douching has been associated with PID. Among the contraceptive practices, the intrauterine device (IUD) is associated with an increased risk, primarily in the first few months after insertion. In contrast, combination birth control pills containing estrogen and progesterone and barrier methods are slightly protective against non-chlamydial PID and should therefore be recommended over IUDs to contracepting women. Young, nulliparous women, particularly if they are sexually active with more than one partner, should be encouraged to use condoms[1,2,11].

Once PID develops it has an unpredictable effect on the reproductive performance of the woman. Therefore the best way to handle PID at present is to prevent it. This can be accomplished by educating the population at risk in sexual practices and identifying and treating the asymptomatic infectious male who is most often responsible for spreading the disease. Because the symptoms are frequently absent and the disease often progresses without any clinical signs, preventive measures are mandatory. In our experience, prevention of the disease is possible by the routine and regular testing of young sexually active people (both male and female) for the presence of sexually transmitted bacteria (Figure 1).

SYMPTOMS AND DIAGNOSIS

More than half of women with PID will develop scarring of the adnexa without any symptoms of the disease[2]. These cases are most commonly associated with *Chlamydia* infection. The Centers for Disease Control, recognizing this new observation, has recommended the following classification for PID:

(1) *Salient, asymptomatic PID* The patient is not aware of any genital tract infection. Adnexal scarring occurs without the patient's knowledge. The first contact with these women is at the time of their work-up for tubal-factor infertility;

(2) *Atypical PID* The following few symptoms present which are not characteristic of pelvic infection: midcycle bleeding, spotting, irregular periods, sometimes mild, low abdominal discomfort. These cases are frequently overlooked both by physicians and patients;

(3) *Acute PID* This form is most commonly seen in patients presenting to emergency rooms throughout the country. These women are acutely ill, have moderate to severe low

abdominal pain, cervical motion tenderness and adnexal swelling and tenderness, making the diagnosis usually easy and accurate in this group;

(4) *PID residual syndrome* This is the end-stage of the disease. The patients usually have extensive pelvic adhesions, adnexal scarring, unilateral or bilateral tubal blockage, hydrosalpinx or pyosalpinx, and chronic pelvic pain.

Laparoscopy is the diagnostic procedure of choice. Only visual inspection of the pelvis can either confirm or rule out the infection with acceptable probability. The reddened, thick, tortuous, and hyperemic tube is the diagnostic sign for acute PID. There is usually straw-yellow-colored fluid in the cul-de-sac and, in some cases, the fimbriated end secretes a mucus-like material. The fimbriae may be blunted. In the more advanced cases, scarring of the pelvic organs and adhesions are visualized[13].

It is estimated that about 20% of women with laparascopically proven salpingitis will have classic symptoms of PID, and about two-thirds of women with PID can be identified based on clinical symptoms only. The advent of PCR technology has greatly aided bacterial identification. This method is capable of amplifying bacterial DNA. In a small study of women with high-risk sexual behavior, we found PCR to be at least one hundred times more sensitive than the conventional *Chlamydia* culture[14].

Tumor necrosis factor-α, a cytokine produced by macrophages, is usually elevated in the infected adnexal tissue of women with PID. The presence of high levels of this cytokine may indicate an upper genital tract infection[15]. Another important cytokine, interferon-γ is also elevated in the peripheral blood of women with adnexal infection[16]. In a very important study, Arno and associates[17] found significantly higher concentrations of interferon-γ in cervical secretions of women with positive *Chlamydia* cultures, when compared to culture-negative controls. The blood interferon levels were similar in both groups. This finding may indicate the presence of an early localized immune response to *Chlamydia* at the cervical level without any signs of systematic immune activation. Treatment at this point should result in complete resolution without any sequelae.

Recently we succeeded in developing a lymphocyte proliferation assay to *Chlamydia* heat shock protein. The presence of an elevated lymphocyte response to this protein confirms the operation of an immunological mechanism that may lead to extensive tissue damage. We now have in our laboratory several epitopes of the recombinant human heat shock protein that have entirely identical amino acid sequences with certain parts of the *Chlamydia* heat shock protein (Table 1).

In a small study we found that women whose lymphocytes developed sensitivity to these human epitopes (due to previous *Chlamydia* infection) almost always developed tubal damage after treatment[18,19]. Other, less specific, blood tests include estimated sedimentation rate and C-reactive protein measurements. Both have very low predictive values.

DIAGNOSTIC ULTRASOUND

Ultrasound has been gaining acceptance in the diagnosis of PID. Since the advent of the modern endovaginal probes, more detailed information can be obtained about the texture and consistency of the pelvic organs. Using the transvaginal route, high-frequency transducers can be positioned in

Table 1 Epitopes of the 57 kDa chlamydial heat shock protein present in the human heat shock protein

Source	*Amino acid position*	*Sequence*
Chlamydia	45–59	GSPQVTKDGVTVAK
Human		GSP**K**VTKDGVTVAK
Chlamydia	85–96	AGDGTTTAVLA
Human		AGDGTTTAVLA
Chlamydia	144–153	IAQVATISAN
Human		IAQVATISAN
Chlamydia	276–288	AVKAPGFGDRRK
Human		AVKAPGFGD**N**RK
Chlamydia	367–379	ERLAKLSGGVAV
Human		ERLAKLS**D**GVAV
Chlamydia	402–412	HATIAAVEEGI
Human		HA**R**IAAV**AA**GI

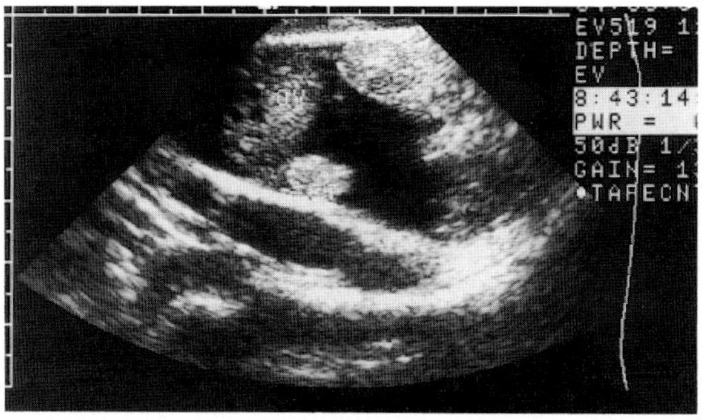

Figure 2 Transvaginal sonogram of acute salpingitis showing excess fluid in the pelvis. The ovary (OV) and Fallopian tube (FT) appear normal

close proximity to the pelvic structures, without loss of resolution. Utilizing gray-scale imaging with this method, Patten and colleagues successfully diagnosed inflammation in 25 of 27 cases[20]. We have found that using color ultrasound in some cases can enhance the visualization of both normal and abnormal tissues. Encouraged by the pioneering work of Timor-Tritsch and Rottem[21], sonographers now make an effort to examine the tubes during sonography of the pelvis. This task is relatively easy when there is a considerable amount of free fluid in the pelvis (Figure 2). This occurs during the midcycle under normal circumstances and, also, in an acute pelvic infection. At the onset of PID, however, there is a minimal amount of fluid in the cul-de-sac and the examination is quite difficult. To optimize visualization, the examination of the tubes should be carried out with the patient placed in a slightly reversed Trendelenburg position. We also found push–pull movements of the transducer, as described by Timor-Tritsch, very useful. Bilateral tubal visualization can be accomplished, even without an increase in the amount of pelvic fluid, with this method.

The ovaries are relatively easy to find on transvaginal examination in premenopausal women. Mehta and associates[22] report a 95% success rate in visualizing at least one ovary in women on oral contraceptives. The ovaries have a characteristic appearance of an echogenic mass and they are usually located in the vicinity of the internal iliac vessels. The usual presence of several follicles facilitates identification. The most significant ovulatory changes – the presence of the leading follicle, follicular rupture, and the formation of the corpus luteum, can all be recognized in the active ovary. In two perpendicular planes the three ovarian diameters (longitudinal, transverse, and anteroposterior) can be measured and the volume calculated. We use the following formula, suggested by Campbell and co-workers[23], for volume determinations:

$$\text{Ovarian volume} = 4/3 \times \pi \times d_1/2 \times d_2/2 \times d_3/2$$

where d_1, d_2 and d_3 are the three ovarian diameters.

Transvaginal sonography also makes the visualization of postmenopausal ovaries easier. In a prospective study of menopausal women, Fleischer and co-workers[24] detected both ovaries in 60% of patients and at least one ovary was visualized in 85% of the patients. They also found transvaginal sonography very accurate in detecting adnexal masses. Comparing transabdominal and transvaginal sonography, Andolf and Jörgensen[25] concluded that, because of the limited field, large ovarian and uterine masses may not be adequately assessed by using only transvaginal sonography. They recommend the combined transvaginal–transabdominal approach to evaluate these cases. For smaller adnexal masses and for assessing the endometrium, transvaginal sonography seems superior.

In our opinion the infected ovary, which is usually swollen, enlarged, and contains multiple cystic structures, is best visualized with transvaginal sonography. A tubo-ovarian abscess, which always represents a complex adnexal mass, is best evaluated by combining the transabdominal and transvaginal approach. By the use of this technique, the extent of the mass will be clearly determined and the change in structure and size accurately followed during the treatment.

Because the inflammatory process in the ovary involves both structural and vascular changes we also studied the use of color Doppler ultrasound as an adjunct to imaging ovarian and uterine blood flow in pelvic infection. Many studies have assessed flow-related functional changes of the uterus and the ovaries. For example, color Doppler was used to study follicular morphology and flow patterns in the periovulatory period[26,27].

These studies have demonstrated that the resistance to flow in the uterine arteries is least during the midluteal phase and that, around ovulation, the resistance to uterine blood flow may markedly change during the course of one day.

Significant variations in resistance to flow have been described in the active ovary as well. These changes were attributed to angiogenesis in the corpus luteum, however. Ovarian blood flow was longitudinally studied during the entire menstrual cycle of infertile patients and normal controls by Kurjak and associates[28]. Patients with infertility had increased resistance in the active ovary when compared to controls. Kurjak and associates and Bourne and colleagues used this method to measure blood flow impedance in ovarian tumors to screen for malignancy[26,29,30]. Examining large groups of women, both investigators were successful in identifying all cases of ovarian cancer at an early stage. Schulman and co-workers (personal communication) have argued for the cost effectiveness of ovarian screening in low risk women provided the study also includes screening for endometrial cancer at the same time.

Using a transvaginal 2-dimensional real-time and pulsed Doppler method, Scholtes and associates[31] performed serial studies of the uterine and ovarian arteries in healthy women in a donor insemination program. They found a significant difference in uterine artery impedance between the left and the right side on only day 21 of the cycle. There was, however, a decreased resistance to flow in the artery of the dominant ovary developing the corpus luteum on days 13, 16, and 21. These results indicate that the uterine arteries are only marginally involved in the blood flow changes accompanying ovulation and that the lower impedance in the dominant ovary is most likely caused by neovascularization of the corpus luteum. Tinkanen and Kujansu[32] studied uterine artery impedance in women with tubo-ovarian abscess. They found significantly lower resistance indices in the acute phase when compared with healthy controls. When the disease subsided, the indices returned to normal. This suggests that the infection-induced vasodilatation can cause increased blood flow.

We believe that ovarian blood flow may also be affected by an inflammatory process in the pelvis. This hypothesis is based on two factors. First, the ovary is in close proximity to the tube which is the primary focus of infection in PID; and second, because of its anatomical location, the ovary shares a significant part of its blood supply with the ipsilateral tube.

The ovary receives its blood supply from the ovarian and the uterine arteries. These vessels reach the ovary through the infundibulopelvic and the ovarian ligaments. They anastomose alongside the ovary and give off numerous small branches into the mesosalpinx to supply the tube. The ovarian artery can be readily identified on longitudinal section in the infundibulopelvic ligament, next to the artery (Figure 3).

Ovarian parenchymal blood flow can be obtained both from the active and the inactive ovary late in the follicular phase. We found that the resistance in the ovarian parenchymal blood vessels varied in the acute phase of PID (Figures 4 and 5) but almost invariably was increased in the chronic, more advanced, stage, when significant tissue damage had already developed (Figure 6). In a study of 42 women with suspected PID, the intraovarian blood flow was measured with color Doppler ultrasound, prior to the diagnostic laparoscopy. Fourteen patients had negative findings or pathology. The remaining 28 women had PID with some degree of permanent tissue damage in all cases (PID residual syndrome). The intraovarian resistance was found to be increased in all but two patients, as indicated by a higher pulsatility index (PI) with a range of 0.9–2.8. The PI in the controls ranged between 0.4 and 1.1. The difference was statistically significant[33].

Clinical and ultrasound appearance of acute pelvic inflammatory disease

Infection reaches the tubes and the ovaries in an ascending fashion. There is a characteristic way that the detectable signs appear on transvaginal sonograms during the course of the disease. Initially, the sonographic findings may be entirely normal, except for fluid collection in the pelvis or in the uterine cavity. This latter may be the only sign of endometritis. As the infection progresses, an increased number of changes can occur in the pelvic organs with characteristic sonographic

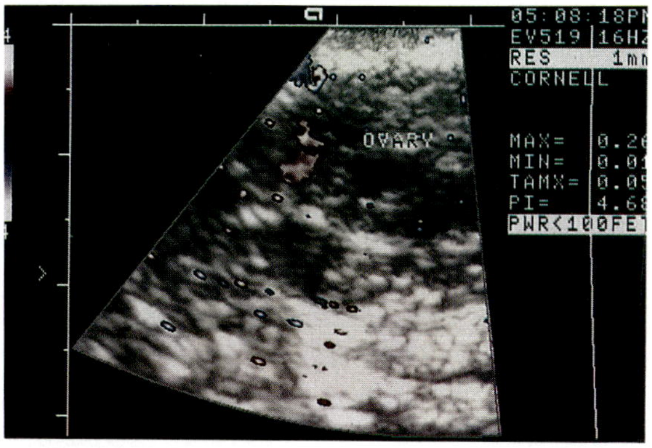

Figure 3 Transvaginal sonogram demonstrating the ovary with the ovarian artery clearly seen by color Doppler

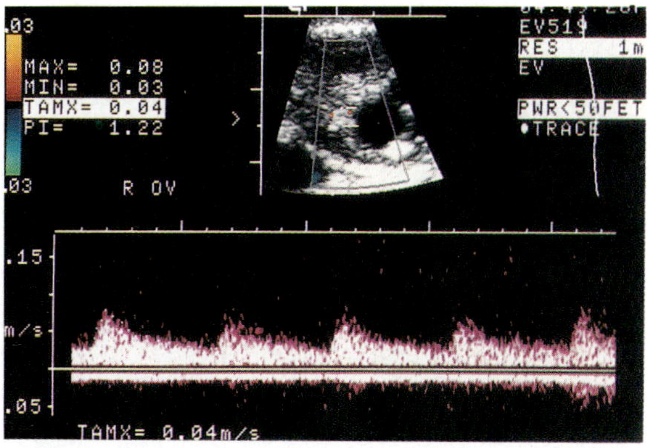

Figure 5 Color Doppler ultrasound scan of the ovary in acute salpingitis. Note the increased pulsatility index (PI), suggesting decreased parenchymal ovarian blood flow

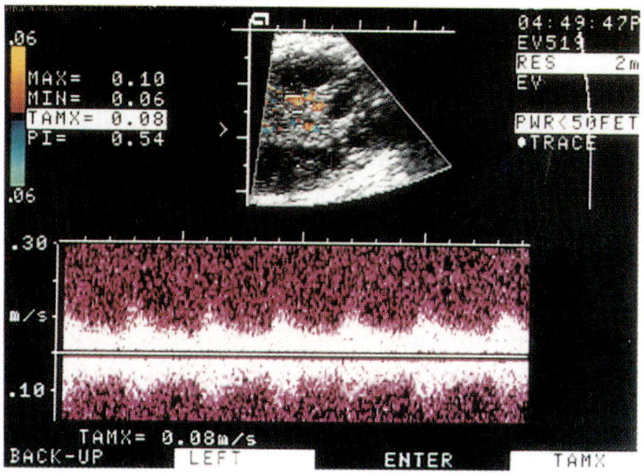

Figure 4 Color Doppler ultrasound scan of the ovary in acute salpingitis. Note the polycystic ovarian appearance and the low pulsatility index (PI)

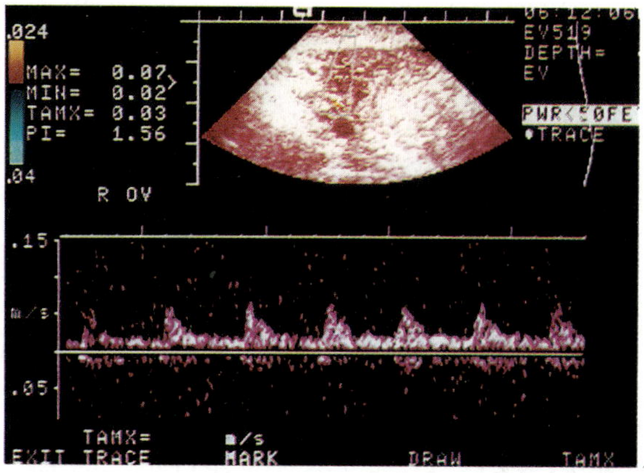

Figure 6 Color Doppler ultrasound scan in a patient with pelvic inflammatory disease and extensive scarring. Note the high pulsatility index (PI)

features[34]. Visualization of the Fallopian tubes greatly improves the accuracy of the diagnosis.

Because their echogenicity is the same as that of the surrounding organs, the normal tubes are hard to visualize by sonogram unless there is a significant fluid accumulation in the pelvis[21]. Large amounts of fluid will make evaluation possible, even of the fimbriated end. However, fixed tubes that are already adherent to the ovarian surface will be difficult to investigate (Figure 7).

Hyperemia, swelling, tortuosity, and purulent exudate from the lumen and the serosal surfaces of the tubes are the main characteristics of acute PID. Of 12 women with laparoscopically proven acute salpingitis, we could identify fluid collection by ultrasound in the lumen of one or both tubes in ten cases within 72 hours following onset of the symptoms (Figure 8). Tubal swelling was documented in all patients as represented by an ampullary diameter of greater than 10 mm. The intraluminal exudate was gradually absorbed and the diameter was rapidly decreased after antibiotic treatment was begun. Blood vessels in the tubal wall can be identified by color Doppler in this early phase of the disease. The ovaries are enlarged, globular, and may contain multiple cysts. The cysts are infected follicles. A larger,

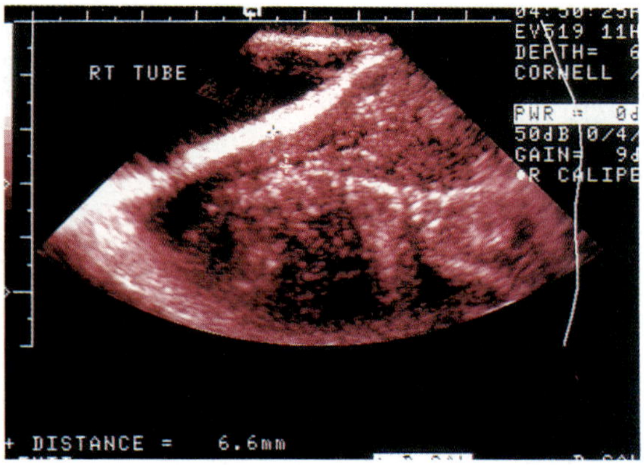

Figure 7 Vaginal ultrasound scan of Fallopian tube in acute salpingitis. Note the fluid collection in the lumen near the fimbriated end

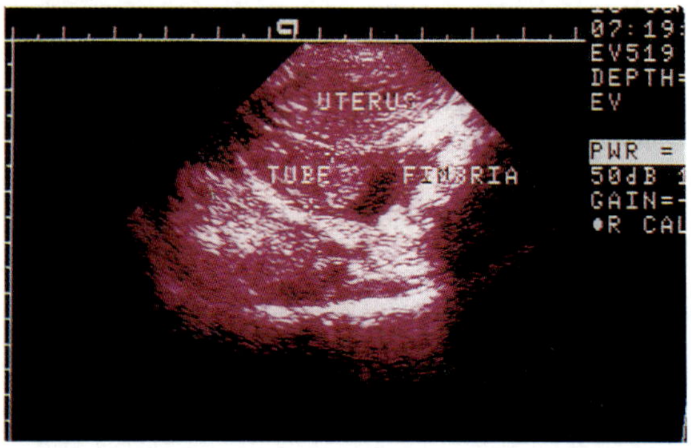

Figure 8 Vaginal ultrasound scan of the tube with acute salpingitis, showing fluid accumulation in the lumen proximal to the fimbriated end

debris-filled cavity most likely represents an infected corpus luteum. The margins may be indistinct due to the accompanying perioophoritis. We found no characteristic changes in resistance indices of the uterine and ovarian arteries of women with acute salpingitis. Intraovarian parenchymal blood flow indices, however, varied between low and slightly elevated values (PI, 0.4–1.5).

Clinical and ultrasound appearance of tubo-ovarian abscess

Tubo-ovarian abscess is the most severe form of an acute infection. Symptoms are relatively severe, even in the earlier cases. The continuous spillage of purulent material from the tube reaches the ovarian surface and neighboring structures (e.g. bowel, omentum). The end result is a complex adnexal conglomerate with hypoechoic, septate sonographic appearance. The initial impression is that of a solid mass, but the acoustic enhancement and the total absence of blood flow confirms the presence of complex fluid. The external margins are irregular and indistinct. This is because the ovary is usually tightly adherent, either to the uterus or to the pelvic sidewall. Sometimes it is difficult to identify the ovary or tube within the mass. The tube may be dilated and partially filled with fluid, as shown by the fluid–debris levels. Part of the mass may appear in the cul de sac, which contains echogenic pus as well (Figure 9).

The more advanced the disease, the more ill-defined the tubo-ovarian abscess becomes, with complete loss of anatomic landmarks. The full extent of the process at this point is best determined by transabdominal ultrasound[34] (Figures 10 and 11). The abscess cavities can be safely drained under sonographic guidance. This procedure usually enhances recovery. Periappendiceal and diverticular abscesses, endometriomas, benign and malignant ovarian tumors, and ectopic pregnancy have to be considered in the differential diagnosis. When conservative management is elected, the regression of the mass is best followed by serial ultrasonography.

Clinical and ultrasound appearance of chronic pelvic inflammatory disease residual syndrome

This condition can develop as a consequence of an acute infection or even in patients without any clinical evidence of salpingitis. The obstruction of the fimbriated end results in fluid collection in the tube, thus producing hydrosalpinx. This appears as a tubular anechoic structure on sonogram. The absence of blood flow on color Doppler helps differentiate the hydrosalpinx from a large blood vessel. Thickened mucosal folds and nodular projections into the lumen are characteristic sonographic signs (Figure 12). The appearance of internal echoes in the distended lumen with absence of blood flow suggests pyosalpinx. The

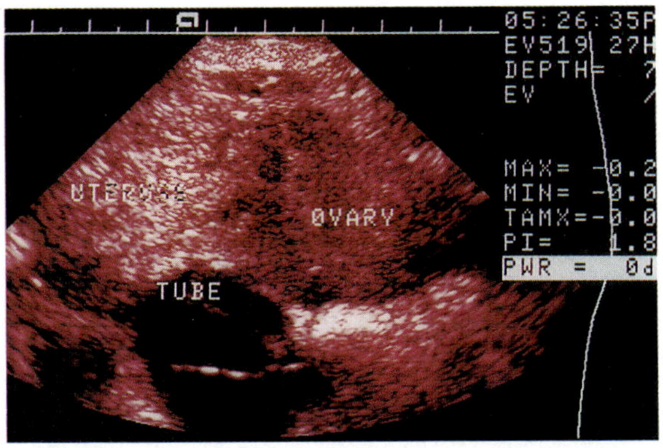

Figure 9 Vaginal ultrasound scan of a tubo-ovarian abscess, showing dilated, fluid-filled tube, an ovary with indistinct borders and cystic appearance, adherent to the posterior wall of the uterus, representing a complex adnexal mass

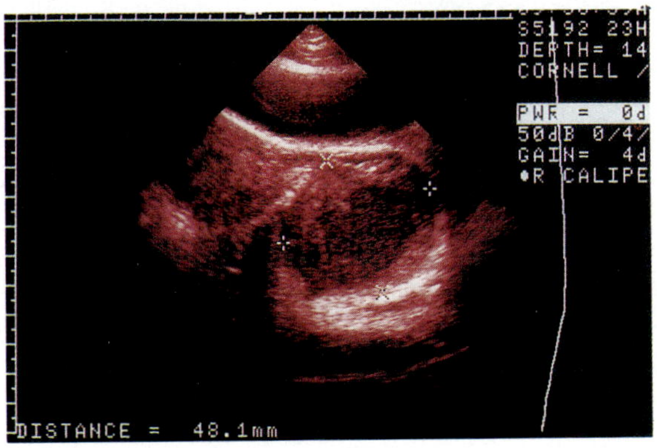

Figure 10 Abdominal ultrasound scan of patient with a tubo-ovarian abscess; fully developed stage. The extent of the mass is best determined by abdominal sonogram; note posterior acoustic enhancement and complex fluid in the ovary

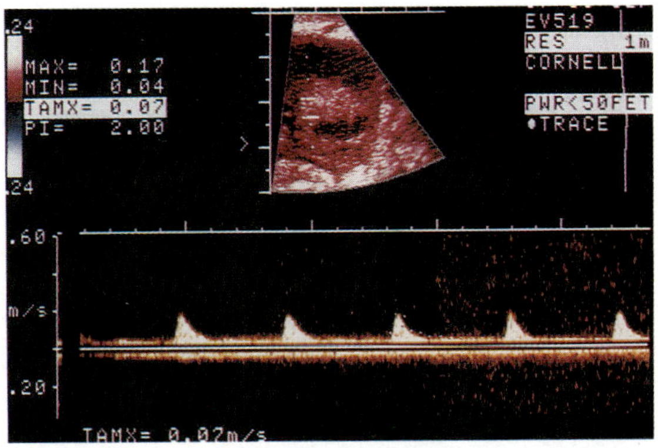

Figure 11 Vaginal Doppler ultrasound scan of a tubo-ovarian abscess with high pulsatility index (PI) due to scarring in a complex adnexal mass

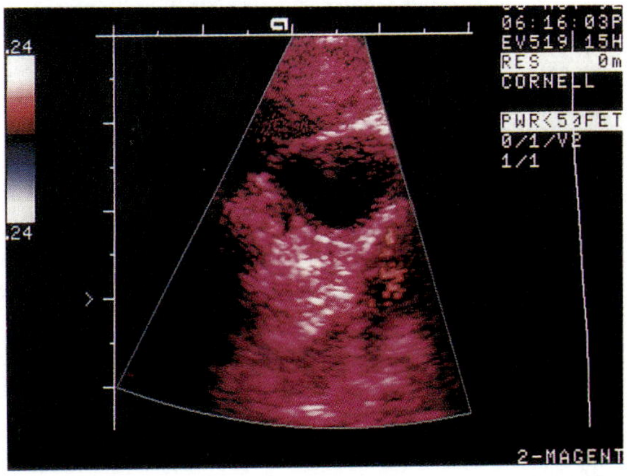

Figure 12 Vaginal ultrasound scan of early hydrosalpinx, with tubal wall thickened. Note the papillary projections in the lumen, representing the deteriorating endosalpinx

adjacent ovary may be recognized with its convex border slightly compressing the wall of the anechoic fluid-filled hydrosalpinx (Figure 13). Loss of mobility in the different pelvic organs can occur because of extensive adhesions. The ovarian parenchymal blood flow is almost invariably decreased as indicated by elevated PI values (Figure 7). The ovarian volume is normal or increased. This latter is probably attributable to the sclerotic capsule around the scarred parenchyma. Follicles are scarce, and the corpus luteum is frequently absent in the second half of the cycle, indicating the loss of ovulatory function.

Hysterosalpingo–contrast sonography

This is a relatively new application for transvaginal or transabdominal color Doppler. The method involves the injection of contrast material into the uterine cervix and monitoring its flow within the cavity of the uterus and the tubes by Doppler ultrasound. Several studies indicate that this technique is comparable to a hysterosalpingogram[35]. In the evaluation of women with tubal factor infertility it does not require the use of ionizing radiation, as does hysterosalpingography, and it allows for the examination of the entire

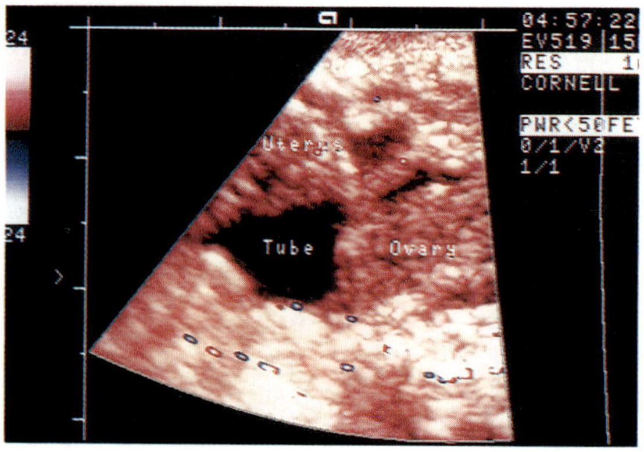

Figure 13 Vaginal ultrasound scan of patient with chronic hydrosalpinx. The convex ovarian border is seen protruding in the ovarian lumen

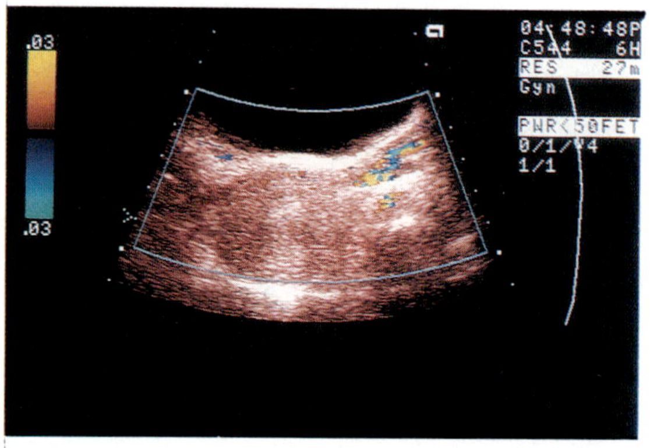

Figure 14 Abdominal hysterosalpingosonography showing a patent tube with normal flow in the proximal portion

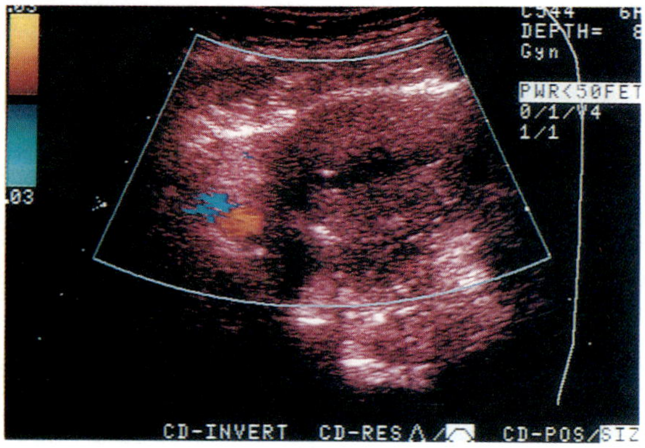

Figure 15 Abdominal hysterosalpingosonography showing a patent tube with normal flow in the fimbriated end

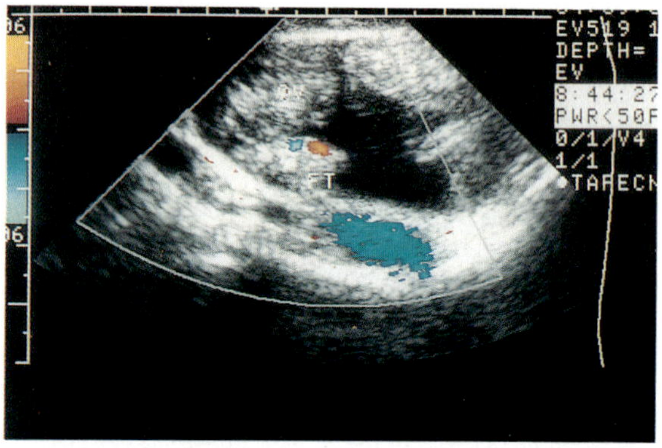

Figure 16 Abdominal hysterosalpingosonography in a patient with salpingitis. Color Doppler indicates intact flow through the fimbriated end

pelvis by sonogram as a part of the procedure (Figures 14 and 15). A ballooned catheter is secured within the uterine cervix and the contrast medium, SH U 454 (Schering AG, Berlin), is injected directly into the endocervical canal. The vaginal or the abdominal transducer is used to track the movement of the contrast material and to establish tubal patency. Color Doppler hysterosalpingo–contrast sonography is capable of visualizing the tube in its entire length, thereby documenting its patency or any partial or total obstruction. The uterine cavity can also be well visualized. It is easy to obtain information regarding the shape and size of the cavity, myomas, and pathology. There is only minor discomfort associated with the procedure. In some centers, the procedure is now combined with falloposcopy for direct visualization of the tubal lumen and, if obstruction is found, catheterization and recanalization under ultrasound observation is attempted. In a small study of infertility patients with tubal obstruction, Lisse and Sydow[36] reported a 91% success rate for tubal catheterization and an 84% success rate in recanalization of at least one tube. Of their 16 patients who underwent recanalization, five (31%) became pregnant within 6 months. It is possible that the mere dislodging of intraluminal debris and the breaking down of filmy adhesions in the normal or minimally-distressed tubes contributes to the increased pregnancy rate following the procedure. In our experience, hysterosalpingo–contrast sonography can be useful in the management and follow-up of PID patients as well.

To avoid even the possibility of exacerbating or causing a flareup of the infectious process we use Vibramycin solution instead of contrast material. In the early phase of the infection of the ovaries and the tubes, a significant amount of low viscous material may accumulate near the fimbriated ends. This is especially characteristic of chlamydial salpingitis. On laparoscopy, the fluid had the appearance of a 'sticky exudate' protruding through the blunted fimbriae. In some cases of excessive exudate we successfully used hysterosalpingosonography to safely remove this material (Figure 16). After the intrauterine and intratubal application of Vibramycin solution, the distended tube regains its normal appearance and shrinks back to its original caliber. The procedure can also be used in the more advanced stages of the disease, to assess tubal status. There is evidence to show that tissue damage in PID may be caused by a hypersensitivity reaction to chlamydial heat shock protein.

In a small study of 14 women with *Chlamydia* salpingitis, we performed hysterosalpingosonography three months after the laparoscopic diagnosis. Bilateral tubal patency was documented in all cases at the time of the surgery. At the time of three months' follow-up, bilateral tubal obstruction was shown in two patients, and unilateral blockage in three. The remaining nine women had normal hysterosalpingosonographic studies. All women who developed tubal obstructions during the follow-up period had positive lymphocyte reactions against the conserved epitopes of human heat shock protein, which were homologous to the identical parts of the *Chlamydia* heat shock protein. The results supported the hypothesis that, beyond a certain stage, *Chlamydia* PID may become an autoimmune process that causes tubal and ovarian damage through a delayed hypersensitivity reaction to *Chlamydia* heat shock protein. The disease can progress without the presence of the bacterium.

CONCLUSIONS

Ultrasound with color Doppler has proved to be a useful tool in the diagnosis and management of pelvic inflammatory disease. Color Doppler readily identifies the engorged blood vessels of the pelvic organs in the acute phase, it helps differentiate between dilated vessels and fluid-filled hydrosalpinx and it can be useful in the differential diagnosis of tubo-ovarian abscess. Examining ovarian involvement and function by measuring intraovarian resistance in the acute phase reflects the rapidly changing patterns of the disease at this stage. The increased resistance in the chronic phase is most likely consistent with extensive scarring. This condition may have long-term effects on the endocrine function of the ovary. It is worth noting that there is increased intraovarian resistance in premature ovarian failure and after prolonged use of oral contraceptives as well. Hysterosalpingosonography with or without contrast material is valuable to assess tubal status at any stage of the disease. This method allows for more detailed visualization of pelvic structures, especially when the transvaginal approach is used. Ovarian position, volume and architecture can be evaluated during the course of the infection. Using ultrasound has shown us that most women who acquire pelvic inflammatory disease will end up with permanent damage of some extent to their reproductive tract. The best tool for managing pelvic inflammatory disease is prevention. The mechanism and diagnosis of the disease is summarized in Figure 1. There is a male-to-female vector in the transmission of the bacteria that cause pelvic inflammatory disease. This is because of the difference in sexual behavior between the sexes. Any preventive effort that ignores the role of the male sex partners as the main source of sexually transmissible bacteria will fail to achieve its goal. Regular bacteriological screening of the sexually active male and female populations is the only effective way to identify the disease at the earliest possible stage and to prevent its consequences.

In our view, color Doppler ultrasound, in conjunction with ultrasound imaging, can be invaluable to a clinical program emphasizing diagnosis, management, and prevention of pelvic inflammatory disease.

References

1. Expert Committee on Pelvic Inflammatory Disease (1991). Research directions for the 1990s. *Sex. Trans. Dis.*, **18**, 46–64
2. Gales, W. and Wasserheit, J. N. (1991). Genital chlamydial infections: epidemiology and reproductive sequelae. *Am. J. Obstet. Gynecol.*, **164**, 1771–81
3. Toth, M., *et al.* (1993). Pregnancy outcome following pelvic infection. *Infect. Dis. Obstet. Gynecol.*, **1**, 12–15
4. Weström, L. (1980). Incidence, prevalence and trends of acute pelvic inflammatory disease and its consequences in industrialized countries. *Am. J. Obstet. Gynecol.*, **138**, 880–92
5. Licciardi, F., *et al.* (1992). Relation between antibiotics to *Chlamydia trachomatis* and spontaneous abortion following *in vitro* fertilization. *J. Assist. Reprod. Genet.*, **9**, 207–10, 215
6. Campbell, L. A., *et al.* (1993). Detection of *Chlamydia trachomatis* deoxyribonucleic acid in women with tubal infertility. *Fertil. Steril.*, **59**, 45–50
7. Battiger, B. E., *et al.* (1989). Association of recurrent chlamydial infection with gonorrhea. *J. Infect. Dis.*, **159**, 661–9
8. Draper, D., *et al.* (1980). *In vitro* modeling of acute salpingitis caused by *Neisseria gonorrheae*. *Am. J. Obstet. Gynecol.*, **138**, 996–1001
9. Morrison, R. P., *et al.* (1992). Immunology of *Chlamydia trachomatis* infection: immunoprotective and immunopathogentic responses. *Adv. Host Defense Mech.*, **8**, 57–84
10. Morrison, R. P., *et al.* (1989). *Chlamydia* disease pathogenesis. The 57 KD chlamydial hypersensitivity antigen is a stress response protein. *J. Exp. Med.*, **170**, 1271–83
11. Aral, S. O. (1992). Behavioral aspects of chlamydial infections: their epidemiology, prevention, and control. *Second Meeting, European Society for Chlamydia Research*, Lidingo, Sweden. Division of STD/HIV Prevention, Centers for Disease Control, Abstr.
12. Witkin, S. S., *et al.* (1993). Detection of *Chlamydia trachomatis* in semen by the polymerase chain reaction in male members of infertile couples. *Am. J. Obstet. Gynecol.*, **168**, 1457–62
13. Sellors, J., *et al.* (1991). The accuracy of clinical findings and laparoscopy in pelvic inflammatory disease. *Am. J. Obstet. Gynecol.*, **164**, 113–20
14. Robo, L., *et al.* (1990). Diagnosis of *Chlamydia trachomatis* cervical infection by detection of amplified DNA with a unique immunoassay. *J. Clin. Microbiol.*, **28**, 1968–73
15. Toth, M., *et al.* (1992). *In vivo* tumor necrosis factor production in women with salpingitis. *Surg. Gynecol. Obstet.*, **174**, 359–62
16. Grife, J. A., *et al.* (1989). Interferon-β in the diagnosis and pathogenesis of pelvic inflammatory disease. *Am. J. Obstet. Gynecol.*, **160**, 26–30
17. Arno, J. N., *et al.* (1990). Interferon β in endocervical secretions of women infected with *Chlamydia trachomatis*. *J. Infect. Dis.* **162**, 1385–9
18. Witkin, S. S., *et al.* (1993). Cell-mediated immune response to the recombinant 57-KDa heat shock protein of *Chlamydia trachomatis* in women with salpingitis. *J. Infect. Dis.*, **167**, 1–5
19. Witkin, S. S., *et al.* (1991). Increased induceability of inflammatory mediators from peripheral blood mononuclear cells of women with salpingitis. *Am. J. Obstet. Gynecol.*, **165**, 719–23
20. Patten, R. M., *et al.* (1990). Pelvic inflammatory disease: endovaginal sonography with laparoscopic correlation. *J. Ultrasound Med.*, **9**, 681–9
21. Timor-Tritsch, I. E. and Rottem, S. (1987). Transvaginal ultrasonographic study of the Fallopian tube. *Obstet. Gynecol.*, **70**, 42–8
22. Mehta, A. E., *et al.* (1992). Noninvasive diagnosis of resistant ovary syndrome by ultrasonography. *Fertil. Steril.*, **57**, 56–61
23. Campbell, S., *et al.* (1982). Real-time ultrasonography for determination of ovarian morphology and volume. *Lancet*, **1**, 425–6
24. Fleischer, A., *et al.* (1990). Transvaginal sonography of postmenopausal ovaries with pathologic correlation. *J. Ultrasound Med.*, **9**, 637
25. Andolf, E. and Jörgensen, C. (1990). A prospective comparison of transabdominal and transvaginal ultrasound with surgical findings in gynecologic disease. *J. Ultrasound Med.*, **9**, 71–5
26. Bourne, T., *et al.* (1989). Transvaginal color flow imaging: a possible new screening technique for ovarian cancer. *Br. Med. J.*, **299**, 1367–70
27. Collins, W., *et al.* (1991). Ovarian morphology, endocrine function and intrafollicular blood flow during the peri-ovulatory period. *Hum. Reprod.*, **6**, 319–29
28. Kurjak, A., *et al.* (1991). Transvaginal color flow Doppler in the assessment of ovarian and uterine blood flow in infertile women. *Fertil. Steril.*, **56**, 870–3
29. Kurjak, A., *et al.* (1989). Transvaginal color ultrasound for the assessment of pelvic circulation. *Acta Obstet. Gynecol. Scand.*, **68**, 131–5
30. Kurjak, A., *et al.* (1991). Evaluation of adnexal masses with transvaginal color Doppler ultrasound. *J. Ultrasound Med.*, **10**, 295–7

31. Scholtes, M. E. W., *et al.* (1989). Uterine and ovarian flow velocity waveforms in the normal menstrual cycle: transvaginal Doppler study. *Fertil. Steril.*, **52**, 981–5
32. Tinkanen, H. and Kujansu, E. (1992). Doppler ultrasound studies in pelvic inflammatory disease. *Gynecol. Obstet. Invest.*, **34**, 240–2
33. Toth, M., *et al.* (1992). Color Doppler ultrasound in the diagnosis of pelvic inflammatory disease. *Annual Meeting of the Infectious Diseases Society for Obstetrics and Gynecology*, Abstr. 7, San Diego
34. Spirtos, N. J., *et al.* (1982). Sonography in acute pelvic inflammatory disease. *J. Reprod. Med.*, **6**, 312–9
35. Schef, R. and Deichert, U. (1991). Hysterosalpingo-contrast sonography of the uterus and Fallopian tubes. *Radiology*, **178**, 213–5
36. Lisse, K. and Sydow, P. (1991). Fallopian tube catheterization and recanalization under ultrasound observation: a simplified technique to evaluate tubal patency and proximally obstructed tubes. *Fertil. Steril.*, **56**, 198–201

Polycystic ovarian syndrome and the current contribution of ultrasound

13

J. Beires, N. Montenegro and D. Pignatelli

The polycystic ovarian syndrome (PCOS) encompasses a series of clinical situations and is in fact a very heterogeneous disease. In addition, other diseases, sometimes described as being independent, differ very slightly from the classic one. Examples of these are multifollicular ovaries, hyperthecosis and the Hairan syndrome (hyperandrogenism, insulin resistance and acanthosis nigricans). This is also true for the simple division of PCOS cases into type I (classic form) and type II (in which the adrenal gland's contribution has greater relevance)[1–5]. There is also a significant association with other situations such as congenital adrenal hyperplasia, Cushing's syndrome, hypothyroidism, hyperthyroidism, acromegaly, hyperprolactinemia and all states of insulin resistance.

Table 1 Characteristics of polycystic ovarian syndrome

Amenorrhea/oligomenorrhea
Chronic anovulation/irregular ovulation
Infertility
Hyperandrogenism/hirsutism
Acne
Bilateral multicystic ovaries
Hyperestrogenemia
Obesity
Bilaterally enlarged ovaries
Elevated LH/FSH ratio
High prolactin levels
Galactorrhea
Dopamine deficiency
Insulin resistance

CHARACTERIZATION OF THE SYNDROME

As initially described by Stein and Leventhal[6], the polycystic ovarian syndrome was defined by the simultaneous presence of amenorrhea, hirsutism and infertility. Other signs and symptoms such as obesity and acne have also been frequently associated with the syndrome. The main characteristics of the syndrome are summarized in Table 1. After the initial description, it was noted that oligomenorrhea and dysfunctional hemorrhages were more frequently found than amenorrhea.

OVARIAN CHANGES

The changes found in the ovaries include thickening and fibrosis of the capsule and the presence of many atretic-appearing follicles underneath[7]. The ovaries, as seen by laparotomy, laparoscopy or ultrasound, have numerous cysts of small dimensions which probably correspond to those follicles; according to some authors, the definition of polycystic ovaries should include ten or more cysts, 2–8 mm in diameter[8]. They may also have larger cysts simultaneously. Histologically, hyperplasia of the theca cells is prominent[9].

PCOS is generally found with ovaries of increased size[4,10,11], but they may have normal dimensions and in our experience this is not rare[12] (although the average volume of the ovaries of PCOS cases is significantly greater than that of normal ovaries).

Initially, the ovarian disease was confirmed by laparotomy. Then there was a period in which it was essentially 'assumed'. Ultrasonography has necessarily become increasingly important in the diagnosis and study of this disease. This method, which has gained increased popularity and is now being used with greater frequency, allows direct and non-invasive visualization of the ovaries. The first trustworthy studies of the frequency of polycystic ovaries have been made possible. In 1986, it was shown that 26% of women with amenorrhea and 87% of those with oligomenorrhea had polycystic ovaries[8]. Polycystic ovaries were later reported to exist in 25% of normal women[13] and, surprisingly, 34% of a Mediterranean population[12].

HORMONAL ALTERATIONS

Polycystic ovaries are frequently associated with characteristic hormonal alterations. The basal levels of luteinizing hormone (LH) are typically increased in a high percentage of cases[14,15]. A fixed increase of LH without the normal variations of the menstrual cycle[16] and a relative suppression of follicle-stimulating hormone (FSH) are generally observed.

An elevated LH/FSH ratio (arbitrarily considered >2 or >3) is one of the fundamental criteria for including cases in this syndrome. However, one quarter to one half of patients with polycystic ovaries have LH/FSH ratios below 3 and many have ratios below 2[17,18].

Hyperplasia of the theca cells results from the LH stimulus of the follicle cells[15,19,20]. It probably also occurs due to insulin action on these cells (as well as on the stroma cells)[21] because insulin levels are frequently elevated in these women.

Theca cell and stromal hyperplasia results in the second hormonal characteristic of PCOS: hyperandrogenemia. Hirsutism is a direct consequence of this hyperandrogenism and it is one of the most important clinical markers of PCOS. Nevertheless, polycystic ovaries and even hyperandrogenism may occur without hirsutism[22]. Hyperandrogenism results in the premature termination of follicular development[23,24]. A deficiency of estradiol production results from deficient aromatization of androgens in the granulosa layer[25]. This is a consequence of follicular non-development[26] and lack of FSH stimulation of the granulosa cells[19,20].

Although estradiol is produced in smaller quantities by each follicle individually, the total secretion is still quite substantial[27]. Even if that was not the case, however, women with PCOS would not be estrogen deficient. The reduction in sex hormone-binding globulin (SHBG) associated with high levels of androgens leads to an increase in the levels of free estrogens[28,29]. In addition, the increase of estrone production from androgens, mainly from androstenedione[15,30], may result, at least partially, from the augmentation of adipose tissue.

ULTRASOUND IN POLYCYSTIC OVARIES

Ultrasonography was used for the first time as a technical aid for gynecological diagnosis by Ian Donald about 35 years ago, but it only gained its widespread use in the last 20 years. It is now widely employed for the diagnosis of pelvic pathology, giving a great deal of information about pelvic anatomy.

It also plays a fundamental role in the study of female infertility by giving detailed visualization of ovarian and uterine structures and allowing non-invasive observation of its functional alterations.

Many attempts have been made over the years to define typical ultrasound patterns which would characterize gynecological syndromes. This is particularly true in the case of PCOS.

The first description of the ultrasonographic aspects of the ovaries of patients with PCOS was made by Kratochwil in 1972[31]. He defined them as having a typically round shape and symmetrically increased volume. Later, in 1981, in addition to confirming the symmetrical increase in ovarian volume, Swanson[32] mentioned the presence of small ovarian cysts, 2–6 mm, and pointed out their diagnostic importance as well as the technical difficulty in their visualization. Afterwards, different opinions started to emerge[33–35], drawing attention to the variability of the different parameters used in the ultrasonographic characterization of PCOS (volume, shape, presence of cysts). Hann and colleagues[33], for example, stated that 29% of the patients clinically included in the PCOS group had normal ultrasound characteristics. Nicolini and associates[34] stated that only 34% had increased volume. Yeh and co-workers[35] reported that the roundness index is a useless concept, unrelated to what is observed.

Various ultrasonographic classifications of PCOS have been described in the literature. Comparetto and colleagues[36] classified PCOS by relating the follicular cysts to the ovarian stroma. This is difficult to calculate and has almost no diagnostic value. Hann and associates[33] divided the PCOS characteristics into three patterns: (1) ovaries with only small cysts; (2) hypoechogenic ovaries without cysts; and (3) isoechogenic ovaries without cysts. Orsini and colleagues[37] divided the PCOS characteristics into four patterns: (1) enlarged cystic ovaries; (2) enlarged solid ovaries; (3) normal-sized cystic ovaries; and (4) normal-sized solid ovaries. We believe that these classifications are not very useful in a study protocol of PCOS.

One of the principal criteria for the ultrasonic diagnosis of PCOS is the presence of morphologically identical, multiple small cysts (2–8 mm) which sometimes appear in healthy women[38,39] but are found in greater numbers in cases of PCOS (Figure 1). Although the lower limit (2 mm) has been referred to by many authors using transabdominal ultrasound, our experience tells us that this technique only allows visualization of follicles greater than 4–5 mm. Only the use of transvaginal ultrasound has permitted the detection of such small cysts.

Transvaginal ultrasound provides a clearer picture because the probe is placed closer to the pelvic structures and a higher frequency is used (5–10 MHz), increasing the resolution and so the image quality. This allows visualization of small cysts and a more detailed description of the ovarian stroma (Figure 2). Furthermore, the bladder is empty during examination and so distortion of the pelvic anatomy is avoided (Figure 3). It also avoids some difficulties of conventional ultrasound, namely the adiposity found in many of the cases.

The ovary is a dynamic organ which is greatly influenced by age, hormonal stimuli and reproductive state[40]. The comprehension of these dynamics is crucial for the interpretation of eventual pathology. A functional cyst is one of the most frequently observed anomalies in pelvic ultrasound, resulting from simple follicular cysts, corpus luteum cysts and hemorrhagic cysts. Its size is variable and its main characteristic is its transitory nature.

The incidence of ovulation in PCOS is much lower than that in the general population and when it does occur, it does so at irregular intervals.

Another parameter used by various authors to define the ultrasonic pattern of PCOS is volume[38,41]. Ovarian volume is usually calculated using a simplified formula for an ellipsoid (0.5233 × length × width × thickness). Mean ovarian volumes in normal women varying between 6.5 and 10.0 cm^3 have been reported[34,35]. It has been our experience[12] that normal Portuguese women have an average ovarian volume of only 3.1 ± 1.3 cm^3.

Volume may vary according to age as well as to phase of the menstrual cycle, being larger in the ovary which contains the ovulatory follicle[38]. Although the ultrasonic demonstration of bilateral and symmetrically increased volume of the ovaries has been described as one of the criteria for the diagnosis of PCOS[6], this characteristic is not present in a large proportion of cases[12,33–35]. However, what most authors usually mean is that, on average, the volume is augmented[12,42], and not that every individual case has increased ovarian volume.

Great variation in shape was also found in the patients with PCOS (Figure 4). The original idea that the majority of these ovaries would have a round shape was not proved[35].

Other points to be considered in the ultrasound study of PCOS are related to the stromal hyperplasia and endometrium thickness. Stroma has been reported usually to be hypertrophied[13,43,44] and it has higher echogenic intensity[45]. This probably reflects the direct action of both LH and insulin.

Transvaginal ultrasound also allows good characterization of the endometrium which has in the majority of these cases a thickness greater than 5 mm (double layer) and a homogeneous texture (Figure 5). The demonstration of a thickened endometrium is also in favor of the diagnosis of PCOS because it may be considered a consequence of increased estrogen levels.

DOPPLER BLOOD FLOW EVALUATION

Recently, transvaginal color Doppler blood flow evaluation of pelvic circulation has been regarded as a promising tool by extending the range of ultrasound from a morphological to a functional role[46]. It allows the study of vascular parameters such as flow velocity and blood flow impedance

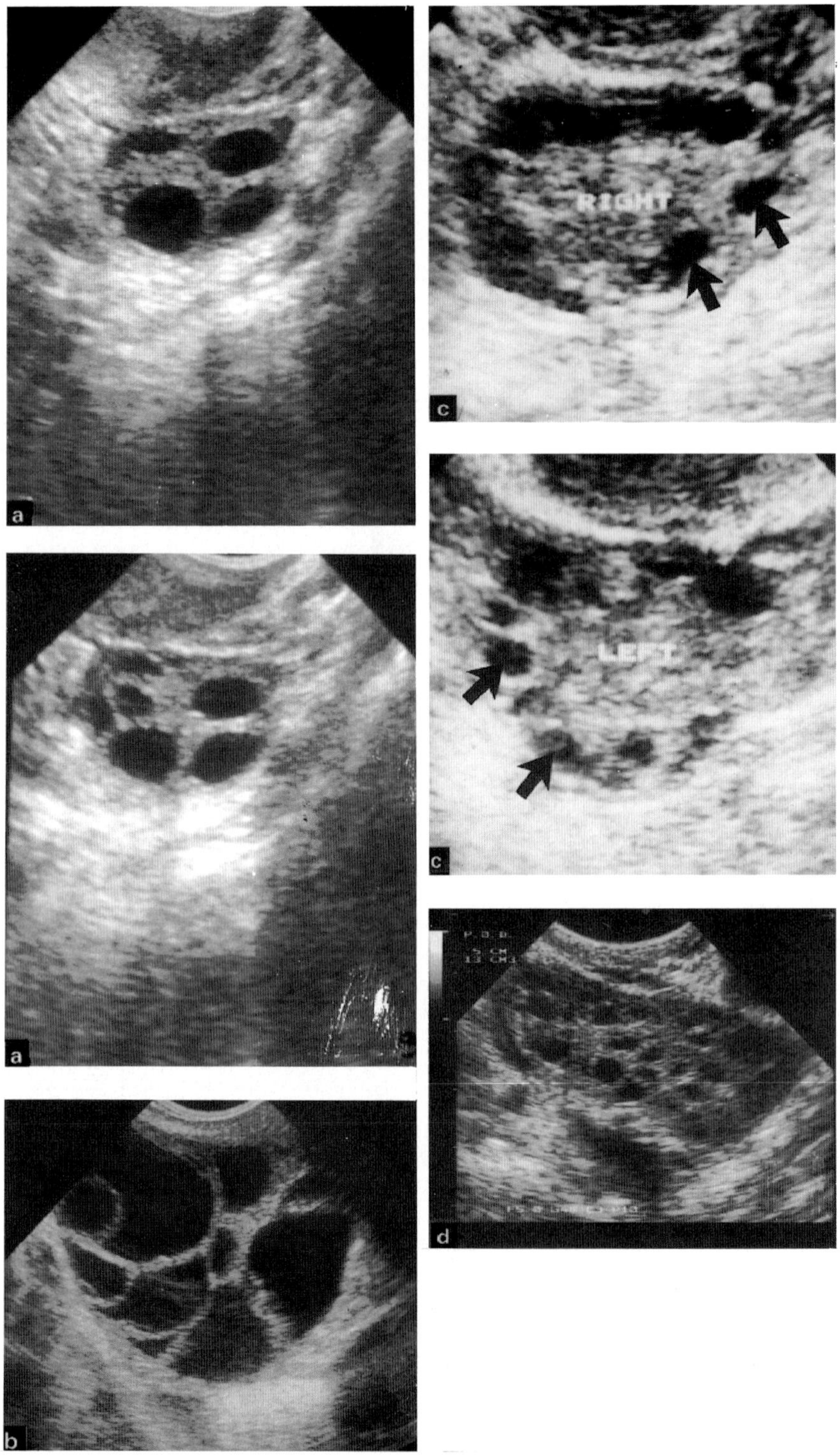

Figure 1 (a) Normal ovaries which contain functional follicular cysts; (b) hyperstimulated ovary, with large cysts and decreased stroma; (c) polycystic ovaries, with multiple small cysts near the periphery (arrows); (d) polycystic ovaries with cysts dispersed throughout the parenchyma

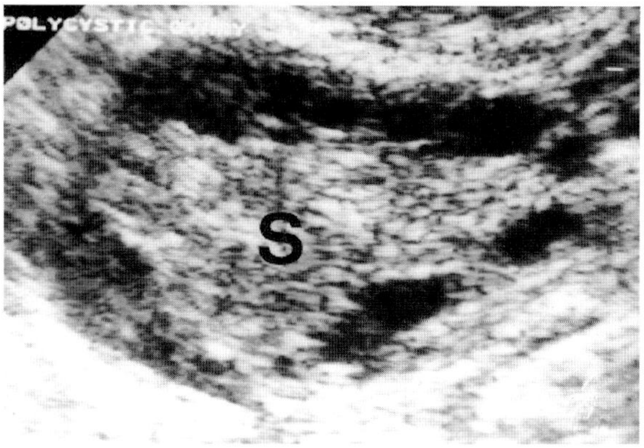

Figure 2 Polycystic ovary with high-density stroma (S)

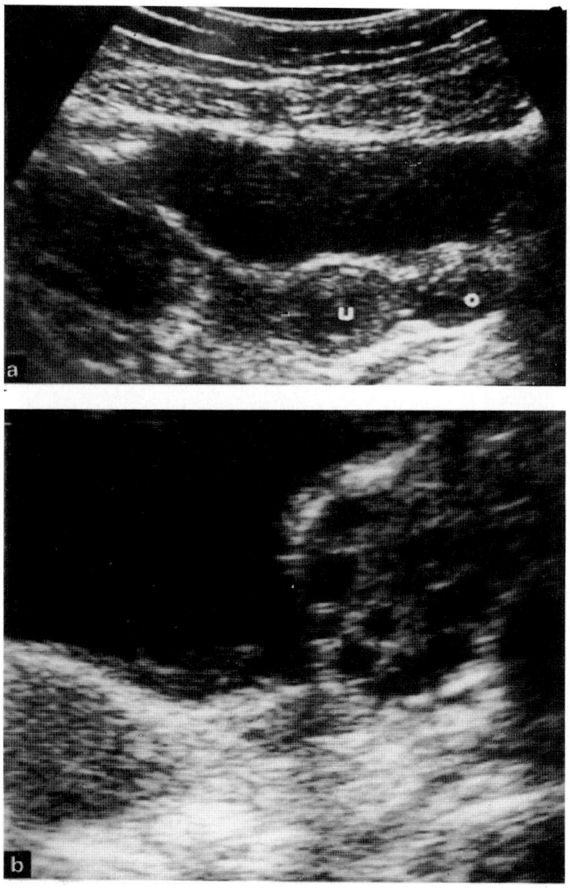

Figure 3 Transabdominal ultrasound scans; (a) poor image quality; (b) distortion due to full bladder

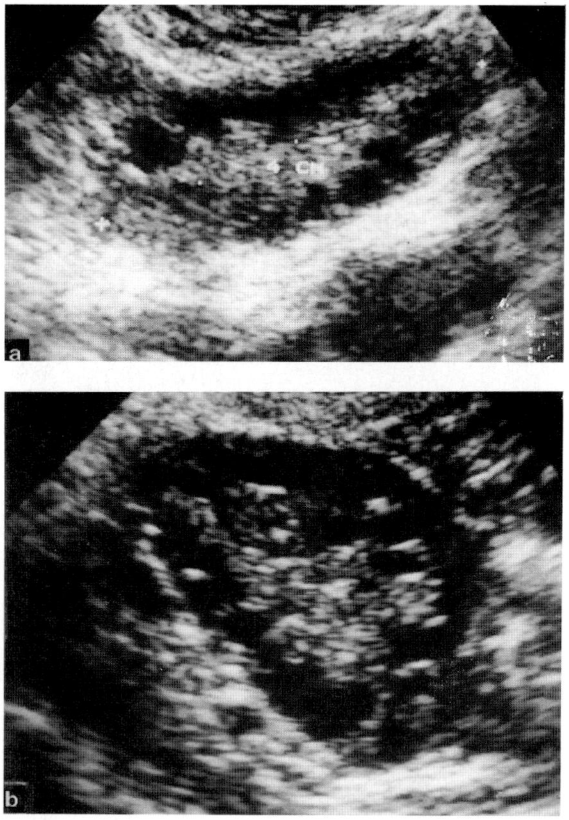

Figure 4 Polycystic ovaries. Note the different shapes (a, b)

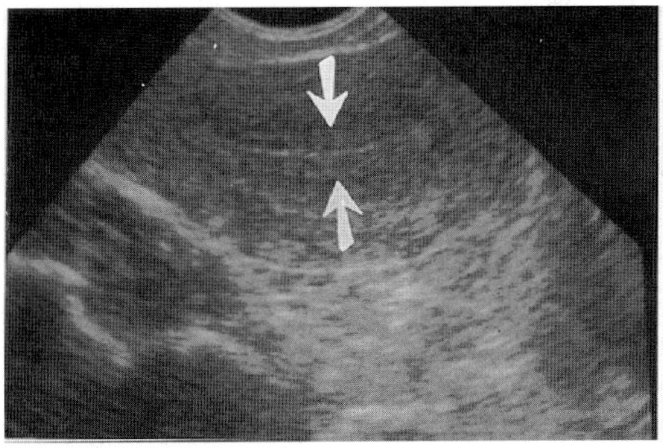

Figure 5 Thickened endometrium (arrows) in polycystic ovarian syndrome

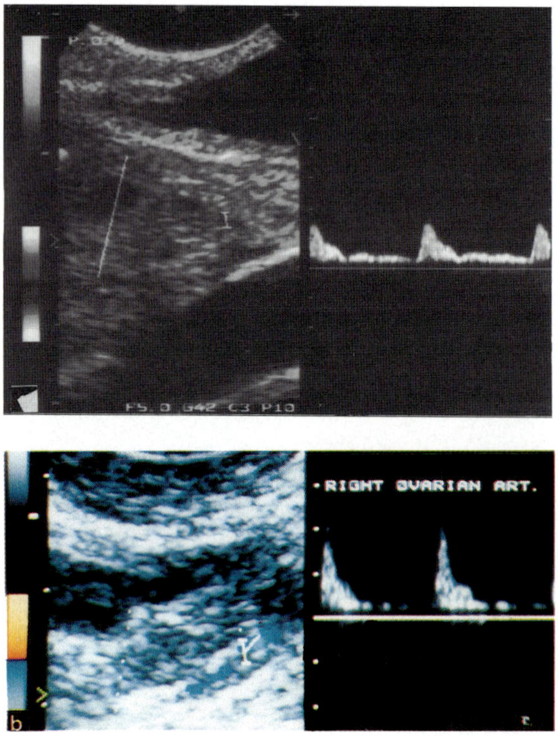

Figure 6 Transvaginal color Doppler blood flow evaluation of the ovarian (a) and stromal (b) arteries in polycystic ovarian syndrome

and the assessment of the relationships between alterations in these patterns and the normal and abnormal ovarian and uterine functions[47,48]. All of the major pelvic vessels have characteristic 'waveform signatures'[48] (Figure 6). Ovarian blood flow patterns change during the normal menstrual cycle as reported in the literature[49–53]. In the proliferative phase a high resistance flow is seen. On the other hand, in the secretory phase a low resistance blood flow is observed in the artery supplying the corpus luteum[51–53]. This postovulatory profile can also be found very soon after successful fertilization and during the first weeks of pregnancy[54,55].

Color Doppler has also proved to facilitate the detection of small vascular areas in the ovarian stroma and it may eventually be used to quantify blood flow parameters in these vessels[52].

Perhaps, in the future, this technique may also be useful in the study of PCOS and also shed some light on its pathogenesis. What we have found so far with respect to the resistance indices of the ovarian artery and its branches in some of these patients (unpublished) appears to be quite interesting but requires further investigation. In the majority of cases with clinical, ultrasonographic and hormonal findings suggestive of the disease, we found a high resistance/low velocity pattern in both the ovarian and stromal arteries. However, in some of the cases that were followed longitudinally, high diastolic flow patterns were found. This could be due to a recent or imminent ovulation in a sporadic ovulatory cycle.

CONCLUSION

From all of these studies, we concluded that polycystic ovaries exist in many situations, and if looked for with the newer generation of ultrasound equipment, they may be seen in a high percentage of normal women.

The broadening of the criteria to consider, in classifying each case, has almost made this disease a non-disease. It is our belief that one should 'go back' and be very precise in the definition of the syndrome: anovulation is a necessary part of the definition and it must be proved, for example by progesterone determination around days 21–23 of the cycle. Since the finding is chronic in this syndrome, the evaluation should be repeated at least two or three times. The second most important demonstration is the existence of polycystic ovaries. This is where ultrasound is crucial. We suggest that increased ovarian volume is not necessary for the definition but instead, the number of small cysts and increased stromal density should be evaluated initially as well as the existence of normal (non-atrophic) endometrium, which is a sign of the existence of estrogens in appreciable quantities. Ultrasound evaluation should be performed in the follicular phase if it is not possible to perform repeated examinations at different times.

Perhaps PCOS is not a primary ovarian disease. The ovaries and ovarian functions are like a window that allows observation of a complex interior through its consequences.

Doppler blood flow evaluation of both ovarian and stromal arteries is still under investigation. These data must be correlated with the classical signs in an attempt to define the disease correctly.

After case selection, the hormonal alterations, metabolic factors and stressful events should be exhaustively looked for and studied in a strict chronobiological integration. Nothing is interpretable if one does not correctly analyse everything that surrounded it at the time it occurred. We also feel that prospective studies starting before adrenarche are very important so that the true primary event can be discovered.

Only after a concise definition of the typical syndrome can one look for variants; for example, one in which the ovaries are polycystic but ovulate; or one in which there are both anovulation and polycystic ovaries, but LH is not elevated; or one in which there is no hyperandrogenemia, or hyperinsulinemia; and so on.

Perhaps, we will then conclude that between normal women and those having PCOS there exists a continuum of clinical conditions that may be relevant to the understanding of female physiology, especially the hypothalamic–pituitary–ovarian axis and its relationship with the environment, nutrition, brain function, adrenal influences, and other factors.

ACKNOWLEDGEMENT

The authors wish to thank Dr Alice Coimbra Peixoto for her invaluable co-operation in the preparation of this chapter.

References

1. Mahesh, V., Greenblatt, R., Aydar, C., *et al.* (1962). Secretion of androgens by the polycystic ovary and its significance. *Fertil. Steril.*, **13**, 513
2. Kahn, C., Flier, J., Bar, R., *et al.* (1976). The syndromes of insulin resistance and acanthosis nigricans. *New Engl. J. Med.*, **294**, 739–45
3. Tucker, M., Adams, J., Mason, W. and Jacobs, H. (1984). Infertility, megalocystic and polycystic ovaries: differential response to LHRH therapy. *Ups. J. Med. Sci.*, **89**, 43–6
4. Adams, J., Franks, S., Polson, D., Mason, H., Abdulwahid, N., Tucker, M., Morris, D., Price, J. and Jacobs, H. (1985). Multifollicular ovaries: clinical and endocrine features and response to pulsatile GnRH. *Lancet*, **2**, 1375–8
5. Venturoli, S., Porcu, E., Fabbri, R., Paradisi, R., Gammi, L., Passarini, M., Orsini, L. and Flamigni, C. (1986). Ovarian multifollicularity, high LH and androgen plasma levels and anovulation are frequent and strongly linked in adolescent irregular cycles. *Acta Endocrinol.*, **111**, 368–72
6. Stein, I. and Leventhal, M. (1935). Amenorrhea associated with bilateral polycystic ovaries. *Am. J. Obstet. Gynecol.*, **29**, 181–91
7. Coney, P. (1984). PCOD: current concepts of pathophysiology and therapy. *Fertil. Steril.*, **42**, 667–82
8. Adams, J., Polson, D. and Franks, S. (1986). Prevalence of polycystic ovaries in women with anovulation and idiopathic hirsutism. *Br. Med. J.*, **293**, 355–9
9. Green, J. and Goldzieher, J. (1966). The polycystic ovary. IV. Light and electron microscope studies. *Am. J. Obstet. Gynecol.*, **91**, 173–81
10. Jaffe, R., Abramowicz, J., Eckstein, N., Vagman, I., Fejgin, M. and Ayalon, D. (1988). Sonographic monitoring of ovarian volume during LHRH analogue therapy in women with PCOS. *J. Ultrasound Med.*, **7**, 203–6
11. Di Carlo, C., Shoham, Z., MacDougall, J., Patel, A., Hall, M. and Jacobs, H. (1992). Polycystic ovaries as a relative protective factor for bone mineral loss in young women with amenorrhea. *Fertil. Steril.*, **57**, 314–19
12. Pignatelli, D. and Beires, J. (1990). A comparison of echographic and hormonal studies in PCOS and in normal females. *J. Endocrinol. Invest.*, **13** (Suppl. 2), 214
13. Polson, D., Wadsworth, J., Adams, J. and Franks, S. (1988). Polycystic ovaries – a common finding in normal women. *Lancet*, **1**, 870–2
14. Rebar, R., Judd, H., Yen, S., Rakoff, J., Vandenberg, G. and Naftolin, F. (1976). Characterization of the inappropriate gonadotropin secretion in polycystic ovary syndrome. *J. Clin. Invest.*, **57**, 1320–9
15. Mckenna, T. (1988). Pathogenesis and treatment of polycystic ovary syndrome. *N. Engl. J. Med.*, **318**, 558–62
16. Yen, S., Vela, P. and Rankin, J. (1970). Inappropriate secretion of FSH and LH in PCOD. *J. Clin. Endocrinol.*, **30**, 435–42
17. Hull, M. (1987). Epidemiology of infertility and PCOD: endocrinological and demographic studies. *Gynecol. Endocrinol.*, **1**, 235–45
18. Lobo, R. (1989). Androgen excess in women. In Soules, M. (ed.) *Controversies in Reproductive Endocrinology and Infertility*, p. 59–77. (New York: Elsevier)

19. Goldzieher, J. (1981). Polycystic ovarian disease. *Fertil. Steril.*, **35**, 371–94
20. Seibel, M. (1984). Towards understanding the pathophysiology and treatment of PCOD. *Semin. Reprod. Endocrinol.*, **2**, 3
21. Barbieri, R., Makris, A., Randall, R., Daniels, G., Kistner, R. and Ryan, K. (1986). Insulin stimulates androgen accumulation in incubations of ovarian stroma obtained from women with hyperandrogenism. *J. Clin. Endrocrinol. Metab.*, **62**, 904–10
22. Mckenna, T., Moore, A., Magee, F. and Cunningham, S. (1983). Amenorrhea with cryptic hyperandrogenemia. *J. Clin. Endocrinol. Metab.*, **56**, 893–6
23. McNatty, K., Moore-Smith, D., Makris, A., Osathanondh, R. and Ryan, K. (1979). The microenvironment of the human antral follicle: interrelationships among the steroid levels in antral fluid, the population of granulosa cells and the status of oocyte *in vivo* and *in vitro*. *J. Clin. Endocrinol. Metab.*, **49**, 851–60
24. Erickson, G. (1982). Follicular maturation and atresia. In Flamigni, C. and Givens, J. (eds.) *The Gonadotropins: Basic Science and Clinical Aspects in Females*, p. 177–85. (London: Academic Press)
25. Erickson, G., Hsueh, A., Quigley, M., Rebar, R. and Yen, S. (1979). Functional studies of aromatase activity in human granulosa cells from normal and polycystic ovaries. *J. Clin. Endocrinol. Metab.*, **49**, 514–19
26. Goldzieher, J. and Green, J. (1962). The polycystic ovary. Clinical and histological features. *J. Clin. Endocrinol. Metab.*, **22**, 325–38
27. Laatikainen, T., Apter, D., Paavonen, J. and Wahlstrom, T. (1980). Steroids in ovarian and peripheral venous blood in PCOD. *Clin. Endocrinol.*, **13**, 125–34
28. Anderson, D. (1974). SHBG. *Clin. Endocrinol.*, **3**, 69–96
29. Lobo, R., Granger, L., Goebelsmann, U. and Mishell Jr, D. (1981). Elevation of unbound serum estradiol as a possible mechanism for inappropriate gonadotropin secretion in women with PCO. *J. Clin. Endocrinol. Metab.*, **52**, 156–8
30. Yen, S. (1980). The polycystic ovary syndrome. *Clin. Endocrinol.*, **12**, 177–207
31. Kratochwil, A., Urban, G. and Friedrich, F. (1972). Ultrasonic tomography of the ovaries. *Ann. Chir. Gynaecol.*, **61**, 211–14
32. Swanson, M., Sauerbrei, E. and Cooperberg, P. (1981). Medical implications of ultrasonically detected polycystic ovaries. *J. Clin. Ultrasound*, **9**, 219–22
33. Hann, L., Hall, D., McArdle, C. and Seibel, M. (1984). Polycystic ovarian disease: sonographic spectrum. *Radiology*, **150**, 531–4
34. Nicolini, U., Ferrazzi, E., Bellotti, M., Travaglini, P., Elli, R. and Scaperrota, R. (1985). The contribution of sonographic evaluation of the ovarian size in patients with PCOD. *J. Ultrasound Med.*, **4**, 347–51
35. Yeh, H., Futterweit, W. and Thornton, J. (1987). PCOD: ultrasonographic features in 104 patients. *Radiology*, **163**, 111–16
36. Comparetto, G., Gullo, D., Venezia, R. and Mogavero, G. (1982). Proposal for a purely echographic classification of the PCOS. *Acta Steril. Fertil.*, **13**, 79–94
37. Orsini, H., Venturoli, S., Lorusso, R., Pluchinotta, Y., Paradisi, R. and Bovicelli, L. (1985). Ultrasonic findings in polycystic ovarian disease. *Fertil. Steril.*, **43**, 709
38. Grant, E. (1992). Benign conditions of the ovaries. In Nyberg, D., Hill, L., Bohm-Vélez, M. and Mendelson, E. (eds.). *Transvaginal Ultrasound*, pp. 187–207. (St Louis: Mosby Year Book)
39. Merril, J. (1963). The morphology of the prepubertal ovary. *South. Med. J.*, **56**, 225–31
40. Hall, D., Hann, L., Ferruci, J., Black, E., Braitman, B., Cowley, W., Nikoui, N. and Kelley, J. (1979). Sonographic morphology of the normal menstrual cycle. *Radiology*, **133**, 185–7
41. Parisi, L., Tramonti, M., Casciano, S., Zuvli, A. and Gazzarrini, O. (1982). The role of ultrasound in the study of PCOD. *J. Clin. Ultrasound*, **10**, 167–72
42. Venturoli, S., Paradisi, R., Sabiotti, E., Barnabé, S., Porcu, E., Fabbri, R. and Flamigni, C. (1983). Ultrasound study of ovarian morphology in women with PCOS before and during treatment with an oestrogen/progestagen preparation. *Arch. Gynecol.*, **234**, 87–93
43. Cano, A., Bonilla-Musoles, F. and Millet, A. (1992). El ovario poliquístico. In Bonilla-Musoles, F. (ed.) *Tratado de Endosonografia en Obstetricia y Ginecología*, pp. 231–48. (Barcelona: Ediciones Cientificas y Técnicas)
44. Kurjak, A. and Jurkovic, D. (1987). The value of ultrasound in the initial assessment of gynecological patients. *Ultrasound Med. Biol.*, **13**, 401–19
45. Pache, T., Hop, W., Wladimiroff, J., Schipper, J. and Fauser, B. (1991). Transvaginal sonography and abnormal ovarian appearance in menstrual cycle disturbances. *Ultrasound Med. Biol.*, **17**, 589–93
46. Fleischer, A. (1991). Ultrasound imaging – 2000: assessment of utero-vaginal blood flow with transvaginal color Doppler sonography; potential clinical applications in infertility. *Fertil. Steril.*, **55**, 684–91
47. Kurjak, A., Zalud, I., Jurkovic, D., Alfirevic, Z. and Miljan, M. (1989). Transvaginal color Doppler for the assessment of pelvic circulation. *Acta Obstet. Gynecol. Scand.*, **68**, 131–5
48. Bourne, T. (1991). Transvaginal color Doppler in gynecology. *Ultrasound Obstet. Gynecol*, **1**, 359–73
49. Scholtes, M., Wladmiroff, Y., Van Rijen, H. and

Hop, W. (1989). Uterine and ovarian flow wave forms in the normal menstrual cycle: a transvaginal Doppler study. *Fertil. Steril.*, **52**, 981–5

50. Steer, C., Campbell, S., Pampiglione, J., Kingsland, C., Mason, B. and Collins, W. (1990). Transvaginal color flow imaging of the uterine arteries during the ovarian and menstrual cycles. *Hum. Reprod.*, **5**, 391–5
51. Hata, K., Hata, T., Senoh, D., Makihara, K., Aoki, S., Takamiya, O. and Kitao, M. (1990). Change in ovarian arterial compliance during the human menstrual cycle by Doppler ultrasound. *Br. J. Obstet. Gynaecol.*, **97**, 163–6
52. Mercé, L., Garcés, D., Barco, M. and De La Fuente, F. (1992). Intraovarian Doppler velocimetry in ovulatory, dysovulatory and anovulatory cycles. *Ultrasound Obstet. Gynecol.*, **2**, 197–202
53. Sladkevicius, P., Valentin, L. and Marsal, K. (1993). Blood flow velocity in the uterine and ovarian arteries during the normal menstrual cycle. *Ultrasound Obstet. Gynecol.*, **3**, 199–208
54. Schaaps, J. and Soyeur, D. (1989). Pulsed Doppler on a vaginal probe. *J. Ultrasound Med.*, **8**, 315–20
55. Montenegro, N., Beires, J. and Carrera, J. (1993). Quantitative and combined color Doppler and hormonal assessment of the first trimester pregnancy. In Kurjak, A. (ed.) *Transvaginal Color Doppler*, 2nd edn., pp. 95–104. (Carnforth, UK: Parthenon Publishing)

Normal and abnormal ovarian circulation

14

S. Kupesic and A. Kurjak

Over the last 5 years there has been a large increase in the number of studies on the normal and abnormal ovarian vascularity. Transvaginal color Doppler opened up exciting new possibilities for better understanding of the physiology and pathophysiology of ovarian blood flow, resulting in a number of completely new diagnostic parameters. This chapter will investigate the relationship between ovarian vascularity and ovarian perfusion in normal cycling women and patients with benign, borderline and malignant gynecological tumors. Finally, the vexed question of the role of color Doppler in the assessment of ovarian circulation will be addressed.

OVARIAN VASCULAR ANATOMY

For adequate application of Doppler technology in studies on hemodynamics, it is important to be familiar with the vascular anatomy of the ovary, which consists of an arterial, venous and lymphatic system. Although the near future may render the Doppler assessment of the lymphatic system possible, it is not so at the moment. Similarly, evaluation of the venous flow is feasible, but the technique has not been standardized. Therefore, the first objective of our research is to study arterial anatomy and blood flow changes which reflect functional activity and pathological circumstances in the most intensive form.

The ovarian vascular system can be divided into extrinsic and intrinsic vascular systems. The extrinsic vascular system consists of arteries that start from big abdominal trunks before they enter into the ovary and the homologous venous system. The intrinsic vascular system is formed by vessels which enter into the gland from the ovarian hilus, giving rise to the microcirculation and posteriorly causing venous drainage[1]. Although we are dealing with a topographical division, as the adjacent systems together constitute one vascular system, it is interesting from a functional point of view. The cyclic changes of ovarian vascularization are manifest most intensively in the intrinsic vascular system.

Extrinsic vascular system

The pattern of the ovarian blood supply is similar in all mammals, although it grows more complex closer to the top of the phylogenetic scale[1]. The extrinsic vascular system of the human ovary is shown in Figure 1.

Arteries

The ovary receives its arterial vascularization from two sources: the ovarian artery and the utero-ovarian branch of the uterine artery[2]. These arteries anastomose, forming an arch parallel to the ovarian hilus, and constitute the vascular genital arcade. The ovarian artery emerges from the abdominal aorta beneath renal arteries. From there, it obliquely descends and, crossing the ureter and iliac vessels, enters into the infundibulopelvic ligament. The artery approaches the ovary at its upper pole. At this level, the external tubarian artery, which does not participate in the vascularization of the ovary, branches off. The other artery involved in blood perfusion of the ovary is the utero-ovarian. This artery begins from the uterine artery at the altitude of the uterine horn and goes to the lower pole of the ovary. Both arteries anastomose directly or through branches which enter into the ovary by the front or the ovarian hilus. Although embryological evolution apparently demonstrates that the principal share of blood in the ovary originates

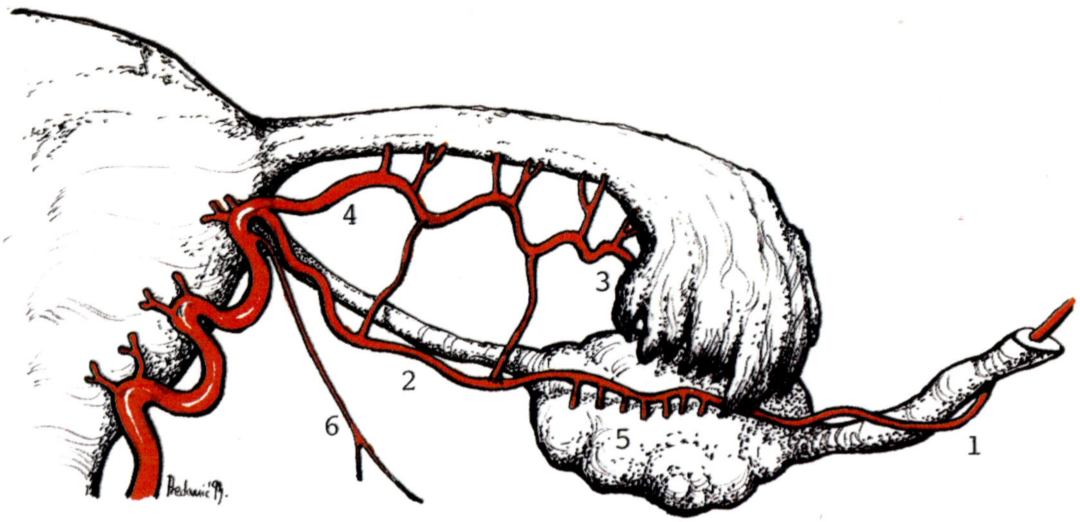

Figure 1 Extrinsic vascular system of the ovary. 1, ovarian artery; 2, utero-ovarian artery; 3, external tubarian artery; 4, internal tubarian artery; 5, ovarian branches in the hilus of the ovary; 6, artery of the round liagment

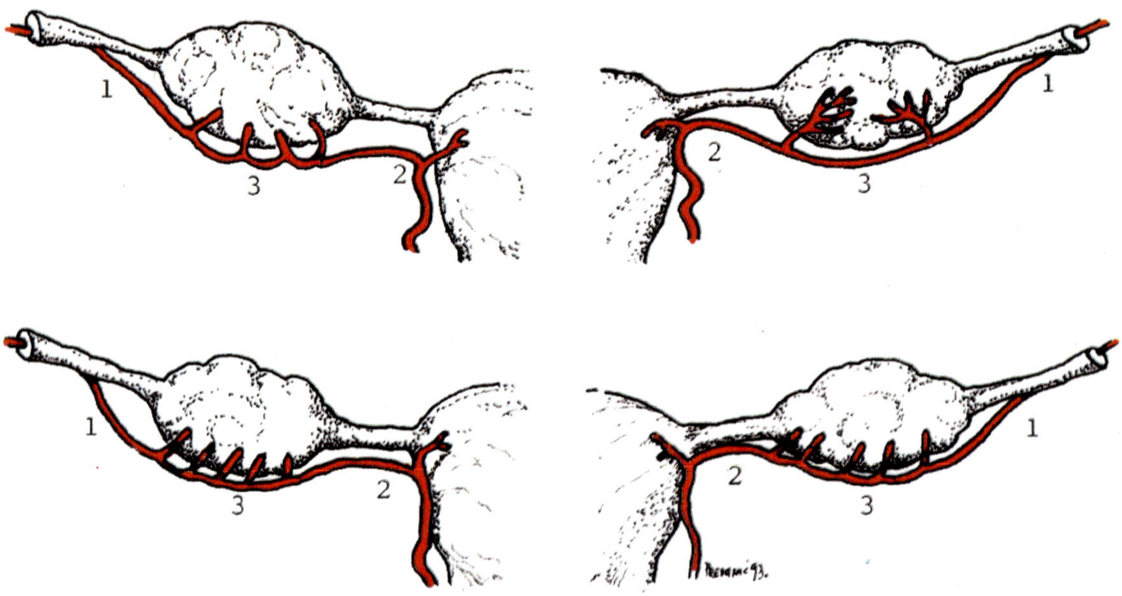

Figure 2 Topographic types of anastomoses between ovarian and utero-ovarian arteries. 1, ovarian artery; 2, utero-ovarian artery; 3, ovarian branches

from the ovarian artery, the importance of supply by the utero-ovarian artery seems to be related to the type of anastomosis. Topographically, between two arteries, four types of anastomoses are observed, with equal or dominant participation of one of them (Figure 2).

Veins

Ovarian veins leave the ovary at the level of the hilus, giving rise to the pampiniform plexus, with its many characteristic interconnections. Anastomosing with veins coming from the uterus, it forms a utero-ovarian vein, consisting of two canals, interconnected by numerous anastomoses[3]. Both canals ascend to the abdomen and end by joining together into a single utero-ovarian vein, opening on the left to the renal vein, and on the right to the vena cava.

Intrinsic vascular system (microcirculation)

The ovary has an arterial supply known for its special pattern and obvious functional changes. From the ovarian hilus, arterial branches penetrate the stroma[1] and acquire a tortuous and helicoid pathway (they roll up round their own axis). For such a special pattern, they are named spiral or helical arteries. Getting further into the ovarian stroma, spiral arteries divide more and more and become progressively smaller in diameter. In the cortical zone, the diameter becomes 40–60 μm and, dividing at a right or sharp angle from the principal branch, they successively form arterioles of the first capillary system[3]. The abundance of spiral arteries in the ovarian stroma constitutes an authentic medulla at this stage[1]. The arterial system drains by the agency of a venous system rolled up into a ball, with a diameter larger than that of the arteries (80 μm), called the ovarian bulb.

The spiral pattern of the ovarian arteries plays an important role in the hemodynamics and cyclic structural adaptation of the ovary. The helicoid pathway of the arteries enlarges the surface of friction as blood flows through, increasing resistance and lowering blood pressure, which is necessary to contain the elevated pressure at the entrance of the ovarian artery[1]. An arterial pattern of this kind generates a centrifugal force, rather than a blood circulation which has turbulations in the system. Angular bifurcation of the arterioles contributes to the stability of the flow with minimum energetic waste. Finally, such a structure facilitates accommodation to changes in size, due to development of the follicle and the corpus luteum. When they grow, arteries unwind and become larger, returning to the basal state during follicular atresia or luteal regression[4]. This is vitally important for the understanding of changes in intraovarian Doppler velocimetry.

PHYSICAL PRINCIPLES

Ultrasound imaging has provided a unique method for the non-invasive study of ovarian structural changes. The measurement of blood flow velocity by ultrasound is based on the Doppler effect, which is named after the Austrian physicist Christian Johann Doppler (1803–53). The Doppler effect implies that the frequency of a sound wave emitted from a stationary source and reflected from a moving interface changes according to the velocity and direction of the moving interface[5]. Movements toward the source will increase the frequency of the reflected waves, and movements away from the source will decrease it. The changes of frequency are directly proportional to the velocity of the moving interface. This change of frequency is called the Doppler shift, F. If the ultrasound beam is sent towards a blood vessel, the moving erythrocytes will act as reflectors and cause a change of the reflected sound frequency. The Doppler shift is described by the standard equation:

$$F_D = 2F_0 v \cos\theta / c$$

where v = velocity of the reflector, F_0 = frequency of the emitted sound, c = velocity of ultrasound in the medium, and θ = angle between the insonating sound wave and the direction of the moving reflector.

The Doppler effect can be used to measure mean blood velocity across a vessel area. With two-dimensional ultrasound, all necessary information regarding the angle between the vessel direction and insonating sound and the diameter of the vessel can be obtained. Once the standard form of the Doppler equation is used for quantification of blood volume, the total rate of blood flow in the vessel can be calculated easily by multiplying the average velocity by the cross-sectional area of the vessel:

$$Q = vr^2 / \cos\theta$$

where Q = blood-flow volume, v = mean blood velocity over the vessel cross-sectional area, r = vessel radius, and θ = angle of approach of the Doppler beam to the vessel.

However, quantification of the blood flow can be performed only in the vessels that are demonstrated by ultrasound. The analysis of the blood flow in thin non-visualized vessels can be based on blood flow velocity waveform analysis. Velocity waveform shows the frequency shift vs. time. It represents maximum Doppler shifts throughout the cardiac cycle, thus reflecting the pulsatile nature of blood flow in arterial vessels. Analysis of flow velocity is an alternative method of blood flow assessment. The major advantage of this analysis is angle-independence and there is no need for simultaneous vessel visualization and diameter measurement. More than ten indices have been used for velocity waveform analysis. The A/B ratio, resistance index (RI) and pulsatility index (PI) are predominantly used:

A/B ratio $= A/B$ (peak systole/end diastole)
RI $= (A-B)/A$ ((peak systole − end diastole)/peak systole)
PI $= (A-B)/\text{mean}$ ((peak systole − end diastole)/mean frequency)

Doppler ultrasound has the potential to study patterns of ovarian blood flow and hence identify functional changes[6]. Until recently the use of this method for examination of flow in specific deep vessels has been difficult, since conventional continuous-waveform meters provide confusing signals from flow or tissue movements occurring anywhere along the entire length of the ultrasound beam. The availability of pulsed Doppler instruments has made it possible to sample the signals at a chosen depth and thus to detect flow in any selected deep vessel. Pulsed Doppler combined with real-time ultrasound imaging, the so-called 'duplex' method, allows the precise localization of a deep vessel and positioning of the Doppler sample volume within it[7]. Furthermore, recent technological advances have resulted in transvaginal color Doppler. The system uses pulsed Doppler which performs flow analysis at multiple points along each scan line of echo data[8,9]. Flow information is then color-coded and displayed on an entire corresponding 2-dimensional image. The main advantages of the color system are rapid and definitive determination of the position of small and tortuous normal and newly formed vessels, accuracy of the measurement and precise indication of flow direction and velocity. Red indicates flow towards the transducer, and blue away from the transducer. The brightness of the color is proportional to the velocity of flow within the vessel, whilst turbulent flow may appear as various shades of green. After simultaneous visualization of morphological and blood flow information, a pulsed Doppler range gate is placed over the area of interest to provide flow velocity waveforms which may be analyzed in a conventional fashion.

This new modality carries many safety advantages when compared to the use of transvaginal pulsed Doppler alone[10]. By reducing the time required to find and sample a vessel, the total exposure of the area of interest to ultrasound should be reduced.

COLOR DOPPLER VELOCIMETRY OF THE OVARY

Ovarian artery

The ovarian artery is a tributary of the upper aorta and reaches the lateral aspect of the ovary through the infundibulopelvic ligament[1]. In some patients, these vessels are not clearly visualized and the sample volume should be moved across the ligament and then through the substance of the ovary until the arterial signal is identified. Signals from the ovarian artery are characterized by the low Doppler shifts of a small vessel with low velocity (Figure 3). The waveform shape varies

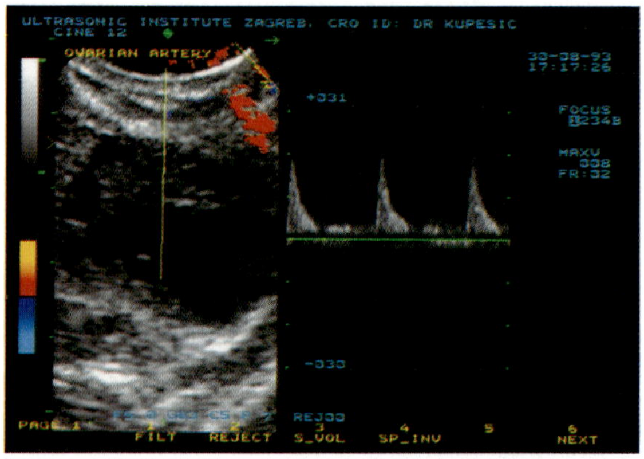

Figure 3 Flow velocity waveforms obtained from ovarian artery during the early proliferative phase of the menstrual cycle

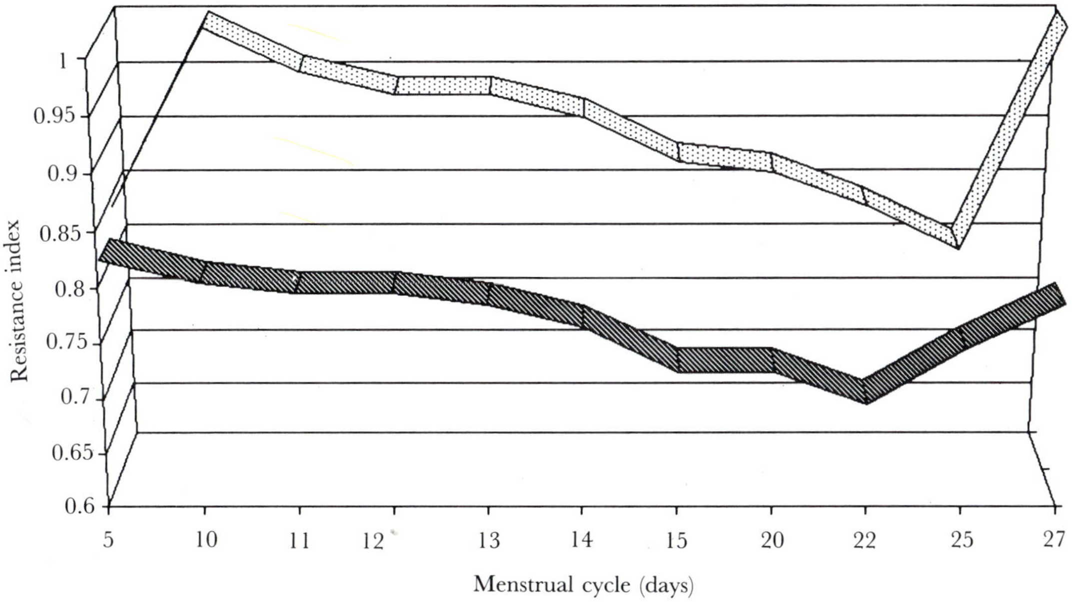

Figure 4 Ovarian artery flow velocity. Resistance index of the 'active' ovary (dark line) and 'inactive' ovary (light line)

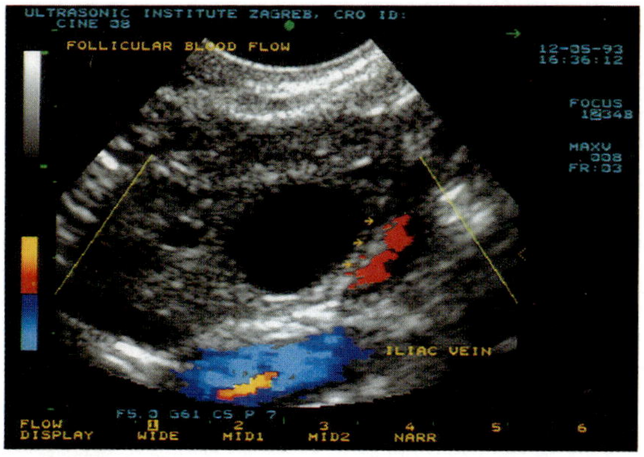

Figure 5 Transvaginal scan demonstrating a ring of angiogenesis around the follicle during the moment of presumed ovulation

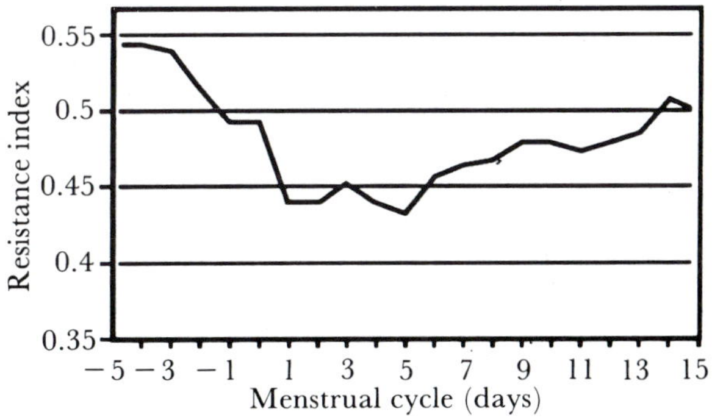

Figure 6 Intraovarian flow velocity

with the state of activity of the ovary. Studies of ovarian artery blood flow velocity waveforms show the difference in the vascular impedance between the two ovarian arteries depending on the presence of the dominant follicle or corpus luteum[11,12]. A longitudinal study of the ovarian artery over the ovarian cycle performed at the Ultrasonic Institute, University of Zagreb, suggested decreased pulsatility and resistance indices, reflecting vascular impedance and implying increased flow to the ovary containing the dominant follicle or corpus luteum. The ovarian artery of the 'inactive' ovary showed low end-diastolic flow or absence of diastolic flow. A rise in end-diastolic flow velocity of the 'active' ovary is most obvious on day 21 and suggests that the corpus luteum acts as a low impedance shunt (Figure 4). The increased blood supply to the functioning corpus luteum is essential for delivery of precursors involved in steroidogenesis and for removal of progesterone[13–15].

Various invasive and non-invasive techniques

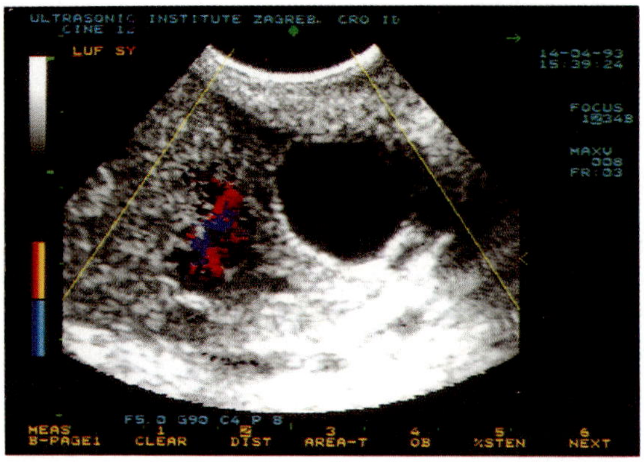

Figure 7 A mature ovarian follicle seen on the left ovary on day 14 of the menstrual cycle. The same finding persisted for a few days and a diagnosis of luteinized unruptured follicle syndrome (LUF SY) was made

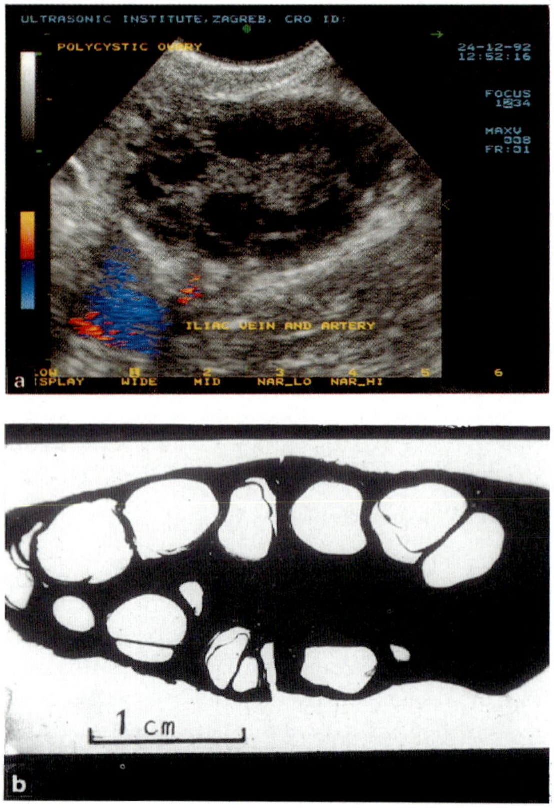

Figure 8 Polycystic ovary. (a) Transvaginal sonogram. A large number of small cystic structures are 'crowded' and stand out from the surface of the enlarged ovarian stroma; (b) histopathological finding

of ovarian blood flow measurement in mammals have been used, including microspheres[13], direct blood collection[16], and implantation of Doppler flow meters[17] and electromagnetic flow meters in cows[14]. These techniques have shown that 80–90% of the blood flow to the ovary is supplied to the corpus luteum[18]. A rapid decrease in ovarian blood flow accompanying luteolysis is noticed in animal models[16]. Prostaglandin $F_{2\alpha}$ is reported to be the active luteolysin, and a reduction of 90% in luteal flow has been reported following its local administration[19]. Patients treated with clomiphene citrate and/or human menopausal gonadotropin at our Institute typically developed multiple follicles bilaterally and both ovarian arteries showed low pulsatility waveforms typical of low impedance.

If pregnancy occurs, the corpus luteum maintains its function for the first trimester of pregnancy and the active waveforms persist during this period. Pregnancy is known to be dependent on a functioning corpus luteum, and Doppler ultrasound is a good means by which to identify this activity. The important clinical applications that follow from this statement are considered further in this chapter.

Intraovarian blood flow

The ovarian artery is a high-pressure system with flow velocity waveforms totally different from intraovarian waveforms. Near the ovarian hilus the penetration vessels are coiled and tortuous. This type of vascularity demonstrates high-resistance blood flow.

The fundamental unit of the ovary is the follicle, which consists of the female germ cell (oocyte) surrounded by a series of specialized cell layers, the granulosa and theca cells. Every month during the woman's reproductive life, one oocyte is released from the single mature follicle that has completed development. A number of biochemical, morphological and vascular changes occur with the cells during this process and a significant proportion of them can be studied by color Doppler. With this modality, areas of vascularity on the follicular rim can be detected when the dominant follicle reaches 10 mm in diameter (Figure 5). The RI is around 0.54 while ovulation approaches (Figure 6). A decline begins 2 days before ovulation and reaches its nadir at ovulation (0.44 ± 0.04)[20]. The increase in the peak systolic blood velocity within the follicle in the presence of a relatively constant RI is a particularly interesting finding that might herald impending ovulation. Increased vascularity on the innermost rim of the follicle[21] may represent the dilatation of new vessels that have developed between the relatively vascular theca cell layer and the normally hypoxic granulosa cell layer of the follicle. Disruption of these vascular changes has profound effects on the oxygen concentration across the follicular epithelium[22,23]. It is hoped that information on ovarian perfusion may be used both to predict ovulation, and to investigate ovulatory dysfunction. We have observed twelve cases of luteinized unruptured follicles with a failure of the peak blood velocity in the preovulatory period (Figure 7). These data support the hypothesis that changes in oxygen tension within the follicular wall are necessary for follicular rupture[21–23]. If the process of oogenesis or ovulation can be inhibited independently from the main pathways of steroidogenesis, then novel methods of avoiding conception may be advised. Steroids that inhibit angiogenesis in the presence of heparin have already been identified[24]. It is apparent that transvaginal sonography with color Doppler facilities can be used to monitor the progress towards these novel contraceptive methods.

The same modality can follow changes of the intraovarian circulatory network in patients with polycystic ovarian syndrome (Figure 8). In a study of 34 oligo- or amenorrheic women with bilaterally increased ovarian volume, thickened ovarian capsule and numerous cystic structures measuring 2–8 mm in diameter, hormonal parameters (LH/FSH ratio > 3, increased androgen level) and intraovarian blood flow were measured. We found no changes in resistance indices of the ovarian arteries and intraovarian parenchymal vessels during the menstrual cycle. High diastolic flow patterns were followed continuously from the ovarian stroma, resulting in the mean resistance index of 0.54. These vascular changes are the possible effect of local hyperandrogenism and/or LH stimulus to (vascular) theca cells.

Color flow is more easily obtainable from ovarian tissue in the luteal phase. The qualitative postovulatory changes in intraovarian flow velocity waveforms are exciting: increased turbulent flow accompanying morphological changes in the intraovarian vascular network[25] and the appearance of numerous arteriovenous shunts during the luteal phase[26] (Figure 9). After ovulation, the RI shows a significant difference from the preovulatory values. Each woman with documented ovulation showed an RI of 0.43 ± 0.04 shortly after ovulation (Figure 10). The RI remained at the low level for 4 to 5 days and then gradually climbed to a value of 0.50, still lower than that seen in the early follicular phase (Figure 6). Luteal conversion can be detected in all the normal ovulatory cycles[20], independently of the corpus luteum identification. Converted blood flow signals are maintained throughout the luteal phase and are not observed on the non-dominant side, or in the patients with anovulatory cycles or luteinized unruptured follicles[27].

Therefore, changes in the intraovarian flow velocity occur before ovulation, implying a complexity of these changes that may involve both angiogenesis and hormonal factors, while postovulatory vascular accommodation is potentially important in the luteal phase. Using transvaginal color Doppler, corpus luteum blood flow, characterized by low impedance and high flow requirements, can easily be detected in normal early pregnancy, ectopic pregnancy and non-pregnant women[28]. It is not clear currently whether inadequate vascularization plays a role in the luteal phase defect and whether luteal flow can be used as an accurate predictor for the evaluation of normal and pathological pregnancy (Figure 11). An interested reader can find more about intraovarian flow in the luteal phase in the chapter on the corpus luteum.

ANGIOGENESIS AND NEOVASCULARIZATION

It was long believed that simple dilatation of existing host blood vessels accounted for increased tumor vascularity[29]. Vasodilatation was generally thought to be a 'side-effect' of tumor metabolites or of necrotic tumor products escaping from the tumor. However, some authors suggested that the

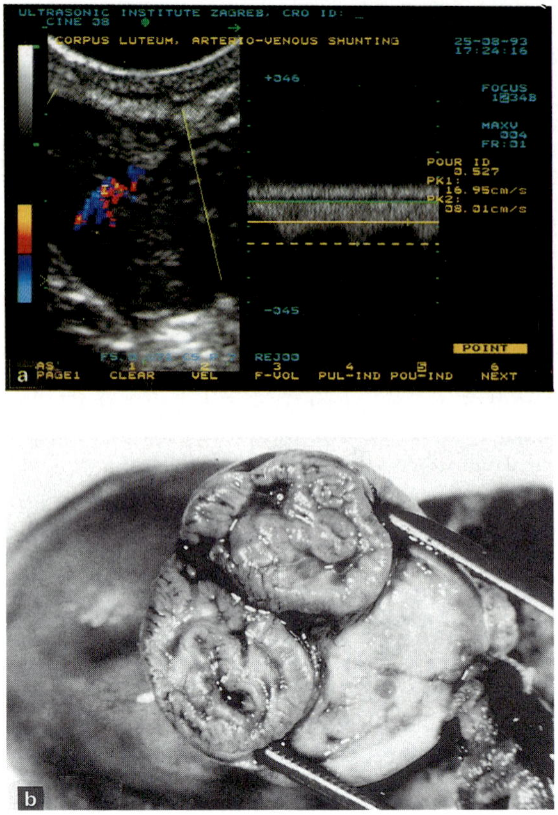

Figure 9 Increased vascularity in the corpus luteum. (a) Transvaginal color Doppler; (b) pathological finding

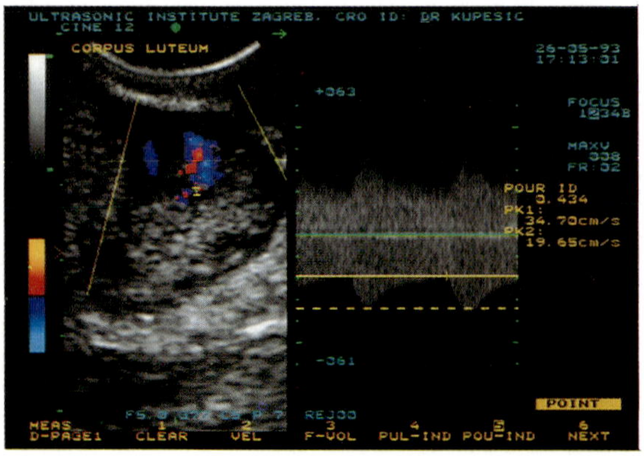

Figure 10 High blood velocity and decreased resistance index represent typical signs of ovulation and early corpus luteum blood flow (right)

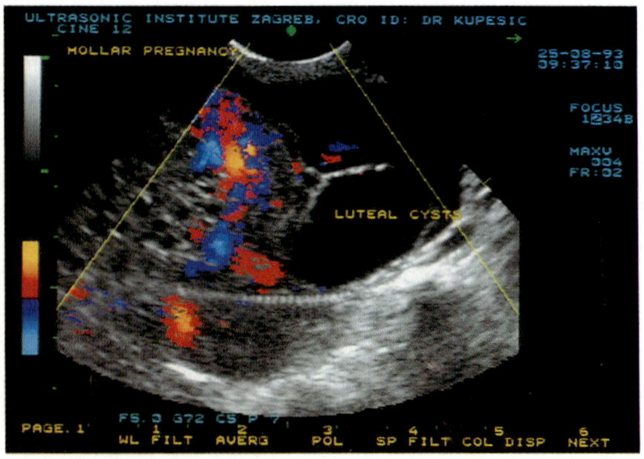

Figure 11 'Hot' areas inside the uterine cavity represent hydatidiform mole. Note luteal cysts of the left ovary with intensive flow in septum

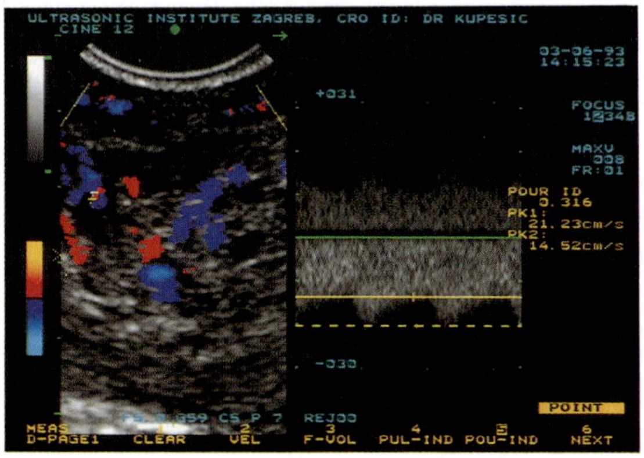

Figure 12 Tumor vasculature seen by transvaginal color Doppler. Pulsed Doppler analysis (right) shows increased diastolic flow and low-resistance blood flow (resistance index = 0.31)

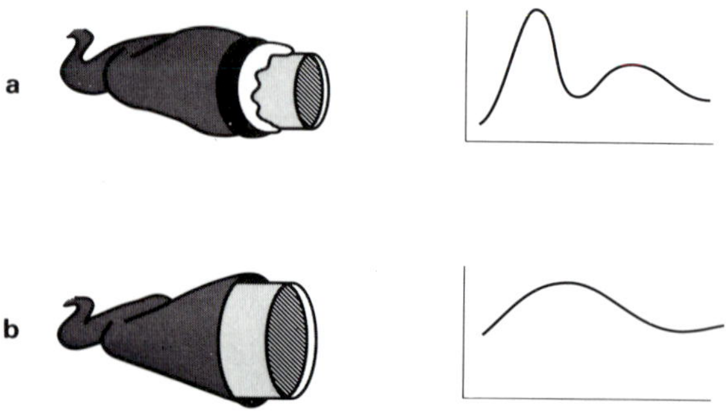

Figure 13 Diagram demonstrating typical Doppler waveforms. (a) Artery (contains muscular tissue). Note high-impedance blood flow and a diastolic notch; (b) tumor vessel (has a paucity or lack of muscular media). Note low-impedance blood flow and lack of a notch

tumor hyperemia could be related to new blood vessel growth. A report published in 1945 revealed that new vessels in the neighborhood of a tumor implant arose from host vessels and not from the tumor itself[30]. After that report, the debate continued in the literature for two more decades about whether tumors were supplied by existing vessels or by neovascularization[31–35].

Angiogenesis and neovascularization are terms that are entering the vocabulary of every ultrasonographer. Angiogenesis occurs during embryonic development and during several physiological and pathological conditions in adult life[36–38]. As mentioned before, angiogenesis is important in the process of ovulation and development of the corpus luteum. It accompanies numerous non-malignant diseases such as acute or chronic inflammation and ectopic pregnancy. However, tumor angiogenesis differs at least in a temporal manner from other types of angiogenesis described. In physiological conditions, angiogenesis is turned off once the process is completed. In non-malignant processes, angiogenesis is prolonged, but still self-limiting.

In contrast, tumor angiogenesis is not self-limiting[39]. Malignant tumor microvasculature does not conform to the vasculature of normal tissues. It contains giant capillaries and arteriovenous shunts without intervening capillaries. Newly formed vessels contain no smooth muscle in their walls, but instead contain only a small amount of fibrous connective tissue[39].

These vascular changes can be detected using color Doppler. Blood flow can be demonstrated throughout diastole, reflecting significantly decreased impedance to flow distal to the point of sampling (Figure 12). Because very similar indices of impedance to blood flow are seen from the preovulatory follicle and corpus luteum, vascular information derived from the premenopausal ovary must always be related to the patient's menstrual cycle. Accordingly, physiological ovarian angiogenic activity could be excluded by carrying out the examination during the early proliferative phase (from the 3rd to the 10th menstrual day). In ovarian lesions which demonstrate low impedance and high diastolic flow, it is important to determine whether the waveform has a diastolic notch. Existence of a notch indicates persistence of an initial resistance from the muscular lining of pre-existing arterioles, and is typical of benign tumors (Figure 13).

Quantitative morphometric studies in induced animal tumors show that vascular volume, length and surface area increase during the early stages of tumor growth, and then decrease after the onset of necrosis[40]. The number of vessels of large diameter increases in the later stages of growth[41]. It is not clear whether the same process happens in cancer metastasis[42] (Figure 14). Tumor cells must gain access to the vasculature in the primary tumor, survive the circulation, stop in the microvasculature of the target organ[43,44], exit from this vasculature[45], grow in the target organ and induce angiogenesis[46].

Small vessels that feed growing ovarian tumors or metastases could not be seen before the transvaginal application of color Doppler. The clinical application of this new modality and characterization of benign and malignant ovarian lesions on the basis of their vascularity have opened exciting avenues in the field of gynecological oncology.

Angiogenesis in benign ovarian tumors

Functional cysts

Functional cysts are the most common source of adnexal masses in women of reproductive age. The two main types of functional cyst, follicle and corpus luteum cysts, are benign and derived from either an unruptured follicle or the cystic degeneration of a corpus luteum, respectively[47]. Typically, these cysts are unilateral and are less than 6 cm in diameter, and during pelvic examination, they feel smooth and cystic. On sonograms, the cysts appear unilocular and fluid-filled, without evidence of solid components or excrescences[48] (Figure 15).

The neovascularization detection rate for these lesions in our study population was 17.8% and the location of vascularization was peripheral or pericystic. Information regarding the Doppler characteristics showed an RI of 0.52 for follicular, and 0.46 for corpus luteum cysts (Table 1). It seems that transvaginal color Doppler is helpful in differential diagnosis of different causes of acute

Table 1 Transvaginal color Doppler in the assessment of benign adnexal masses

Histopathology	*n*	*Color flow* *n*	*Color flow* %	*Resistance index*	*SD*
Functional cysts					
follicular	86	16	18.6	0.52	0.06
corpus luteum	96	24	25.0	0.46	0.08
Dermoid cysts	18	4	22.2	0.48	0.10
Cystadenoma	45	7	15.5	0.50	0.08
Fibroma	5	3	60.0	0.46	0.04
Theca–granulosa cell tumor	1	1	100.0	0.60	
Brenner's tumor	2	1	50.0	0.50	
Endometriosis	103	81	78.6	0.49	0.11
Pelvic inflammatory disease	112	34	30.4	0.54	0.12
All cases	468	171	36.5	0.50	0.08

abdomen and detection of torsion of the functional cyst (Figure 16). Torsion affects blood supply to the ovary both from the ovarian artery and the ovarian branch of the uterine artery. In three patients with symptoms of an acute abdomen, we found color signals and moderate impedance (RI 0.47–0.52) to flow at the periphery of the cyst, above the point of the torsion. Below a morphologically recognized point, no blood supply was detected. Hemorrhage from a ruptured corpus luteum cyst can be severe enough to be mistaken for a ruptured ectopic pregnancy. This new technique enhances our ability to distinguish between these two conditions, and select the patients for surgical intervention when necessary.

Mature teratomas (dermoid cysts)

These occur commonly in women of reproductive age. They contain elements of mature adult structures derived from all three embryonic layers: endoderm, mesoderm and, peripherally, ectoderm[47]. These structures include hair, teeth, bone, skin, and calcified components that give focal, high-amplitude reflectors with acoustic shadowing (Figure 17). Unfortunately, these high-amplitude reflectors may simulate bowel gas; therefore, these lesions may be camouflaged and sometimes even large lesions can go undetected on sonograms. In our study, peripheral arteries were detected in 22.2% of the lesions and had an average RI of 0.48 (Table 1). There was one false-positive result amongst the 18 dermoid cysts that were studied. It was a case of dermoid cyst with actively dividing cells (Figure 18), that showed low-impedance blood-flow signals with a diastolic notch.

Serous and mucinous cystadenomas

These are also common lesions. Serous cystadenomas may be unilocular but are mostly multilocular, with or without papillary growth into the cavity[47,49] (Figure 19). In 19% of benign serous ovarian tumors, a large stromal component was found and, in 4.5%, papillary formations were found inside the cyst wall[49].

Mucinous cystadenomas may attain a huge size, and several have been reported to weigh 45–90 kg. Grossly, they present as rounded or ovoid masses with a smooth capsule that is usually translucent or bluish–whitish gray. Mucinous cystadenomas are thin-walled and mostly multilocular (Figures 20, 21). Papillary formations may be present, but they are less common than in serous cystadenomas. Sonographic evaluation, whether alone or in combination with tumor markers[50,51] cannot determine the nature of the lesion before Doppler assessment. This is not surprising, because it can be difficult to distinguish a benign ovarian tumor from a malignant or borderline one by macroscopic inspection of the specimen or even by microscopic evaluation. It seems that endovaginal color Doppler may increase the reliability of the ultrasonographic diagnosis of serous and mucinous cystadenomas[34,52,53].

In this group of ovarian tumors ($n=45$)

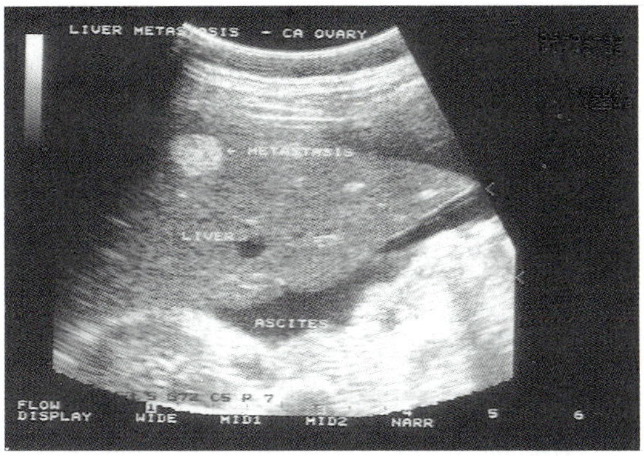

Figure 14 Transabdominal sonogram demonstrating huge ascites surrounding the left liver lobe in a patient with complex adnexal mass. Metastatic nodule is clearly shown

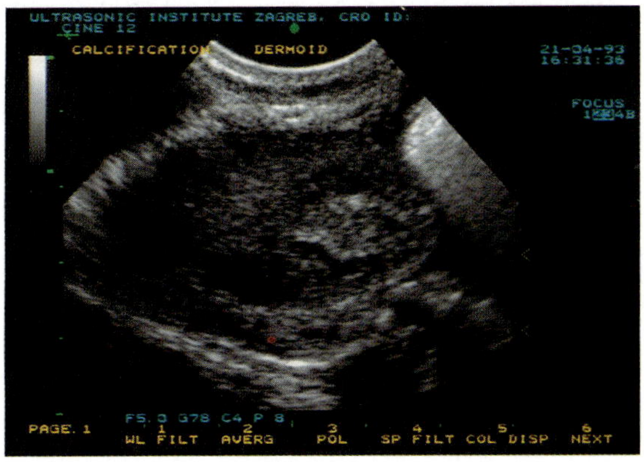

Figure 17 Transvaginal scan showing a dermoid tumor with a completely solid appearance; dense echo represents teeth, a typical finding of this tumor

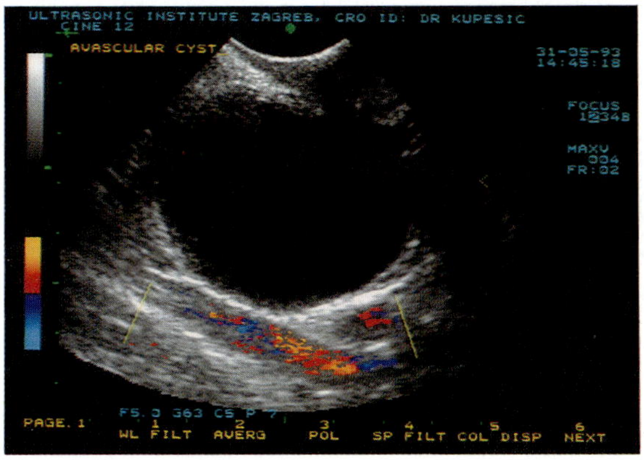

Figure 15 Solitary, avascular ovarian cyst. Color Doppler demonstrates the iliac vessels

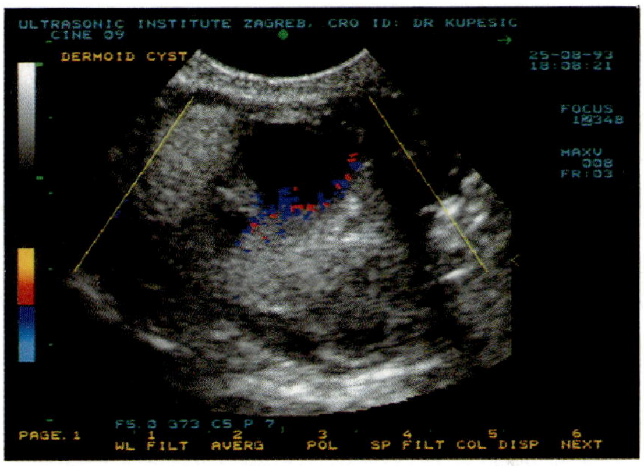

Figure 18 Transvaginal sonogram of complex tumor on the left. Note the echogenicity of the solid tumor parts and a color-coded area. This flow may have low impedance and is typical for cystic teratomas with actively dividing cells

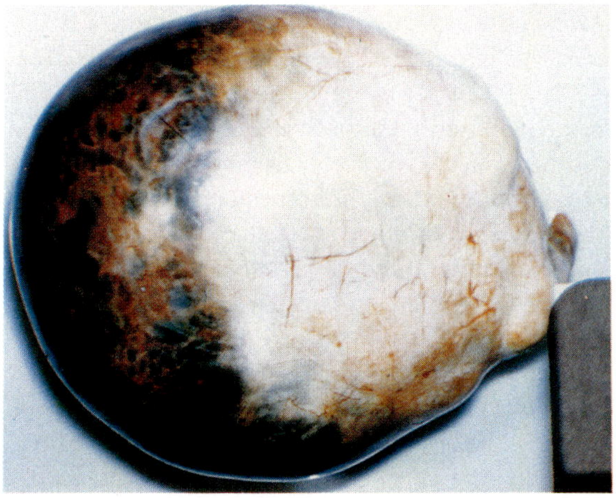

Figure 16 Pathological finding of torsion of a functional cyst

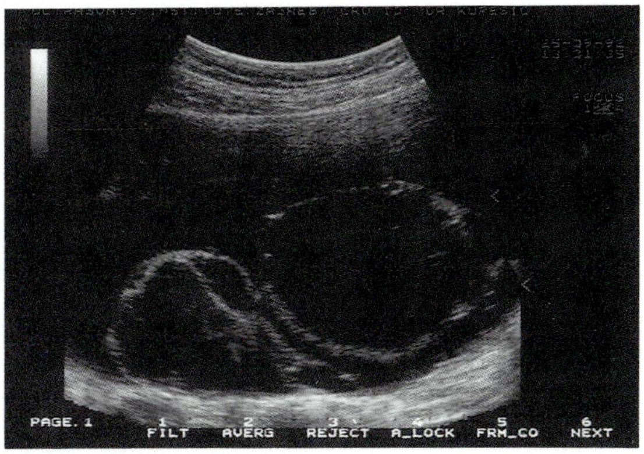

Figure 19 Huge ovoid, multilocular cystadenoma containing anechoic fluid

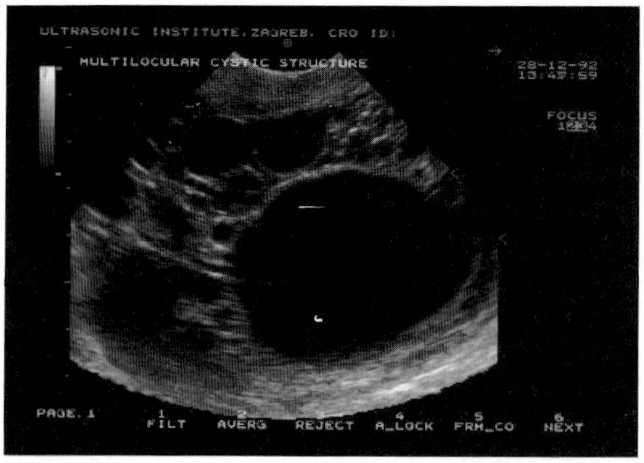

Figure 20 Transvaginal scan demonstrating huge mucinous cystadenoma. The interior is divided into a number of discrete septa or loculi containing a clear viscid fluid

neovascularization was found in seven cases (15.5%). The location of vascularization was an important parameter in reducing the overlap between malignant tumors. Peripheral vessels which originated from pre-existing host vasculature (Figure 22) had an average RI of 0.52 (range 0.48–0.58). Vessels displayed within septae had a mean RI of 0.48 (range 0.45–0.54) (Figure 23, Table 1).

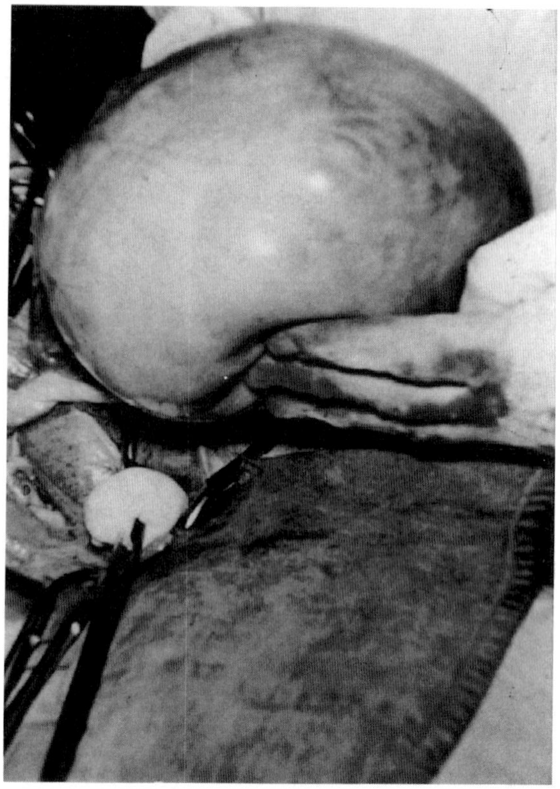

Figure 21 Huge, ovoid, thin walled, multilocular cystadenoma. The fluid contained within the neoplasm was tinged yellow and viscous in quality

Fibromas, thecomas and Brenner's tumors

These are solid, benign tumors found in premenopausal and postmenopausal patients (Figure 24). Small, solid tumors are difficult to detect on sonograms because they are similar in echo texture to the normal ovary[48]. If a solid lesion is observed in the adnexa of a premenopausal woman, it is more likely to be a pedunculated or broad ligament leiomyoma (Figure 25) than a solid ovarian neoplasm.

Transvaginal color Doppler is useful in differentiating fibroids from solid ovarian masses on the basis of their vascularity. Within or on the periphery of the uterine mass, even when it is out of the contour of the uterus, it is possible to detect waveform signals that are typical for the uterine vascular network. In such cases, blood flow is usually similar to normal myometrial perfusion, originating from terminal branches of the uterine artery. On the other hand, small vessels which feed a growing ovarian tumor are of ovarian vasculature origin.

Rarely, solid benign ovarian tumors are associated with ascites and pleural effusions, a situation called Meigs' syndrome[49] (Figure 26). CA 125 levels are elevated in approximately 82% of patients with epithelial ovarian cancers[50]. In addition, elevated levels have been reported in a variety of benign pathological conditions, including pelvic inflammatory disease, endometriosis, leiomyomata, and benign stromal tumors with ascites[50,51]. Jones and Surwitt[52] postulated in patients with Meigs' syndrome that the elevated CA 125 level may be attributed to peritoneal reaction and ascites formation rather than to the ovarian tumor. Other reports[50,51] of CA 125 assessment in patients with benign stromal tumors without ascites describe levels less than 35 IU/ml. However, in our own series of 468 proven benign

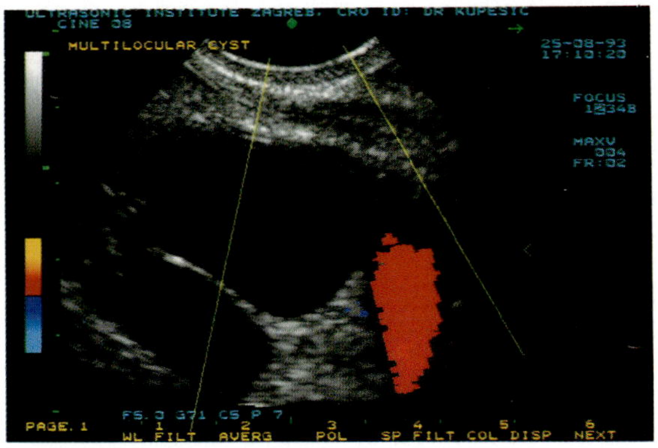

Figure 22 Multilocular cystic ovarian tumor; blood flow detected on the periphery represents vasodilated, pre-existing host vessel

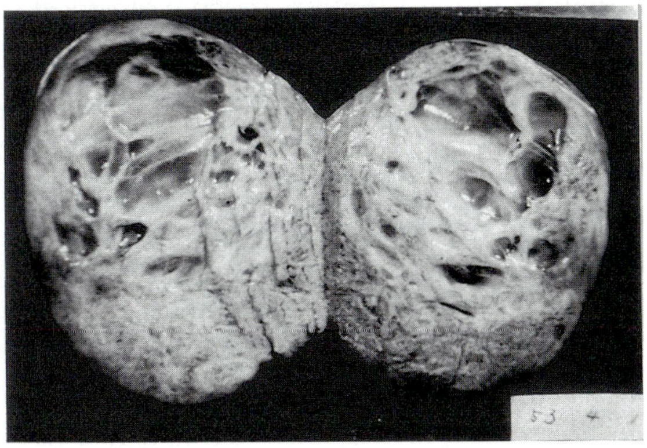

Figure 24 Fibroma – benign, solid tumor of the ovary. It can be difficult to distinguish it from myoma because they have the same echogenicity. The determining factor is whether the ovaries can be visualized

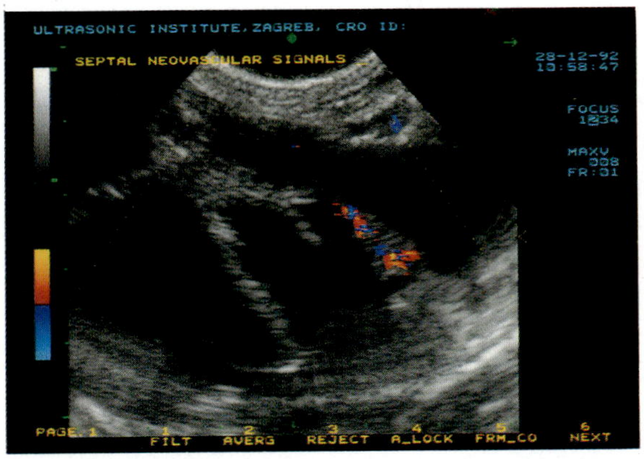

Figure 23 Septal neovascular signals visualized by color Doppler

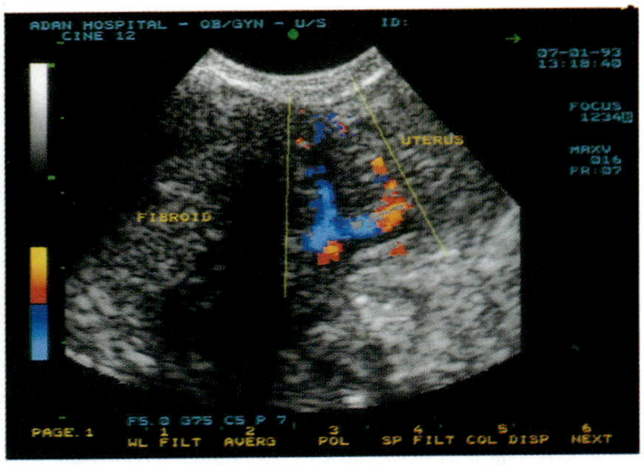

Figure 25 Transvaginal scan showing a mass arising from the uterus. Typical sonographic features of a leiomyoma include a solid and heterogeneous mass showing acoustic attentuation. Superimposed color Doppler demonstrates regularly separated vessels of the intraligamentary fibroid

adnexal masses, we detected low impedance indices (RI = 0.42, PI = 0.78) in a patient with benign stromal neoplasm and elevated CA 125 levels (318 U/ml). Transvaginal sonography demonstrated a complex adnexal mass with a large solid component, while the transabdominal sonogram showed huge ascites (Figure 27). The benign nature of the tumor was confirmed by histopathology.

Endometriosis

Endometriosis is a condition in which abnormal growth of tissue, histologically resembling endometrial tissue, occurs outside the uterus, including on the surfaces of the bowel, bladder, or abdominal wall[53]. The ovary represents a relatively unique site of implantation, as the levels of steroids surpass those in the circulation, and hence this affords an ideal environment for implantation of endometrial growth. It seems that the surface epithelium and the proximity of the tubal ostia influence transplantation production. When endometrial cells enter the ovarian stroma, large endometrial cysts filled with viscous chocolate-colored liquid may be formed (Figure 28). There is usually a well demarcated separation between the endometrial cyst wall and the normal adjacent ovarian stroma. The most prominent vascular

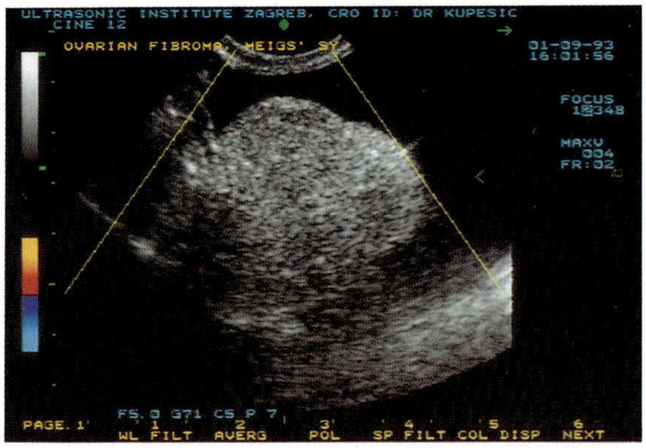

Figure 26 Transvaginal scan demonstrating a case of avascular, solid ovarian tumor associated with ascites. The diagnosis of ovarian fibroma was confirmed after surgery.

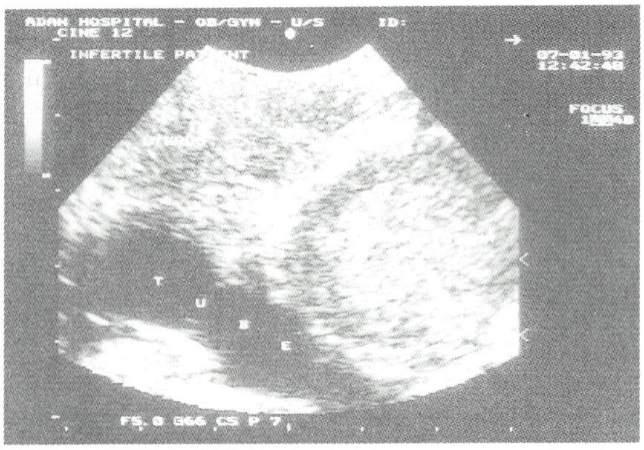

Figure 28 Transvaginal sonogram showing 'chocolate' cyst with homogeneous high-level internal echoes on the left. Note the whole length of the fluid-filled tube below the cyst

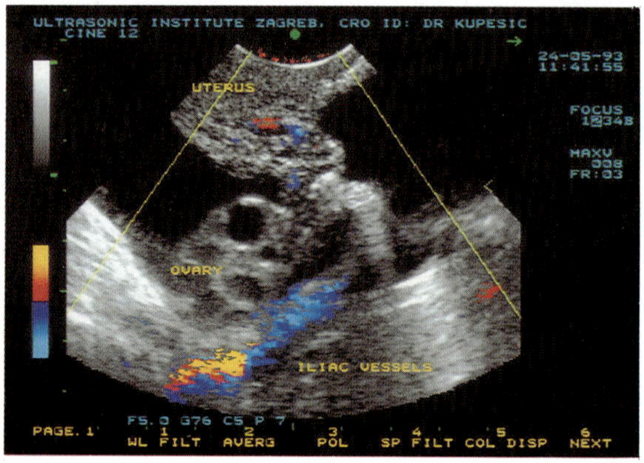

Figure 27 Bizarre appearance of a complex adnexal mass surrounded by marked ascites in a patient with Meigs' syndrome. Color Doppler shows normal pelvic blood flow: iliac and uterine vessels

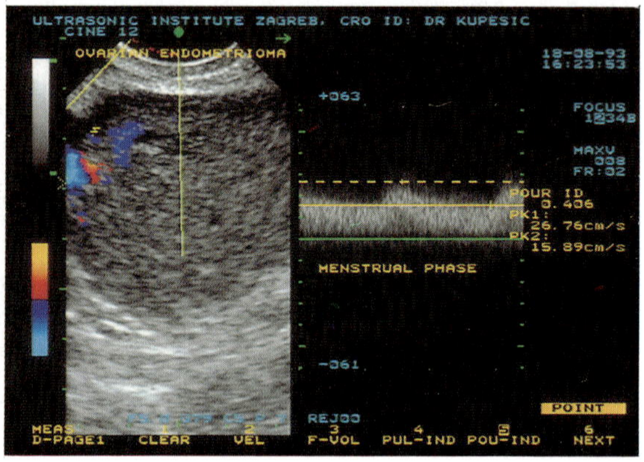

Figure 29 Endometrioma. Color Doppler shows prominent vascularization at the level of the ovarian hilus (left). Pulsed Doppler (right) shows high-velocity and low-resistance flow (resistance index = 0.40) when there was hemorrhage in the menstrual phase of the cycle

area in these common benign cysts is at the level of the ovarian hilus. This type of neovascularization was discovered in 78.6% of endometriomas (Table 1). The RI values measured from this location were usually above 0.45. However, blood-flow indices varied between low (RI = 0.41–0.45) in 20.4% and elevated (RI = 0.51–0.60) in the remaining. It seems that low impedance/high diastolic flow is present when there is a hemorrhage during the menstrual phase of the cycle (Figure 29). Therefore, we recommend study of ovarian endometrioma vascularity during the late follicular phase. It is postulated that the effect of medical treatment is highly dependent upon the metabolically active implants arriving via a blood-supplying network. Conservative treatment has encouraging potential and can be successfully used in patients with an optimal vascular pattern. Surrounding inflammation and fibrotic changes (Figure 30) which may disturb this process can be detected by transvaginal color Doppler. Based on our experience, avascular ovarian lesions must be removed surgically.

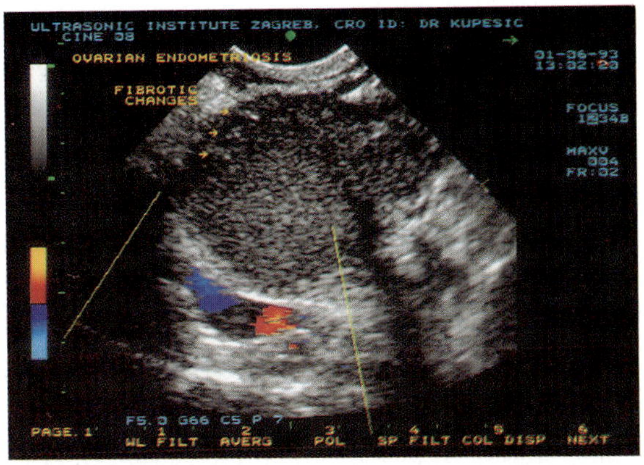

Figure 30 Avascular ovarian endometrioma. The scarification process modifies the vascularization

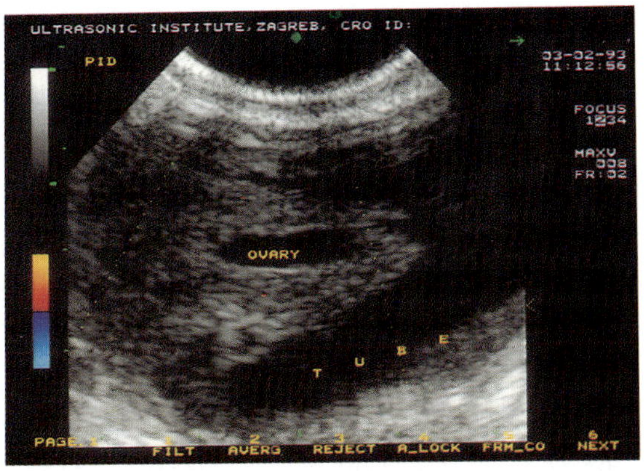

Figure 32 Chronic pelvic inflammation. Transvaginal scan demonstrates avascular encapsulated abscess

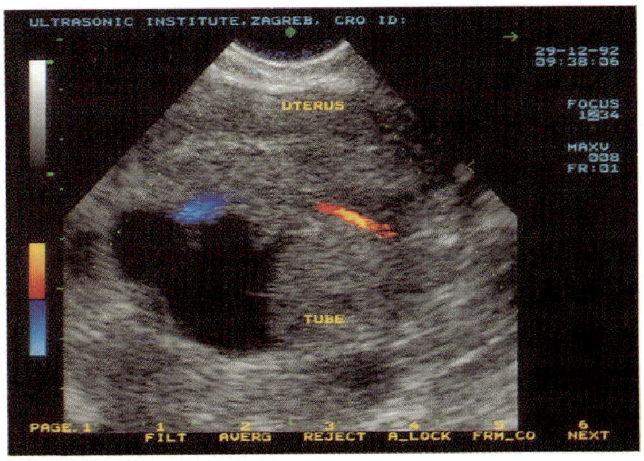

Figure 31 Transvaginal color Doppler demonstrates complex adnexal mass which occupies the pouch of Douglas in a patient with acute pelvic inflammation. Increased vascularity is a response to various bacterial antigens and products

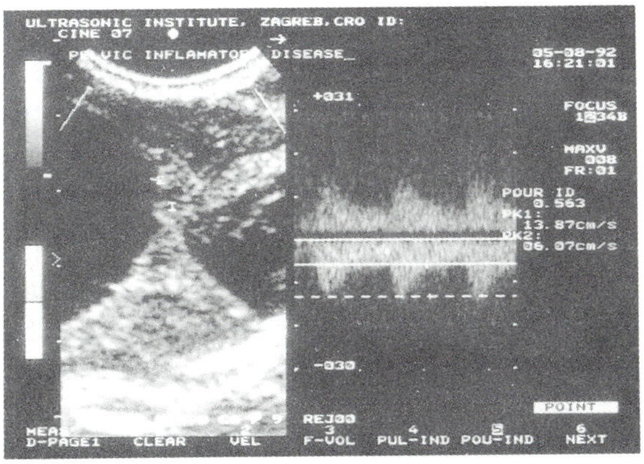

Figure 33 Acute pelvic inflammation: color flow is visualized within the walls of the Fallopian tubes and inflamed ovaries which are filled with multiple cysts (left). Pulsed Doppler (right) shows moderate-resistance flow (resistance index = 0.56)

Pelvic inflammatory disease

Pelvic inflammatory disease is a non-specific term for a variety of findings in the upper female genital tract characterized by inflammation and infection[54]. Endometritis, salpingitis, peritonitis and tubo-ovarian abscess are included in pelvic inflammatory disease. The initiating event in the formation of a tubo-ovarian abscess is believed to be the invasion of the epithelium of the Fallopian tube by a pathogen, causing tissue damage and necrosis, thereby providing an ideal environment for anaerobic invasion and growth[55]. Bacteria produce various factors, such as lysosomal enzymes, exotoxins, surface virulence factors and antigens, that produce an intense inflammatory response and increased vascularization (Figure 31). The consequence of this reaction is edema, that compromises the blood supply in a later stage, and leads to ischemia and necrosis of the wall of the Fallopian tube (Figure 32). This mechanism results in the formation of an inflammatory exudate, or pus, that spills out of the fimbriated ends of the infected Fallopian tubes. A tubo-ovarian abscess is formed when this infected spillage causes an inflammatory process involving Fallopian tubes and other adnexal structures, such as ovaries and broad ligaments. Laparoscopic evaluation is the 'gold standard' for diagnosis, but it is expensive and carries operative and anesthetic risks[56]. Ultrasonography is often used to exclude intrauterine and ectopic pregnancy or to document the presence of an adnexal mass[57]. Sonography shows a predominantly cystic collection with internal echoes that may have multiple loculations. Occasionally, distinction from fluid-filled loops of bowel may be difficult. In this instance, a water enema may be helpful because the movement of water through the bowel will be observed on real-time ultrasound.

Because the inflammatory process in the ovary involves both structural and vascular changes, color Doppler ultrasound can be a useful tool in its diagnosis and management. The early phase of the disease is characterized by edema of the Fallopian tubes and dilatation of the blood vessels in their walls (Figure 33). The mean RI of the tubal artery blood flow in 112 patients with PID was 0.55. The inflamed ovaries were enlarged and filled with multiple cysts which represented infected follicles or corpus luteum cysts. Intra-ovarian vessels could easily be identified and showed a mean RI of 0.52 (Table 1).

It is well known that the sonographic appearance of a complex adnexal mass should be interpreted in the context of the clinical setting. For example, in the febrile patient, a thick-walled mass containing echogenic fluid is likely to be an abscess. In this advanced and most severe form of pelvic inflammatory disease, it is difficult to identify the pelvic anatomy. Ovaries are usually adherent to the pelvic sidewall or to the uterus, and the scarring process can alter their endocrine function and circulation. In a group of 57 patients in this stage of pelvic inflammatory disease, the ovarian parenchymal blood flow showed significantly higher impedance to blood flow (mean RI = 0.68). Based on our experience, dynamic use of color Doppler ultrasound in patients affected with pelvic inflammatory disease is important for accurate diagnosis, follow-up and evaluation of the ovulatory function and ovarian perfusion:

Angiogenesis in borderline tumors

Serous borderline tumors of the ovary account for 21 to 33% of all ovarian serous carcinomas. These neoplasms are characterized by a relatively good prognosis when compared with other ovarian cancers[58]. They exhibit varying degrees of cytological atypia but no evidence of destructive stromal invasion[59]. Such tumors, however, can be associated with extraovarian peritoneal implants in 30–40% of patients[60] and have an increased incidence of bilaterality. Grossly, serous borderline tumors are uni- or multilocular cysts that exhibit endophytic and confluent papillary growth. They differ from serous carcinomas in that they lack significant necrosis and hemorrhage.

Borderline mucinous tumors are mostly thin-walled and multilocular and do not differ significantly from their benign counterparts. They are voluminous masses with a smooth outer surface, although solid areas and papillary formations are reported in approximately 25–60% of lesions[61].

Ultrasonography has been widely used to detect, characterize, and evaluate ovarian tumors. The principle of the diagnostic imaging study is based on macropathology. Thick septae, irregular solid parts within a mass, indefinite margins, presence of ascites, and bowel loops with matter are regarded as malignant patterns[62] (Figure 34). Some authors have reported that ovarian tumors of low malignant potential presented the same patterns as malignant tumors[63]. On the other hand, Achiron and colleagues[64] mentioned that borderline tumors had an appearance similar to that of benign tumors and it was difficult to differentiate them from their benign counterparts. Therefore, assessment of vascular changes and the resistance to blood flow are required in the ovarian tumor presenting either benign or malignant features by conventional ultrasound. Blood flow velocity waveforms obtained from borderline tumors in our study had a relatively high diastolic flow and low RI (0.43 ± 0.07) (Table 2). We speculate that abnormal Doppler features are extracted from large arterioles or sinusoids with no muscles in their walls. This is a possible hemodynamic response to the tumor angiogenesis factor produced from low malignant-potential cells. Therefore, the preoperative assessment of the adnexal mass by ultrasonography has to include the size, consistency and blood flow to determine the likelihood of malignancy. Based on our experience, transvaginal color Doppler provides useful diagnostic infor-

Table 2 Transvaginal color Doppler in the assessment of borderline and malignant adnexal masses

Histopathology	*n*	*Color flow* *n*	*Color flow* %	*Resistance index*	*SD*
Borderline tumors	6	5	83.3	0.43	0.07
Malignant tumors					
Cystadenocarcinoma	38	37	97.4	0.37	0.10
Endometriotic adenocarcinoma	9	9	100.0	0.41	0.02
Germ cell tumor	4	4	100.0	0.36	0.07
Anaplastic ovarian carcinoma	2	2	100.0	0.34	
Metastases to ovary	17	17	100.0	0.38	0.12
All cases	76	74	97.4	0.37	0.06

mation for the differentiation of benign from malignant or borderline ovarian tumors.

Angiogenesis in malignant ovarian masses

In view of the fact that ovarian malignancy is still an insidious and intractable disease, which is usually diagnosed at a late stage, and since there is a rather high incidence of these malignant tumors in the menopause, all means should be used to detect this disease at an early stage. While serum CA 125 is a fair tumor marker in advanced cases and for follow-up, it is not specific and the detection rate is not adequate. The contribution of computer tomography and magnetic resonance imaging is doubtful and their cost is prohibitive. The advent of vaginal ultrasound screening methods for ovarian cancer has made the ovaries more accessible. Dramatic changes in ovarian tissue vascularity during oncogenesis are mediated by numerous angiogenic factors and can be detected by using flow data from color Doppler. Malignant tumor vessels are usually dilated, saccular, and tortuous, and may contain tumor cells within the endothelial lining of the vessel wall. Other features include the presence of arteriovenous shunting (large and direct communications, or microscopic communications in the tumor microcirculation) and bizarre thin-walled tortuous vessels lined by tumor cells that end in amorphous spaces constituting 'tumor lakes' with or without associated necrosis. Arteriovenous shunts are remarkable because of extreme velocities that occur at sites of high-pressure gradients[65]. This type of vessel is usually situated on the periphery of the tumor[66]. New vessels are continually produced on the periphery of the tumor, creating the potential for its proliferation and growth.

The second type of signal, exhibiting little systolic–diastolic variation, is usually present in the central vessels within the malignant tumor[67]. This is, most probably, their response to the angiogenic activity of tumor cells. These vessels have a relative paucity of smooth muscle in their walls in comparison with their caliber and 'behave' more like capillaries than true arteries or arterioles[68]. Vessels deficient in their muscular elements present diminished resistance to flow and thereby receive a larger volume of flow than vessels with high impedance[69,70].

Such abnormal vascular morphology is a valuable marker for tissue characterization. In a group with malignant ovarian masses ($n=70$), neovascularization was demonstrated in 69 cases (98.6%) (Table 2). The RI of these lesions ranged from 0.27 to 0.47, with a mean of 0.37. Our results have shown that malignant ovarian masses are mostly vascularized in the central parts, within septa and papillary projections (Figures 35, 36). The lowest RIs were measured in septal branches (mean RI = 0.36) (Figure 37), whereas the highest RI value of 0.47 was measured in peripheral vessels. In the present study, a lower resistance was observed in central arteries than in peripheral arteries.

It seems that distribution of the vessels and impedance to blood flow is dependent on tumor type and size. Tumors gradually begin to compress their own blood vessels when they continue growing beyond a certain size. The absence of functional lymphatic vessels in the tumor stroma,

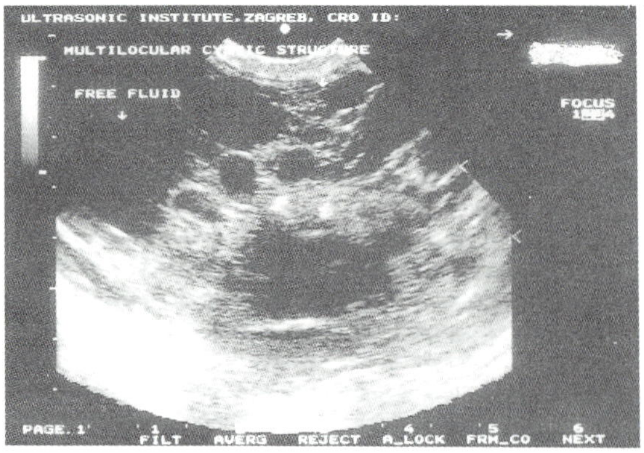

Figure 34 Multilocular voluminous tumor with thick septations, papillary projections and some solid components. Borderline mucinous tumor was confirmed by histopathology

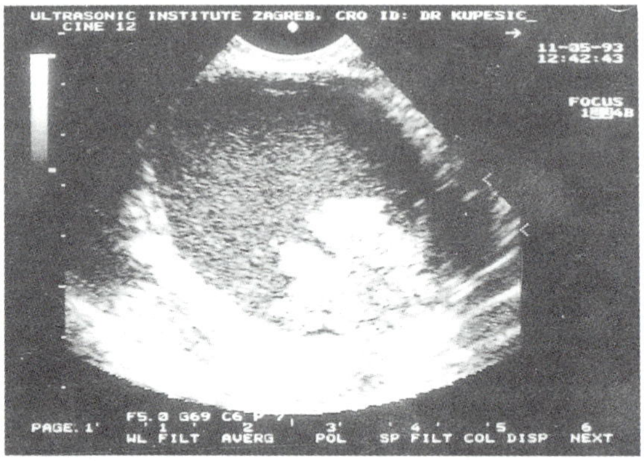

Figure 35 Transvaginal scan of a complex adnexal mass with papillary proliferation. Internal papillary formation is suggestive of malignancy

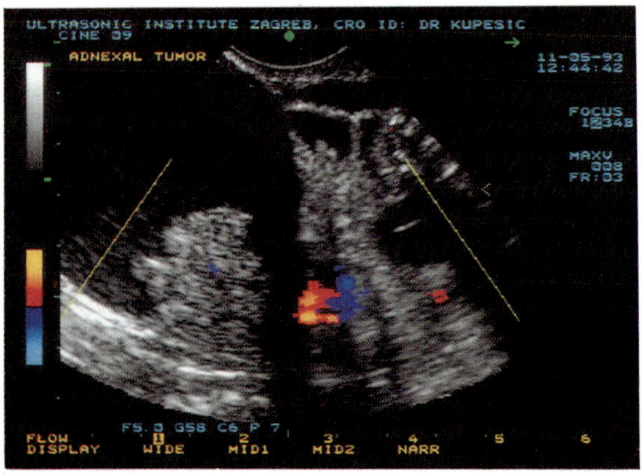

Figure 36 Transvaginal color Doppler shows tumor neovascularization of a papillary proliferation

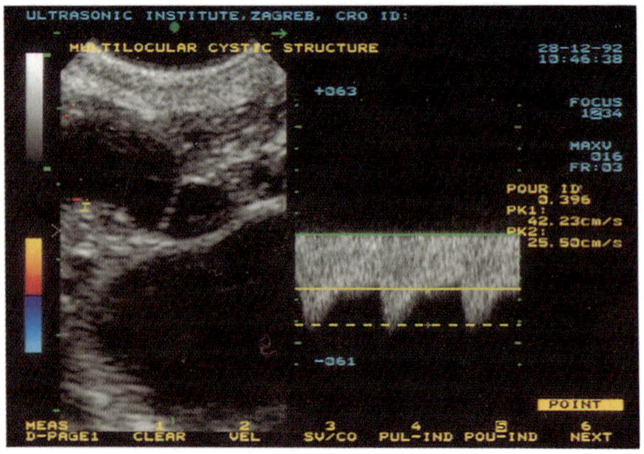

Figure 37 Neovascular signals detected in septal branches (left). Pulsed Doppler (right) is typical for ovarian malignancy. This flow has high velocity and low resistance (resistance index = 0.39), lacking a diastolic notch

and the increase in cell mass and tumor vessel permeability, result in an increase in the interstitial pressure in the tumor core and lead to the occlusion of centrally located tumor vessels[71]. This causes prolonged cessation of flow in the center of the tumor, followed by central necrosis. It seems that low resistance in centrally located vessels is a consequence of a response to the angiogenic activity of the tumor cells and to the differences in necrotic processes. The peak systolic velocities and RI values between benign and malignant tumors occurred in each vessel type. Another important parameter for the assessment of tumor vascularity is the vascular arrangement. Randomly dispersed vessels within the solid part of malignant tumors were seen four times more than regularly separated vessels.

Does benign-to-malignant transformation occur?

Little is known about epithelial neoplasms of the ovary in terms of etiology and pathogenesis. One of the more widely accepted hypotheses for the development of ovarian epithelial tumors is that they are derived from the surface epithelium or mesothelium covering the ovary[72]. It has been postulated that small cystic structures lined by this epithelium become trapped within the ovarian cortex, possibly as the result of repeated ovulations. An inclusion cyst is then formed in the stroma, which is lined initially by benign germinal epithelium. Under the influence of hormonal and other oncogenic stimuli, this benign epithelium undergoes transformation to form a malignant ovarian tumor. Clear trends of increasing risk for ovarian cancer are seen among nulliparous infertile women who have used fertility drugs[73] and among those with a long total duration of premenopausal sexual activity without birth control.

There are two possible explanations for the relationship between ovarian stimulation and development of granulosa cell tumors. First, the granulosa cell tumor is present in the ovary, waiting for the hormonal trigger, and second, increased follicle stimulating hormone concentrations are oncogenic to granulosa cells. Many studies[74,75] suggest that pregnancy, breast feeding, and oral contraceptive use induce biological changes that protect against ovarian malignancy. It is hoped that transvaginal color Doppler will facilitate the study of the complex and sequential process of carcinogenesis. This technique allows precise visualization of the small area of vascularity in the ovarian stroma and follicular rim, and it may be used to monitor the vascular changes in the presence of germinal epithelial inclusion cysts. In this regard, transvaginal color Doppler seems to reveal reliable hemodynamic information even before ovarian lesions appear.

There has been little suggestion in the literature[76] that malignant tumors may arise from the progressive transformation of the epithelium of benign cystic epithelial tumors of the ovary or from low malignant-potential tumors. Plaxe and colleagues[77] examined 50 cases of stage I epithelial ovarian carcinomas for the presence of epithelial atypia adjacent to the invasive tumor. When compared with non-tumor-containing control ovaries, atypia was present in 49 of 50 tumor cases and in no controls. Previous electron microscopic studies[78] described transitions between benign and neoplastic epithelium in serous ovarian tumors. Epidemiological data from a large study screening patients for ovarian cancer[79] reported a significant increase in the frequency of benign epithelial ovarian tumors in first- or second-degree relatives of patients with documented ovarian carcinoma. If benign epithelial cystic tumors are indeed precursors of malignant tumors, then study of intratumoral hemodynamic alterations would become an important strategy to be considered in ovarian cancer control. One might speculate that the transition from inclusion cyst to malignant neoplasm can occur in a relatively short time and the benign phase of tumor growth either might not develop or might not be appreciated clinically. In contrast, if the process occurs slowly, a benign or borderline tumor might result, followed by a malignant tumor only after further steps. Initial evidence suggests that transvaginal color Doppler may be used to monitor the progress towards both objectives.

Undoubtedly, study of ovarian circulation has provided a new, exciting diagnostic field and with further multicentric studies, can offer elucidation of many presently unknown circumstances in complex ovarian physiology and pathophysiology. For the time being, the role of transvaginal color Doppler should not be underestimated or overestimated.

References

1. Reynolds, S. R. M. (1973). Blood and lymph vascular systems of the ovary. In Greep, S. R. (ed.) *Female Reproductive System, Part I*, pp. 261–316. (Washington: American Physiological Society)
2. Ginther, O. J., Diersche, D. K. J., Walsh, S. W. and Del Campo, C. H. (1974). Anatomy of arteries and veins of uterus and ovaries in rhesus monkeys. *Biol. Reprod.*, **11**, 204–19
3. Gillet, J. Y., Koritke, J. G., Muller, P. and Juliens, C. (1968). On the microvascularization of the rabbit ovary. *Compt. Rend. Soc. Biol.*, **162**, 762–6
4. Merce, L. T. A. (1993). Bases anatomicas de la circulacion utero-ovarica. In Merve, L. T. A. (ed.) *Ecografia Doppler en Obstetricia y Ginecologia*, pp. 1–7. (Madrid: Interamericana McGraw–Hill)

5. Gratton, A. D. T., Hodge, C. and Callamander, R. (1990). Basic physics and instrumentation of transvaginal color imaging. In Kurjak, A. (ed.) *Transvaginal Color Doppler*, 1st edn., pp. 9–15. (Carnforth, UK: Parthenon Publishing)
6. Taylor, K. Y. W., Burns, P. N., Woodlock, J. P. and Wells, P. N. (1985). Blood flow in deep abdominal and pelvic vessels: ultrasonic pulsed Doppler analysis. *Radiology*, **154**, 487–93
7. Eik Nes, S. H., Brubakk, A. O. and Ulstein, M. K. (1980). Measurement of human fetal blood flow *Br. Med. J.*, **280**, 283–4
8. Kurjak, A., Zalud, I., Jurkovic, D., Alfirevic, Z. and Miljan, M. (1989). Transvaginal color Doppler for the assessment of pelvic circulation. *Acta Obstet. Gynecol. Scand.*, **68**, 131–3
9. Kurjak, A., Zalud, I., Alfirevic, Z. and Jurkovic, D. (1991). The assessment of pelvic blood flow by transvaginal color Doppler. *Ultrasound Med. Biol.*, **16**, 437–50
10. Bourne, T. H. (1991). Transvaginal color Doppler in gynecology. *Ultrasound Obstet. Gynecol.*, **1**, 359–73
11. Kurjak, A., Kupesic-Urek, S., Schulman, H. and Zalud, I. (1992). Transvaginal color Doppler in the assessment of ovarian and uterine blood flow in infertile women. *Fertil. Steril.*, **56**, 870–3
12. Scholtes, M. C. W., Wladimiroff, J., van Rijen, H. J. M. and Hop, W. C. J. (1989). Uterine and ovarian flow velocity waveforms in the normal menstrual cycle; a transvaginal color Doppler study. *Fertil. Steril.*, **52**, 981–5
13. Janson, P. O., Damber, B. E. and Axen, C. (1981). Luteal blood flow and progesterone secretion in pseudopregnant rabbits. *J. Reprod. Fertil.*, **63**, 491–3
14. Ford, S. P. and Chenalult, J. R. (1981). Blood flow to the corpus luteum bearing ovary and ipsilateral uterine horn of cows during oestrous cycle and early pregnancy. *J. Reprod. Fertil.*, **62**, 555–9
15. Taylor, K. J. W. and Burns, P. N. (1985). Duplex Doppler scanning in the pelvis and abdomen. *Ultrasound Med. Biol.*, **11**, 643–7
16. Bruce, N. W. and Hillier, K. (1974). The effect of prostaglandin F on ovarian blood flow and corpus luteum regression in the rabbit. *Nature (London)*, **249**, 176–7
17. Brown, B. W., Emery, M. J. and Mattner, E. (1980). Ovarian arterial blood velocity measured with Doppler ultrasonic transducers in conscious ewes. *J. Reprod. Fertil.*, **58**, 295–300
18. Wary, M. J. and Cook, M. J. (1973). Redistribution of blood flow by prostaglandin F2-alpha in the rabbit ovary. *Am. J. Obstet. Gynecol.*, **117**, 381–5
19. Nell, T. M. and Niswender, G. D. (1981). Luteal blood flow and receptors for LH during PGF2-alpha induced luteolysis: production of PGF2-alpha during early pregnancy. *Acta Vet. Scand.*, **77** (Suppl.), 117–30
20. Kurjak, A. and Kupesic-Urek, S. (1991). Infertility. In Kurjak, A. (ed.) *Transvaginal Color Doppler*, p. 33–8. (Carnforth, UK: Parthenon Publishing)
21. Bourne, T. H., Jurkovic, D., Waterstone, J., Campbell, S. and Collins, W. P. (1991). Intrafollicular blood flow during human ovulation. *Ultrasound Obstet. Gynecol.*, **1**, 53–9
22. Collins, W., Jurkovic, D., Bourne, T. H., Kurjak, A. and Campbell, S. (1991). Ovarian morphology, endocrine function and intra-follicular blood flow during the preovulatory period. *Hum. Reprod.*, **6**, 319–24
23. Sladkevicius, P., Valentin, L. and Marsal, K. (1993). Blood flow velocity in the uterine and ovarian arteries during the normal menstrual cycle. *Ultrasound Obstet. Gynecol.*, **3**, 199–201
24. Inger, D. E., Madri, J. A. and Folkman, J. (1986). A possible mechanism for inhibition of angiogenesis by angiostatic steroids: induction of capillary basement membrane dissolution. *Endocrinology*, **119**, 1768–75
25. Reynolds, S. R. M. (1948). Morphological determinations of the flow characteristics between an artery and its branch with special reference to the ovarian spiral artery in the rabbit. *Acta Anat.*, **5**, 1–6
26. Niswender, G. D., Reiners, T. J., Diekmann, M. A. and Nett, Y. T. M. (1976). Blood flow: a mediator of ovarian function. *Biol. Reprod.*, **14**, 64–81
27. Merce, L. T., Andrino, R., Barco, M. J. and De la Fuente, F. (1990). Cyclic changes of the functional ovarian compartments: echographic assessment. *Acta Obstet. Gynecol., Scand.*, **69**, 327–32
28. Zalud, I. and Kurjak, A. (1990). The assessment of luteal blood flow in pregnant and non-pregnant women by transvaginal color Doppler. *J. Perinat. Med.*, **18**, 215–8
29. Coman, D. R. and Sheldon, W. F. (1946). The significance of hyperemia around the tumor implants. *Am. J. Pathol.*, **22**, 821–6
30. Algire, G. H., Chalkey, H. W., Legallais, F. Y. and Park, H. D. (1945). Vascular reactions of mice to wounds and to normal and neoplastic transplants. *J. Natl. Cancer Inst.*, **6**, 73–85
31. Day, E. D. (1964). Vascular relationships of tumor and host. *Prog. Exp. Tumor Res.*, **4**, 57–9
32. Folkman, J., Long, D. and Becker, F. (1963). Growth and metastasis of tumor in organ culture. *Tumor Res.*, **16**, 453–67
33. Folkman, J., Cole, P. and Yimmerman, S. (1966). Tumor behavior in isolated perfused organs: *in vitro* growth and metastasis of biopsy material in rabbit thyroid and canine intestinal segment. *Ann. Surg.*, **164**, 491–502
34. Folkman, J. and Gimbrone, M. (1972). Perfusion of the thyroid. *Acta Endocrinol.*, **4**, 237–48
35. Folkman, J. (1970). The intestine as an organ culture. In Burdette, J. and Thomas, C. C. (eds.) *Carcinoma of the Colon and Antecedent Epithelium*, pp. 113–27. (Springfield, Illinois: Charles C. Thomas)

36. Folkman, J. and Shing, Y. (1992). Minireview. *J. Biol. Chem.*, **267**, 10931–4
37. Klagsbrun, M. and D'Amore, P. A. (1991). Regulators of angiogenesis. *Annu. Rev. Physiol.*, **52**, 217
38. Folkman, J., Melrel, E., Abernethy, C. and Williams, G. (1971). Isolation of tumor factor responsible for angiogenesis. *J. Exp. Med.*, **133**, 275–8
39. Kurjak, A., Shalan, H., Kupesic, S., Predanic, M., Zalud, I., Breyer, B. and Jukic, S. (1993). Transvaginal color Doppler sonography in the assessment of pelvic tumor vascularity. *Ultrasound Obstet. Gynecol.*, **3**, 137–54
40. Gamil, S. L., Shipkey, F. H., Himmelfarb, E.H., Parvey, L. S. and Rabinowity, J. G. (1976). Roentgenology – pathology correlation study of neovascularization. *Am. J. Radiol.*, **126**, 376–85
41. Jain, R. K. and Ward Hartley, K. A. (1987). Dynamics of cancer cell interaction with microvasculature and interstitium. *Biorheology*, **24**, 117–23
42. Folkman, J. (1985). Tumor angiogenesis. *Adv. Cancer Res.*, **43**, 175–80
43. Netland, P. and Letter, B. (1984). Organ specific adhesion and metastatic tumor cells *in vitro*. *Science*, **224**, 113–5
44. Nicholson, G. L. (1988). Organ specificity of tumor metastasis: role of preferential adhesion, invasion and growth of malignant cells at specific secondary sites. *Cancer Metastasis Rev.*, **7**, 143–88
45. Boxberger, H. J., Pawelety, N., Speiss, E. and Kniehuber, R. (1989). An *in vitro* model study of BS p73 rat tumor cell invasion into endothelial monolayer. *Anticancer Res.*, **9**, 1777–86
46. Weidner, N., Semple, J. P., Welch, W. R. and Folkman, J. (1991). Tumor angiogenesis and metastasis – correlation in invasive breast carcinoma. *N. Engl. J. Med.*, **324**, 1–8
47. Granberg, S., Nostrom, A. and Wikland, M. (1990). Tumors in the lower pelvis as imaged by vaginal sonography. *Gynecol. Oncol.*, **37**, 224–6
48. Hermann, U., Locher, G. and Goldrich, A. (1987). Sonographic patterns of ovarian tumors: prediction of malignancy. *Obstet. Gynecol.*, **69**, 777–80
49. Luxman, D., Bergman, A., Sagi, J. and David, M. (1991). The postmenopausal adnexal mass: correlation between ultrasonic and pathologic findings. *Obstet. Gynecol.*, **77**, 726–9
50. Jacobs, I. and Basr, R. (1989). The CA 125 tumor associated antigen: a review of literature. *Hum. Reprod.*, **4**, 1–5
51. Inoue, M., Fujita, M., Nakazawa, A., Ogawa, H., Tanizava, O., Sialyl, T. N. and Sialyl, X. I. (1992). CA 19–9, CA 125, carcinoembryonic antigen, and tissue polypeptide antigen in differentiating ovarian cancers from benign tumors. *Obstet. Gynecol.*, **79**, 434–8
52. Jones, O. W. I. and Surwitt, E. A. (1989). Meigs' syndrome and elevated CA 125. *Obstet. Gynecol.*, **73**, 520–1
53. Donnez, J., Nissole, M., Casanas-Roux, F. and Grandejan, P. (1990). Endometriosis: pathogenesis and pathophysiology. In Shaw, R. E. (ed.) *Endometriosis*, pp. 11–31. (Carnforth, UK: Parthenon Publishing)
54. Landers, D. V. and Sweet, R. L. (1985). Current trends in the diagnosis and treatment of tuboovarian abscess. *Am. J. Obstet. Gynecol.*, **151**, 1098–2001
55. Paavoren, J., Teisala, K. and Heinonen, P. K. (1987). Microbiological and histopathological findings in acute pelvic inflammatory disease. *Br. J. Obstet. Gynecol.*, **94**, 454–7
56. Reich, H. and McGlynn, F. (1987). Laparoscopic treatment of tuboovarian and pelvic abscess. *J. Reprod. Med.*, **32**, 747–51
57. Teisal, K., Heinonen, P. K. and Punonen, R. (1990). Transvaginal ultrasound in the diagnosis and treatment of tuboovarian abscess. *Br. J. Obstet. Gynecol.*, **97**, 178–82
58. Nation, J. G. and Krepart, G. V. (1986). Ovarian carcinoma of low malignant potential: staging and treatment. *Am. J. Obstet. Gynecol.*, **154**, 290–3
59. Russell, P. and Merkur, H. (1979). Proliferating ovarian 'epithelial' tumours: a clinico-pathological analysis of 144 cases. *Aust. NZ J. Obstet. Gynaecol.*, **19**, 45–51
60. Julian, C. G. and Woodruf, J. D. (1972). The biologic behavior of low-grade papillary serous carcinoma of the ovary. *Obstet. Gynecol.*, **40**, 860–7
61. Russell, P. (1984). Borderline epithelial tumours of the ovary: a conceptual dilemma. *Clin. Obstet. Gynecol.*, **11**, 259–77
62. Bell, D. A., Weinstock, M. A. and Scully, R. E. (1988). Peritoneal implants of ovarian serous borderline tumors: histologic features and prognosis. *Cancer*, **62**, 2212–22
63. Buy, J. N., Ghossain, M. A., Sciot, T., Bazot, M., Guinet, C. and Prevot, C. (1991). Epithelial tumors of the ovary: CT findings and correlation with US. *Radiology*, **178**, 811–18
64. Achiron, R., Schejter, E., Malinger, G. and Zakud, H. (1987). Observation on the ultrasound diagnosis of ovarian neoplasms. *Arch. Gynecol. Obstet.*, **241**, 183–90
65. Taylor, K. J. W., Ramos, I., Morse, S. S., Fortune, K. L., Hammers, L. and Taylor, C. R. (1987). Focal liver masses: differential diagnosis with pulsed Doppler US. *Radiology*, **164**, 163–5
66. Okuda, H., Muss, H. and Jamasaki, T. (1977). Angiographic demonstration of intrahepatic arterioportal anastomoses in hepatocellular carcinoma. *Radiology*, **122**, 53–5
67. Fleischer, A. C., Rodgers, W. H., Rao, B. K., Keppler, D. M. and Jones, H. W. (1991). Assessment of ovarian tumor vascularity with transvaginal color Doppler sonography. *J. Ultrasound Med.*, **10**, 563–8

68. Jain, R. K. and Ward-Hartley, K. A. (1987). Dynamics of cancer cell interaction with microvasculature and interstitium. *Biorheology*, **24**, 117–20
69. Kurjak, A., Zalud, I. and Alfirevic, Z. (1991). Evaluation of adnexal masses with transvaginal color Doppler ultrasound. *J. Ultrasound Med.*, **10**, 295–7
70. Bourne, T., Campbell, S., Steer, C., Whitehead, M. I. and Collins, W. P. (1989). Transvaginal color flow imaging: a possible new screening technique for ovarian cancer. *Br. Med. J.*, **299**, 1367–70
71. Tekay, A. and Jouppila, P. (1992). Validity of pulsatility and resistance indices in classification of adnexal tumors with transvaginal color Doppler ultrasound. *Ultrasound Obstet. Gynecol.*, **2**, 338–44
72. Cramer, D. W. and Welch, W. R. (1983). Determinations of ovarian cancer risk. II Inferences regarding pathogenesis. *J. Natl. Cancer Inst.*, **1971**, 717–21
73. Willemsen, W., Kruitwagen, R. and Bastiaans, B. (1993). Ovarian stimulation and granulosa-cell tumor. *Lancet*, **341**, 986–8
74. Whittemore, A. S., Harris, R. and Itnyre, J. (1992). Characteristics relating to ovarian cancer risk: collaborative analysis of 12 US case–control studies. *Am. J. Epidemiol.*, **136**, 1184–203
75. Puls, L., Powell, D. E., De Priest, P., Gallion, H., Hunter, J. E., Kryscio, R. and van Naegell, J. R. (1992). Transition from benign to malignant epithelium in mucinous and serous ovarian cystadenocarcinoma. *Gynecol. Oncol.*, **47**, 53–7
76. Fearon, E. R. and Vogelstein, B. (1990). A genetic model for colorectal tumorogenesis. *Cell*, **61**, 759–67
77. Plaxe, S. C., Deligdisch, L. and Dottino, P. L. (1990). Ovarian intraepithelial neoplasia demonstrated in patients with stage I ovarian carcinoma. *Gynecol. Oncol.*, **38**, 367–72
78. Steinback, F. (1981). Benign, borderline and malignant serous cystadenomas of the ovary. *Pathol. Res. Pract.*, **172**, 58–72
79. Bourne, T. H., Whitehead, M. I. and Campbell, S. (1991). Ultrasound screening for familial ovarian cancer. *Gynecol. Oncol.*, **43**, 92–7

Ovarian malignant tumors: transvaginal color Doppler assessment

15

A. Kurjak, S. Kupesic, M. Predanic, H. Shalan, M. Ilijas and K. Maeda

Ovarian malignant neoplasms are the most common gynecological pelvic malignancy in most Western countries[1]. Despite progress in chemotherapy and surgery, its incidence continues to rise with age[2]. In the United States malignant ovarian tumors are the leading cause of gynecological cancer death. Of 20 000 new cases of this disease diagnosed per year in the US, approximately 12 000 women will die[1]. In the United Kingdom, the crude annual rate of the disease is 17.3 per 100 000 women; it is the sixth most common cancer among women[3]. This high rate of mortality from ovarian malignancy can be explained by the paucity of early and specific symptoms. By the time that symptoms do appear, the disease has spread beyond the ovaries in 70–90% of cases[4,5]. A late diagnosis by traditional techniques is probably the main reason for the poor prognosis. The 5-year survival rate is about 20% in advanced disease (stages III and IV)[6]. Malignant ovarian tumors, therefore, present a serious problem in terms of both detection and management. A slight improvement only could be obtained by aggressive surgery, new therapeutic regimens, or new diagnostic tools. Hence, attempts to improve survival and decrease the number of deaths from ovarian cancer have been focused in three areas: prevention, early detection and improved treatment regimens.

For a long time, early detection of localized ovarian cancer has been a matter of chance rather than a triumph of some scientific method. The main problems for early ovarian cancer detection arise from the fact that the ovary is a unique tissue. Ovarian tissue reveals huge histological complexity, which not only gives rise to a great variety of malignancies, but also provides a favorite site for metastasis from other organs. The most frequent cancers are of epithelial origin, accounting for nearly 90% of all cases reported[7]. Ovarian cancers generally begin in the ovaries and frequently spread throughout the entire peritoneal cavity by direct peritoneal dissemination. The capacity of cancer to grow and disseminate makes early diagnosis so important. A cancerous tumor 1 cm^3 in size contains about a billion cells, each potentially capable of originating a new focus of cancer. Discovery of cancer when the tumor is considerably smaller than this should materially increase cure rates[8].

The definitive diagnosis of an ovarian mass also presents a common problem in gynecological patients. If the clinician could accurately differentiate a malignant from a benign mass, patients with masses believed to be malignant could seek proper oncological consultation preoperatively. Furthermore, at the time of operation, the appropriate incision would allow careful staging. Hence, the preoperative diagnosis of malignant ovarian tumors might reduce the need for repeated laparotomies and could lead to referral to or consultation with a gynecological oncologist capable of proceeding with radical procedures[9].

TRANSABDOMINAL SONOGRAPHY

Although Sunden (1964)[10] reported that pathological changes in the ovary could be seen with ultrasound, it was not until almost a decade later that the next report of ultrasound examination of the ovary was published by Kratochwil (1969)[11]. In the early 1980s the ovaries could be identified by tracing the course of their vessels. With the advent of real-time sector scanners, quick and easy identification of the ovary became possible. At that time it was justified to use transabdominal ultrasound for early detection of ovarian cancer in a selected group of women at risk[12]. In 1990

Campbell and co-workers[13] evaluated transabdominal sonography as a screening method for cancer of the ovary. The ovary was evaluated by three criteria:

(1) Deviation from the normal ovarian morphology, which is a uniform hypoechogenic structure with smooth outline;

(2) Calculation of the ovarian volume by the formula:

$$\text{Ovarian volume} = d_1 \times d_2 \times d_3 \times 0.523$$

where d_1, d_2, d_3 are the maximal transverse, anteroposterior and longitudinal diameters of the ovary;

(3) Change in ovarian volume at repeat scan, for which they proposed a cut-off value for a positive screen result.

They obtained a positive result (based mainly on the presence of abnormal morphology) in 338 screens (326 women) from 5479 self-referred asymptomatic women. Five patients with primary ovarian cancer were identified (prevalence 0.09%). The apparent detection rate was 100% and the false-positive rate was 3.5% at first screen and 2.3% overall. The authors concluded that the use of abnormal morphology, or the maximum ovarian volume >96th centile for a positive screen result, together with a defined volume change at rescan, would give a false-positive rate of 3.1% at first screen and 2.0% overall. These results provide a very rational basis for the application and development of ultrasound screening procedures for early ovarian cancer in both pre- and postmenopausal women.

As the pelvis contains many soft-tissue organs having a similar sonographic pattern, a transabdominal probe cannot provide a clear image of the various structures due to the low resolution, unacceptable attenuation of the transmitted pulses and, particularly in obese patients, the ovaries being well outside the focal zone of the transducer[14,15]. Herrman and co-workers[16] described the sonographic patterns of malignant ovarian tumors as a method for prediction of malignancy. The authors assessed the following criteria: the size and location of the tumor, borders of the mass, and presence of free pelvic fluid (ascites). The internal structure of the tumor was considered the most important sonographic criterion for distinguishing benign from malignant disorders; tumors were classified as cystic, complex and solid. Thick septa, irregular solid parts within a mass, indefinite margins, and the presence of ascites and bowel loops containing matter were regarded as malignant patterns. The positive predictive value of transabdominal sonography was low (73%). This was a result of the high number of false-positive cases, due to a significant overlap in the ultrasonic endometriotic cysts and mucinous cystadenomas with ovarian malignancies. Andolf and colleagues[17] in their series of 801 women at risk of developing ovarian cancer examined by transabdominal sonography, had 83% sensitivity and 96% specificity, and they concluded that ultrasound screening for ovarian cancer should not be recommended, even in groups at risk for the disease. The authors could not interpret results in six cases, due to inability of the women to distend their bladders or to poor quality of the sonograms. Such conditions present in transabdominal ultrasound, with its known limitations, are not encountered with the use of transvaginal sonography, as there is no need for bladder distension and the resolution of the sonogram is so good that transvaginal sonography is sometimes termed 'sonomicroscopy'[18,19].

TRANSVAGINAL SONOGRAPHY

Morphological criteria established with transabdominal sonography have been stressed and more accurately described with transvaginal high-resolution sonography. Its superb visualization of adnexal tumors allows precise assessment, and its morphological characteristics allow description through the three categories based on the complexity of tumor appearance. Every category has a relative specificity and should always be viewed within the framework of other clinical findings.

Cystic adnexal lesion

A completely cystic adnexal mass represents the first category and is defined according to the following criteria: anechoic cyst contents, well-defined walls of varying thickness and posterior acoustic enhancement. The commonest type of adnexal mass which meets these criteria is the functional ovarian cyst. These cysts may be demonstrated as bilocular, multilocular and unilocular which is the most frequent finding. Histopathological findings of serous and mucinous cystadenomas are also correlated with these images. They are the commonest ovarian epithelial tumors, having a very specific ultrasonic appearance, expressed mostly as multilocular cysts. Besides the linear internal septa which are more pronounced in the mucinous type, they are usually large and contain clear fluid with a very low echogenic pattern. However, the main characteristic is thin septations, less than 3 mm in diameter. Sometimes it is possible to visualize daughter cysts within a large unilocular cyst. Paraovarian cysts which develop from Gartner's duct have the same appearance as functional cysts and are only occasionally distinguishable from them. Paraovarian cysts can measure only 2–3 cm, but more often grow to be quite large. Hydrosalpinx often also appears as a cystic mass. A smaller hydrosalpinx usually assumes a fusiform shape, but larger ones are of a rather round shape.

The presence of dense echogenic contents of the cysts is usually correlated with mucinous cystadenomas, or more often with endometriomata. The presence of a characteristic homogeneous carpet of low-level echoes in a cystic pelvic mass is an extremely common finding in endometriomas. Kupfer and colleagues reported that this characteristic echogenic pattern was found in 82% of studied cases[20]. The described feature may be seen dispersed throughout the lesion or may involve one or several sites in a multiloculated mass. These low-level echoes probably represent degraded blood products associated with cyclic changes occurring during the menstrual cycle[20]. In comparison with a homogeneous, dense-echoic carpet intracystic pattern, in some cases the presence of an irregular geographic hyperechoic region internally can be caused by a more acute phase of hemorrhage.

Cystic–solid ovarian mass

The second morphological group of adnexal masses comprises predominantly cystic structures containing internal echoes such as septa or any other echogenic material or solid structures with homogeneous or unhomogeneous texture. Serous and mucinous cystadenomas can be found in this group as well as in the previous one. Dermoid cysts – adult teratomas and tubo-ovarian abscesses – are the most frequent finding in the group of benign adnexal lesions. A characteristic pattern of dermoid cysts is the content of hair which is ultrasonically demonstrated as a large number of separated and short, hyperechoic linear structures. However, the appearance of dermoid cysts is extremely variable. Sometimes these cysts contain a core of solid tissue with a highly echogenic focus and posterior shadowing. In some cases, the heterogeneous, solid part of dermoids is so emphasized that it gives the impression of a malignant ovarian mass. A tubo-ovarian abscess can contain echoes or fluid levels representing the layering of purulent debris, or may appear as a heterogeneous, solid tumor containing small cystic structures.

Although the complex tumors with a dominant solid or cystic component include most of the benign ovarian masses described above, malignant ovarian lesions such as cystadenocarcinomas, endometrioid carcinomas, clear cell carcinomas and borderline tumors also exhibit this kind of ultrasonic appearance. Because a significant overlap exists in many echo patterns seen in benign and malignant ovarian neoplasms, criteria for transvaginal ultrasonographic diagnosis were proposed[21]. Echo patterns were categorized as follows:

(1) *Septations* Structures which cross a liquid phase as echogenic bridges measuring from 0.5 mm to more than 1 cm;

(2) *Loculations* Semicircular or circular echogenic structures protruding into the sonolucent contents with interstructural contiguity, or measuring more than 1 cm in length in the case of a solitary structure;

(3) *Solid lesions* Formations occupying more than 25% of the space of the mass;

(4) *Papillae* Echogenic formations protruding into the liquid phase, measuring from 5 mm to more than 2 cm, but not occupying more than 25% of the lesion space;

(5) *Daughter cysts* Semicircular echogenic structures protruding into the liquid phase; and

(6) *Liquid phase* Intratumoral sonolucency of low-level echogenicity or completely sonolucent.

Statistically significant correlation was found between ovarian malignancy and sonographic findings such as the presence of papillae, solid components ($p<0.001$) and thick septa ($p<0.003$).

Solid ovarian neoplasms

Solid ovarian tumors are included in the third category. The commonest benign solid tumor types are ovarian fibromas and some dermoids. They are usually round with hyperechogenic texture, well delineated. Intratumoral vascularization, centrally or peripherally located, is rarely seen. However, in some cases a regularly separated vessel with high vascular impedance to blood flow may be displayed.

In comparison with benign ovarian tumors, malignant tumors with a solid sonographic image are adenocarcinomas and malignant teratomas. They are richly vascularized with areas of neovascularization clearly displayed, mostly within the central or peripheral part of the tumor. Pulsed Doppler assessment of observed vessels shows extremely low vascular impedance to blood flow. In terms of the resistance index, values are below 0.40.

Numerous independent studies have compared ovarian lesions with changes of the normal anatomical structure in a healthy ovary. These lesions can be identified as septations, papillary projections, loculations, solid lesions and liquid phase within cystic structures, daughter cysts and solid lesions[22]. The purpose of these studies was to attempt to discriminate between benign and malignant entities using comparable and reproducible criteria. Based on these features of malignant ovarian masses, many authors tried to create universally accepted scoring systems. Unfortunately, reported results most frequently showed high sensitivity with poor specificity, and vice versa. Bourne and associates[23] presented a prospective study to screen for ovarian cancer in a high-risk group of symptomatic women. A scoring system was based on features of an ovarian lesion such as solid, monocystic or multicystic, loculations (unilocular or multilocular), outline of the cyst (irregular, regular), and on the basis of its anechoic, randomly echoic or uniformly echogenic appearance. The results were promising, but the specificity was not high enough. Other anthors tried to develop better scoring systems but with no more success[24–26]. In a comprehensive review of eight series by Sassone and co-workers[26], a range of sensitivities of 62–100%, specificities of 73–95%, and positive predictive values of 31–88% were revealed. Trying to evaluate their own scoring system in prediction of ovarian malignancy, they used the morphological characteristics of the ovarian masses – the inner wall structure, wall thickness, septal thickness, and echogenicity of the tumor. The authors gave numerical scores to each tumor and used a score of 9 as the cut-off value to differentiate between benign and malignant ovarian lesions. Their scores had sensitivity and negative predictive value of 100% and 100%, respectively. However, the specificity and positive predictive value were 37% and 83%, respectively. This was due to the overlap between benign lesions such as teratomas, tubo-ovarian abscesses, hemorrhagic cysts, and hydrosalpinx with the malignant ovarian tumors. Thus, using the morphology of the tumor alone is not a sufficient parameter to detect malignant ovarian tumors, and even when the authors changed the cut-off value to 10, the test became more specific but less sensitive. They concluded that manipulation of the test performance by varying the choice of the threshold is the advantage of a numerical scoring system in aiming to achieve a precise cut-off value. However, very large series are required to determine a more accurate distribution of scores associated with different disease processes and evaluate whether the scoring system can be improved by assigning different weights to each characteristic. Considering what is the main problem in morphological assessment of tumors, it has become clear that some benign tumors produce an image like that of a malignant tumor. Endometriosis and dermoid cysts frequently produce false-positive results. Is it possible to avoid these false results and increase specificity without a reduction in sensitivity? To fulfil this task, an improvement in transvaginal sonography is required. These new modalities are expressed with pulsed and color Doppler analysis.

Transvaginal color Doppler examination of ovarian malignancy

Great interest among gynecologists has been focused on the process of pelvic tumor angiogenesis. It is now well known that tumor hyperemia is related to new blood vessel growth – neovascularization – as well as to dilatation of previously existing vessels. Viable tumor cells release diffusible angiogenic factors which stimulate new capillary growth and endothelial mitosis *in vivo*[27–29] even when tumor cell proliferation has been arrested by irradiation[30]. In 1971, Judah Folkman proposed a hypothesis that 'once tumor take occurs, every further increase in tumor cell population must be preceded by an increase in new capillaries which converge upon the tumor early growth'[29]. According to this concept, a small focus of tumor cells (containing less than 10^6 cells in a volume of a few cubic millimeters) could not increase indefinitely without the induction of angiogenesis. Furthermore, there is strong evidence that growth of solid tumors beyond a few millimeters in diameter depends on the induction of a functional microcirculation from surrounding host tissue[31]. It is obvious that malignant tumor induces growth of the independent and characteristic vascular network on its own. The tumor vasculature is highly heterogeneous and does not conform to the standard normal vascular organization (i.e. artery to arteriole to capillaries to postcapillary venule to venule to vein). A key difference between normal and tumor vessels is that the latter are dilated, saccular and tortuous, and may contain tumor cells within the endothelial lining of the vessel wall[32]. In addition, unlike normal tissue, with a relatively fixed route between the arterial and venous sides, a tumor may have blood flowing from one venule to another via a series of vessels or directly via an arteriovenous shunt. The vascular network is seemingly developed without purpose, keeps to no set course and shows no progressive diminution in caliber[33]. Newly formed vessels are large capillaries (rather large, endothelium-lined, capillary-like channels), or sinusoids, and contain no smooth muscle in their walls but, instead, only some fibrous connective tissue[34]. Furthermore, due to the peculiar nature of the vasculature, the organization of vessels may be different from one location to another and from one time to the next. As a result, one would expect different routes of blood flow in the well-perfused advancing zone, from the semi-necrotic and necrotic zones. Based on perfusion rates, four regions can be recognized in a tumor:

(1) An avascular (necrotic) region;

(2) An ischemic (semi-necrotic) region;

(3) A stabilized microcirculation; and

(4) An advancing front as a region of tumor hyperemia (Figure 1).

In general, as tumors grow larger, their vascular surfaces are decreased, their intercapillary distance increases and they may develop necrotic foci.

In general, the tumor vasculature consists of (1) vessels recruited from the pre-existing network of the host vasculature, and (2) vessels recruited from the angiogenic response of host vessels to cancer cells. Although the tumor vasculature originates from the host vasculature, its organization may be completely different depending upon the tumor type, its growth rate and its location. The architecture is different, not only between various tumor types, but also between a spontaneous tumor and its transplants[33].

Tumor vasculature develops unpredictably, hence the only possible way to assess its features is by means of angiography and color Doppler sonography. Angiography is an invasive procedure, while transvaginal color and pulsed Doppler sonography is non-invasive and more convenient for the patient. During the transvaginal color Doppler examination, the patient is relaxed, and the procedure does not take more than 15 min. The superb resolution of newly developed transvaginal color Doppler transducers allows accurate assessment of suspicious

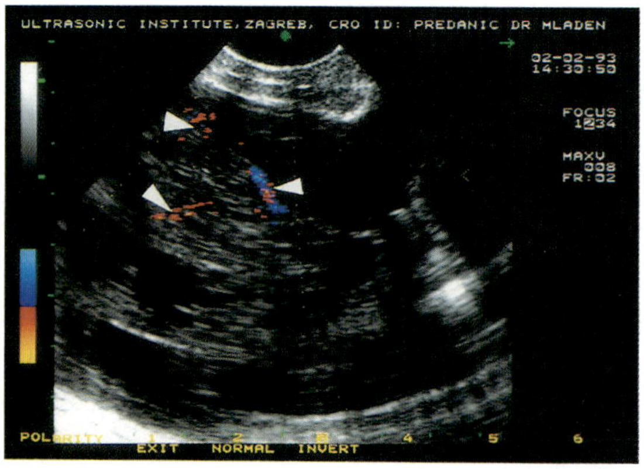

Figure 1 Huge peripheral and central vascularization (arrows) of a malignant ovarian tumor. This vascularized area represents the advancing tumor front and region of tumor hyperemia

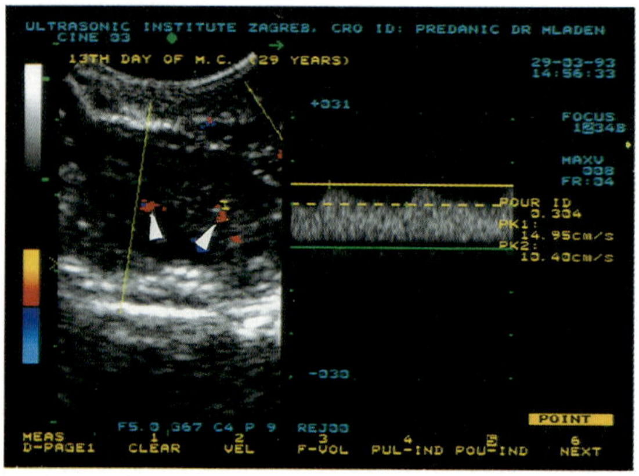

Figure 2 Normal ovary, 4 × 2 cm in diameter. Moderate color Doppler signal within the ovarian stroma (arrows, left), 13th day of menstrual cycle. Pulsed Doppler signal shows low impedance to blood flow (resistance index = 0.304). Length of menstrual cycle was 25 days, hence this early corpus luteum blood flow could be misinterpreted as ovarian malignancy if re-examination was not performed

ovarian masses, as well as precise visualization of their vasculature.

Vessels may be visualized in any part of a malignant ovarian tumor: within the sonographically heterogeneous central part of the mass as well as on its periphery, at the base or within large papillary projections, in the close proximity of cystic mass formations, as well as within the septa. A tumor may consist of many regions, each exhibiting one or other of these vascular patterns.

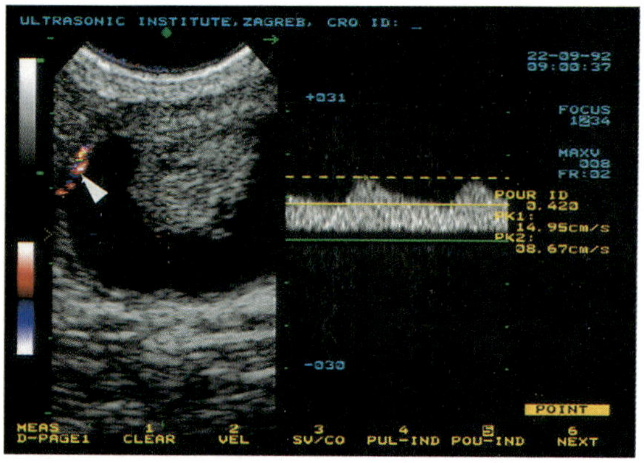

Figure 3 Corpus luteum cyst demonstrated as cystic–solid ovarian mass. Pericystically located vessels (arrow) show moderate vascular impedance to blood flow (resistance index = 0.42). If color and pulsed Doppler technique had not been used, this lesion could have been interpreted as a suspicious mass by black-and-white sonography

Abnormal architecture of malignant tumor vasculature reveals abnormal pulsed Doppler waveform signals. In comparison with pulsed Doppler sonograms obtained in normal tissues and organs, Doppler sonograms gathered from malignant tissues are characterized by low vascular impedance to blood flow, expressed in terms of the resistance index (RI) or pulsatility index (PI), with very low values. These findings are in correlation with results documented in malignant breast tumors. The presence of abnormal flow spectra with very high velocities around the periphery of malignant tumors has been observed[35–37]. High velocity signals in breast cancers have established the hypothesis that such signals result from arteriovenous anastomosis[35]. These results hve been confirmed by several groups[38–40].

The advantages of transvaginal color and pulsed Doppler sonography applied to ovarian tumors were demonstrated for the first time in 1989 by the Zagreb[41] and London[42] groups.

The Zagreb group[41] studied the vascularity of pelvic masses, and observed low impedance intratumoral blood flow in malignant ovarian lesions and other pelvic tumors. In five malignant ovarian tumors, the mean RI value was 0.33 ± 0.08. The results suggested that an increased tumor vascular supply may be accepted as firm evidence of probable tumor malignancy. The London group[42] supported these results. In their study, among 18 women with ovarian tumors, eight were malignant. Pulsatility index values were below 1.0 in seven of eight malignant tumors (0.3–0.9). False-positive results were obtained from bilateral dermoid cysts (PI values of 0.4 and 0.8). They concluded that high vascular impedance to blood flow can be used to exclude the presence of invasive primary ovarian cancer. In another large study, our Institute evaluated 14 317 asymptomatic or minimally symptomatic women for ovarian carcinoma[43]. Among 680 discovered adnexal masses, 624 were benign and 56 malignant tumors. Using an RI value below 0.41 as the threshold value in distinguishing malignant from benign ovarian masses, a sensitivity of 97% and a specificity of 100% were found.

Simultaneously, other groups reported their results with higher RI values obtained from malignant tumors, or with significant overlapping in results between benign and malignant adnexal lesions. Hata and colleagues[44] found moderate vascular impedance to blood flow in eight cases of ovarian cancer (mean RI = 0.50), as well as in four benign lesions. An overlap in results was probably caused by the inability to differentiate blood flow in endometrioid ovarian cysts and corpus luteum cysts from that of carcinoma. In addition, the authors misinterpreted internal iliac artery Doppler signals, in one case, for those within the ovary. In a following study performed by the same authors[45], similar results were found, a mean RI value of 0.50 ± 0.1 from another eight malignant ovarian tumors. Fleischer and coworkers[46] described significant differences between PI values of 32 benign lesions (1.8 ± 0.8) and 11 malignant lesions (0.8 ± 0.6). However, the ranges of benign (4.0–0.7) and malignant (1.5–0.4) masses did overlap. A significant overlap in results using a PI value of 1.0 as the threshold value was confirmed again[47]. Three relatively vascular benign lesions (one immature teratoma, one cystadenoma containing a dermoid cyst, one endometrioma) caused an overlap between the PI values of benign and malignant masses. A large range in RI and PI results as well as significant overlapping published in these papers pose some questions. When more than one signal is obtained, which RI values should be used – the smallest or the highest? Abnormal signals represent reduced vascular impedance to blood flow due to tumoral neovascularization. Hence, the lowest index value should be considered as a reference value for abnormal angiogenesis and possible malignancy.

Weiner and colleagues[48] published results with PI values of the intraovarian or intratumoral blood vessels below 1.0 in all 15 malignant cases. A mean PI of 0.52 (range 0.2–2.6) in malignant ovarian masses and 1.17 for benign ovarian tumors were found by Timor-Tritsch and associates[49] in their most recent report. In all cases of malignant ovarian tumors, blood flow was obtained in terms of color Doppler. In comparison with these papers, Kawai and colleagues[50] suggested a PI cut-off value of 1.25 obtained after the assessment of 13 benign and 11 malignant lesions. Although there are different opinions about cut-off values, as well as different RI or PI ranges for malignant ovarian tumors, all authors agree that recognition of angiogenesis as a reference point for malignant changes within the ovary has proved to be a highly sensitive parameter. Given that the neovascularization is an obligate event in malignant change, this may enable us to observe the earliest stages in ovarian oncogenesis. However, one must be aware of the possibility that angiogenesis may be detected in some cases of transient cyclic pituitary activation[51], as well as in ovarian inflammation. Observed differences between malignant and benign angiogenesis in terms of maximum vascularity (color flow) obtained with transvaginal color Doppler was investigated by Reynolds and colleagues[52]. They investigated the expression of platelet-derived endothelial cell growth factor (PD-ECGF) in ovarian tumors and found that the highest level of expression of PD-ECGF was in the malignant tissues and the lowest in the postmenopausal and follicular phase ovarian tissues. PD-ECGF was also overexpressed in a corpus luteum. These results demonstrated overexpression of PD-ECGF in ovarian cancer and suggest that a stromal component is the source. It is possible that analysis of PD-ECGF levels in ovarian cyst fluid or serum may prove useful and an additional diagnostic test for further evaluation of ovarian malignant tumor angiogenesis.

Table 1 Comparison of color Doppler results in discrimination of malignant from benign ovarian tumors

					Mean value ± SD and range	
Authors	*n*	*M/B*	*Index*	*Cut-off value*	*Malignant*	*Benign*
Kurjak *et al.*[41]	20	5/15	RI	0.40	0.33±0.08	–
Bourne *et al.*[42]	18	8/10	PI	–	0.3–0.9 (5.5)*	3.2–7.0
Kurjak *et al.*[43]	680	56/624	RI	0.40	0.28–0.40	>0.40 (0.39)*
Fleischer *et al.*[46]	43	11/32	PI	1.00	0.8±0.6 (0.5–1.4)	1.8±0.8 (0.7–4.0)
Fleischer *et al.*[47]	26	3/23	PI	1.00	0.7±0.2 (0.7–1.0)	1.9±0.7 (0.6–2.8)
Campbell *et al.*[67]	7	7/0	PI	–	0.61 (0.40–0.96)	–
			RI	–	0.46 (0.33–0.78)	–
Weiner *et al.*[48]	53	17/36	PI	1.00	0.75–0.81	–
Kawai *et al.*[50]	24	9/15	PI	1.25	0.93±0.65	1.45±0.05
Hata *et al.*[54]	20	8/12	RI	–	0.50±0.12	0.88±0.22
Timor-Tritsch *et al.*[49]	94	16/78	PI	–	0.52	1.17
			RI	–	0.39	0.64
Tekay and Jouppila[53]	72	11/61†	RI	0.60 0.50	0.4–0.6	0.4–1.0
			PI	–	0.5–0.9	0.5–3.5
Kurjak *et al.*[57]	83	29/54	RI	0.40	0.37±0.08	0.62±0.11
Zanneta *et al.*[56]	60	23/37	PI	–	0.79	1.45
			RI	–	0.49	0.79

*Value for one case in parentheses; †8 malignant+3 borderline tumors; PI, pulsatility index; B, benign ovarian lesions; M, malignant ovarian lesions

However, a recent publication[53] has suggested that in an assessment of tumor angiogenesis, practical cut-off values for either the pulsatility or resistance indices to assist in differentiating between malignant or benign lesions, do not exist! In the group of 72 patients, with 51 benign, eight malignant and three borderline tumors, the mean PI of tumor blood vessels was 1.2, 0.7 and 0.6, respectively. The corresponding mean RI values were 0.6, 0.5 and 0.5. The differences were not significant and the overlap between the malignant and benign lesions was large. Further, Hata and associates[54] recently suggested that transvaginal color Doppler ultrasound does not provide more useful diagnostic information than transvaginal sonography, magnetic resonance imaging (MRI) and CA 125 measurement for differentiation of malignant from benign ovarian tumors. Although they found a difference in RI values between malignant (0.50±0.1) and benign (0.69±0.18) ovarian neoplasms, the sensitivity and specificity did not differ from those obtained by MRI and CA125 measurement. Similar results were presented by Valentin and Sladkevicius[55]. They claim that ultrasound morphology of the tumor is a better discriminator between benign and malignant tumors than any tested Doppler (color and pulsed Doppler) variable. The ultrasound morphology correctly identified all the malignant tumors with a false-positive rate of 27% in 149 women with 28 malignant and 121 benign ovarian masses. Color and pulsed Doppler were useful only in discrimination between benign and malignant multilocular cysts with some solid components, reducing the false-positive rate to 17–23%, depending on which Doppler variable and which cut-off value was used. They concluded that the present technique of Doppler velocimetry adds little to the differential diagnosis of extrauterine pelvic masses.

A review of the results (mean RI or PI, range, number of patients and benign/malignant tumors) collected from previously mentioned articles is presented in Table 1. In almost all papers, PI and RI values and cut-off points were used for discrimination of benign and malignant tumors. Assessment of ovarian malignancy based on only one parameter – the pulsed Doppler

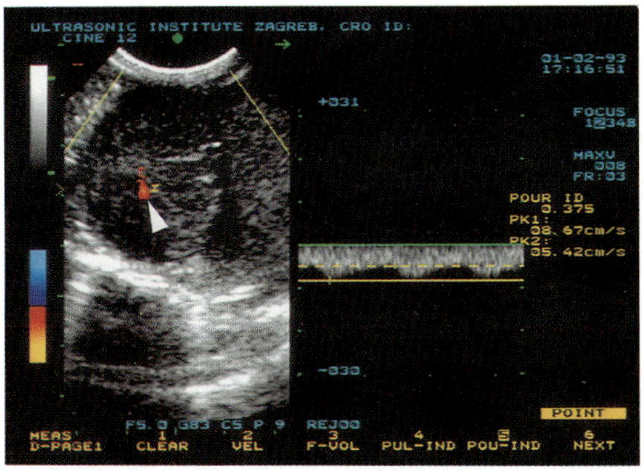

Figure 4 Color Doppler signal in central part of solid–cystic ovarian mass (endometrioid cystadenocarcinoma) (arrow). Low resistance (resistance index = 0.375) is shown in analyzed vessel (right)

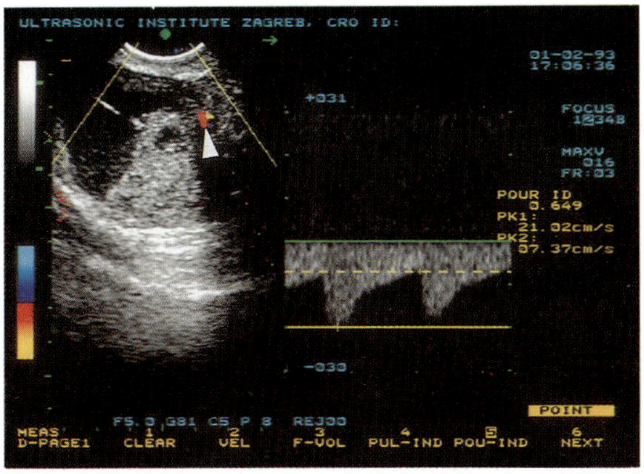

Figure 5 Same ovarian mass as in Figure 4 (endometrioid cystadenocarcinoma), but at its periphery (arrow) high vascular impedance to blood flow was demonstrated (resistance index = 0.65, right)

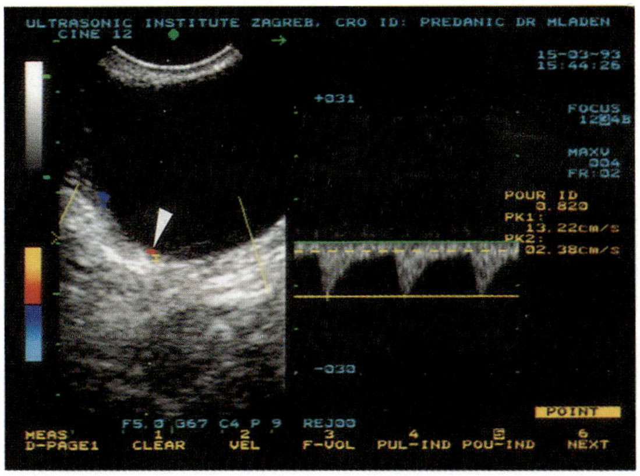

Figure 6 Simple ovarian cyst in a premenopausal patient. Benign vascularization, with single vessel (pericystically located, arrow) and high vascular impedance to blood flow (resistance index = 0.82)

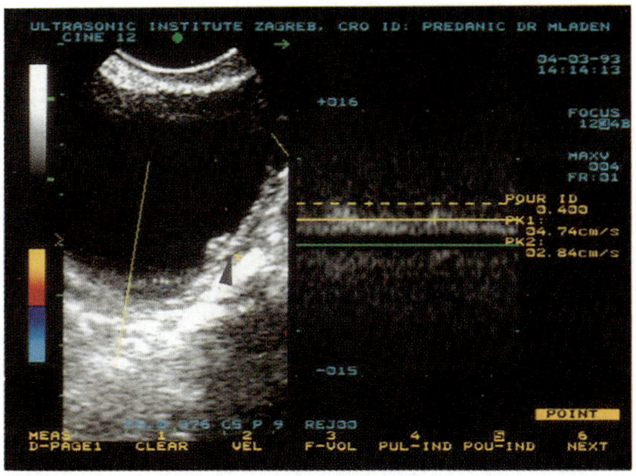

Figure 7 Cystic ovarian lesion with small papillary projection attached to its upper wall (left). Pulsed Doppler signal (right) from the vessel (arrow) at the base of papillary projection. Impedance to blood flow was low (resistance index = 0.40)

sonogram and its value – may be the cause of a large overlap in results between benign and malignant ovarian masses such as is published in some papers. Very often, a corpus luteum, corpus luteum cyst or functional cyst (Figures 2 and 3) may produce false-positive results. Hence, where a large team of ultrasonographers is included in the study, the interobserver variation is larger, and if all patients with hormonal distress or dysfunction are not excluded from the study, a large range of results as well as a large overlap can be expected. Is it possible to reduce the percentage of false-positive and false-negative results? Now, the only acceptable solution is multiparameter assessment of tumor vasculature.

Ultrasonically visualized tumor vasculature in different ovarian mass areas can be categorized in a few idealized types of vascularization by its location. Fleischer and colleagues[46] suggested that, macroscopically, tumor vasculature could be categorized as peripheral and central. Although this classification is not appropriate and is anatomically incorrect, it may help in the location of ultrasonically detectable vessels within

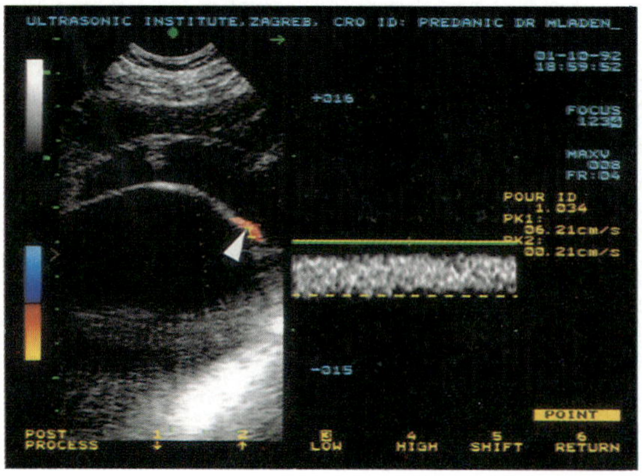

Figure 8 Serous cystadenoma with low malignant potential (assessed histologically as borderline tumor). Color Doppler signal was obtained within septum (arrow); however, pulsed Doppler shows characteristic blood flow pattern of vein (peak systolic velocity was very low, 6.2 cm/s)

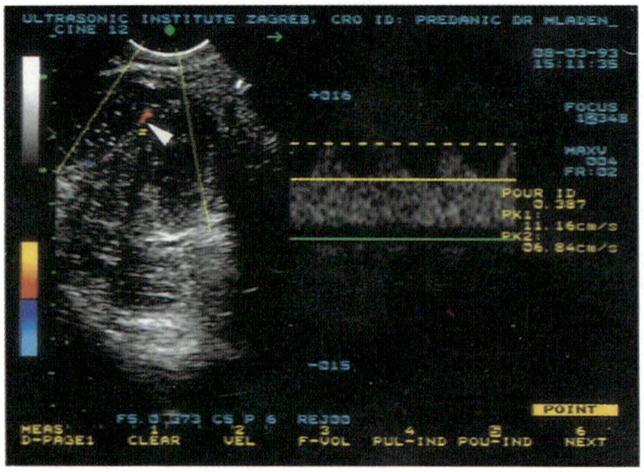

Figure 10 Color Doppler sonography shows blood flow signal within thick septum of mucinous cystadenocarcinoma (arrow). Resistance index = 0.387, indicating malignancy (right)

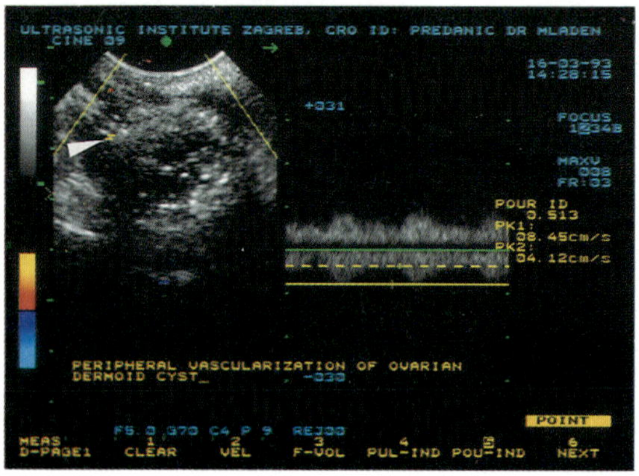

Figure 9 Solid ovarian tumor – ovarian dermoid. Pulsed Doppler waveform analysis shows moderate to high vascular impedance to blood flow (resistance index = 0.52) in peripherally located vessel (arrow)

the tumor. The authors reported that in malignant masses, peripheral arteries had an average PI of 1.1 (range 0.4–2.0), central vessels a mean PI of 0.6 (range 0.5–0.9) and septal arteries a mean PI of 0.5. It is proposed that peripheral vessels within tumor tissue originate from pre-existing host vasculature, while central vessels develop as a response to tumor cells' angiogenic activity and/or due to necrotic processes. Vessels displayed within septa or papillae represent specific intratumoral branches. A similar classification was proposed by the Zagreb group[58,59]. Location of the intratumoral vessels as central, peripheral, pericystic, within papillary projections and septa, were suggested (Figures 4–8). Our results showed that benign adnexal masses were mostly vascularized in the pericystic and peripheral location (Figure 9), while in malignant tumors, central vascularization with low RI values was more frequent (Figure 10). Significant differences between benign and malignant ovarian lesions in terms of the RI are presented in Figure 11. Differences between benign and malignant ovarian tumors in terms of vascular locations and vascular impedance to blood flow are presented in Figures 12–28. In their most recent paper, Fleischer and co-workers[60] studied 25 malignant and 25 benign ovarian lesions. They achieved statistical significance between these entities in terms of vessel location, impedance and waveform shape. Malignant masses typically were characterized by centrally located vessels that had low impedance without a diastolic 'notch' in the waveform. However, maximum systolic velocities were statistically similar in benign and malignant lesions. The mean blood flow velocities in peripheral arteries of the malignant tumors were around 21 cm/s, and in central arteries, 11 cm/s. In our recent study, we could not achieve any significant difference between benign and malignant adnexal tumors[59] (Figure 29). Relatively high velocities in most of the malignant ovarian

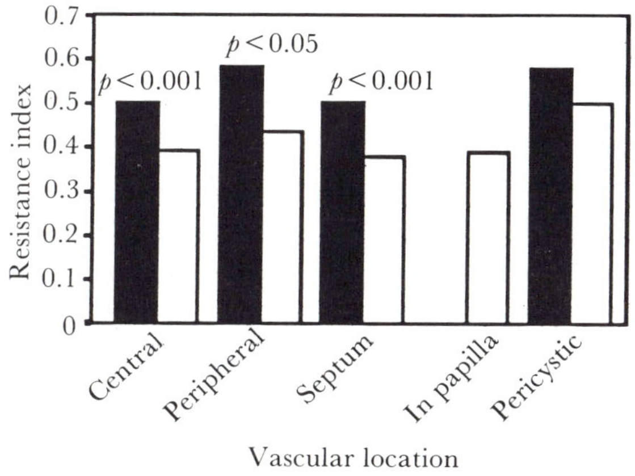

Figure 11 Comparison of mean resistance index values between benign (white bars) and malignant (solid bars) ovarian tumors

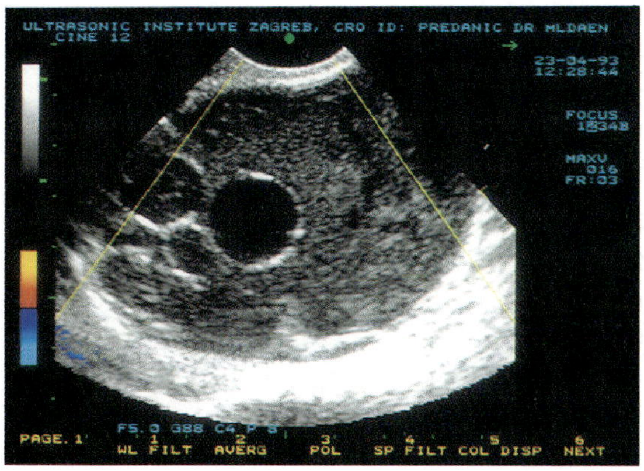

Figure 13 Large avascular ovarian endometriotic cyst with homogeneous intracystic echoes. Note the cystic anechoic areas which represent acute hemorrhage

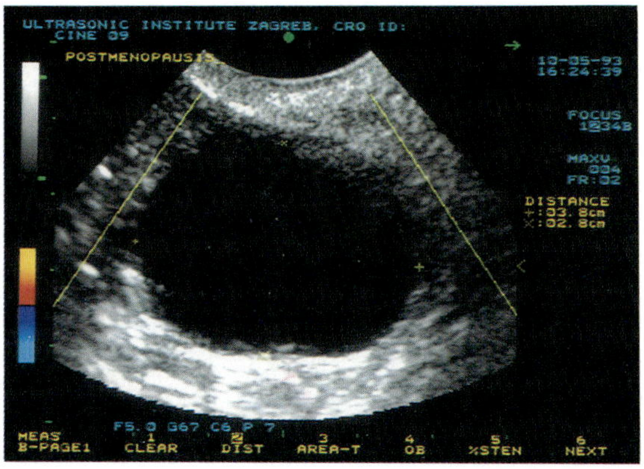

Figure 12 Simple benign ovarian cyst in a postmenopausal patient aged 53 years. Note smooth walls of ovarian cyst and absence of cyst vascularization

Table 2 Assessment based on combination of morphological and color Doppler system results

Assessment	*Morphological*	*Color Doppler*
Benign lesion	benign	benign
Questionable mass (benign tumor with possibility of malignant alteration)	malignant	benign
Suspicious mass (tumor in early stage of developing malignancy)	benign	malignant
Malignant lesion	malignant	malignant

tumors and a statistically significant difference observed in the blood flow velocities of benign versus malignant ovarian tumors were presented by Valentin and Sladkevicius[55]. However, in the group of multilocular cysts with solid parts, the results between benign and malignant lesions totally overlapped. It is possible that in some cases of malignant ovarian tumors, high velocities may be found, although we believe that because of the specific vascular ovarian network, velocities can usually not be higher than 50–70 cm/s, a very high velocity even for a main uterine artery. Hence, further investigations in terms of blood flow velocities are required although it is not likely that significant results will be achieved.

Another important parameter in the assessment of tumor blood vessels is their arrangement[58,59]. Vessels were categorized as no vessel seen, regularly separated (single) vessels and randomly dispersed (diffuse) vessels. In malignant ovarian masses, diffuse arrangement of vessels, mostly localized centrally, were more frequent than in benign lesions. Furthermore, in benign ovarian masses, single vessels were mostly peripherally and pericystically located. All these three parameters: RI, vessel location and arrangement, were the skeleton of the latest published color and pulsed Doppler scoring system[58]. In this way, high sensitivity of 97% and specificity of 100% were achieved. False-negative results are

Table 3 Comparison of color Doppler results in discrimination of malignant from benign ovarian tumors

Authors	*n*	*M/B*	*Index*	*Cut-off value*	*Sensitivity* (%)	*Specificity* (%)	*PPV* (%)	*NPV* (%)	*Accuracy* (%)
Kurjak *et al.*[41]	20	5/15	RI	0.40	100	97	87	100	98
Kurjak *et al.*[43]	680	56/624	RI	0.40	96	99	98	99	99
Fleischer *et al.*[46]	43	11/32	PI	1.00	B: 90	83	95	71	92
					M: 100	83	73	100	100
Fleischer *et al.*[47]	26	3/23	PI	1.00	B: 90	83	95	71	92
					M: 100	83	73	100	100
Weiner *et al.*[48]	53	17/36	PI	1.00	94	97	97	94	–
Kawai *et al.*[50]	24	9/15	PI	1.25	–	–	–	–	96
Timor-Tritsch *et al.*[49]	94	16/78	PI	–	94	99	94	–	–
			RI	–	94	99	94	–	–
Tekay and Jouppila[53]	72	11/61*	RI	0.60	82	72	35	96	74
				0.50	46	89	42	90	82
			PI	–	–	–	–	–	–
Kurjak *et al.*[57]	83	29/54	RI	0.40	90	95	96	95	–
Kurjak and Predanic[58] (scoring system)	174	38/136	RI	–	97	100	100	99	99
Zanneta *et al.*[56]	60	23/37	RI	0.56	87	94	–	–	91
			PI	1.00	95	89	–	–	91

*Eight malignant and three borderline tumors; M, malignant ovarian lesions; B, benign ovarian lesions; PPV, positive predictive value; NPV, negative predictive value; RI, resistance index; PI, pulsatility index

usually caused by borderline tumors in the early stage of malignant alteration, when they cannot be detected owing to lack of neovascularization. However, the color Doppler scoring system helps to reduce the false-negative and false-positive results obtained by transvaginal sonography. After all, the main attitude of the authors was that both scoring systems, morphological and color/pulsed Doppler combined (Table 2), should be used for precise assessment of the adnexal lesions. In the group of adnexal masses suspected of being malignant, 'suspicious' represents those tumors that resemble a normal ovary, but in which color Doppler sonography detects areas of neovascularization. This finding represents ovarian lesions in an early stage of malignant alteration. Lesions are 'questionable' if they are suspected of being malignant and color Doppler does not reveal any areas of neovascularization. These lesions are considered benign with the potential for malignant alteration. Patients with 'suspicious' and 'malignant' lesions should be operated on after one re-examination, whereas the 'questionable' group should be followed up by transvaginal color Doppler sonography. In a study performed by Bonilla-Musoles and co-workers[61], seven malignant and 101 benign ovarian masses were evaluated by transvaginal color Doppler sonography and preoperative puncture and aspiration, for establishing the cytological diagnosis. The aim of the study was to assess whether it was possible to avoid unnecessary surgery (benign cases) due to cytological diagnosis. No significant differences were observed between cytological and histopathological findings in cases that went to surgery. They concluded that, owing to the high percentage of unsatisfactory cytological results (20%) with cyst aspiration, vaginal and color Doppler sonography seemed to be more efficient in distinguishing between benignity and malignancy. So, it is clear that very high sensitivity and specificity in distinguishing benign from malignant ovarian lesions may be achieved. A review of statistical results in terms of sensitivity, specificity, positive and negative predictive value and accuracy are presented in Table 3. There is a large range in the published results, but the mean values, extracted from the table, for specificity of 86.6%, sensitivity of 88.2%, and accuracy of 92.5%, are very promising and with the standardization of color and pulsed Doppler criteria, averaging of results should be expected.

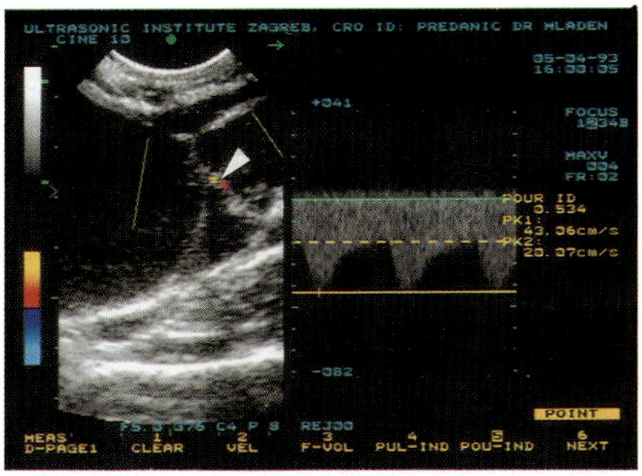

Figure 14 Multilocular endometrioid cyst. Single vessel arrangement (arrow) is seen within the tiny septa. Pulsed Doppler waveform signal shows moderate to high vascular impedance to blood flow (resistance index = 0.53)

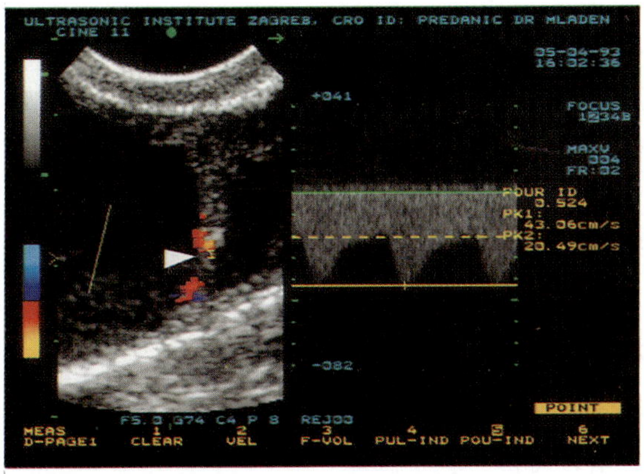

Figure 15 Another scan of the same multilocular endometrioid cyst as in Figure 14. Now, rich vascularization of the septa can be seen (arrow). Vascular impedance to blood flow was moderate to high (resistance index = 0.52, right)

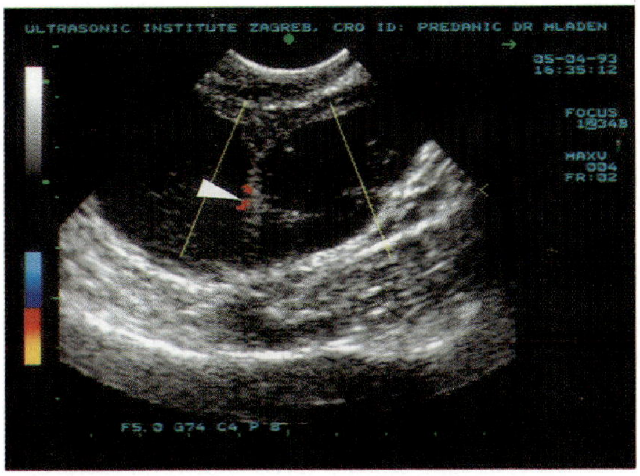

Figure 16 Small bilocular mucinous cystadenoma. Cystic walls are smooth, and subtle intracystic echoes can be observed. Note the septal vascularization (arrow)

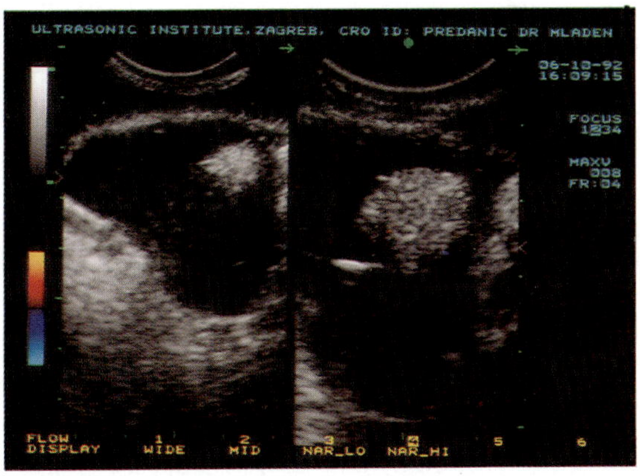

Figure 17 Adult ovarian teratoma, a cystic–solid ovarian structure in which color Doppler shows no area of vascularization

The main advantage of transvaginal color Doppler sonography can be found in its application for the screening of the postmenopausal group of patients for the early stage of ovarian cancer (FIGO stage Ia). Our ignorance about the premalignant stage of ovarian cancer has led to an aggressive approach when an ovarian enlargement is detected. A 10-year study from 1975–85 suggested that when a postmenopausal woman is operated upon for an ovarian neoplasm, the rate of malignancy may be as high as 47%[61]. The rate in women aged 30–49 years was 14–35%. The emergence of pelvic ultrasound examination has led to interventions for ovarian neoplasms resulting in rates of only one malignancy per ten operations[62,63]. This is potentially alarming, unless removal of benign neoplasms can reduce the eventual development of malignant disease. An optimum situation would dictate that surgery should not be performed for benign disease, except under conditions of a randomized clinical trial. Recently, few transvaginal[64] and transvaginal color and pulsed Doppler[65] studies with promising results were published. Our group

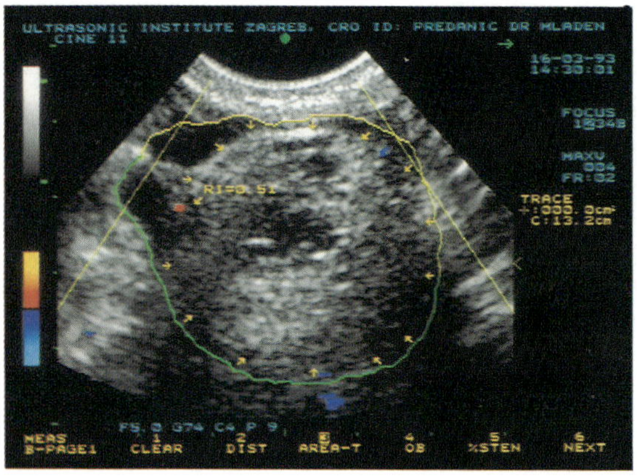

Figure 18 Characteristic presentation of a dermoid – solid ovarian tumor. Note the subtle vascularization presented as a single vessel arrangement located at its periphery (arrow)

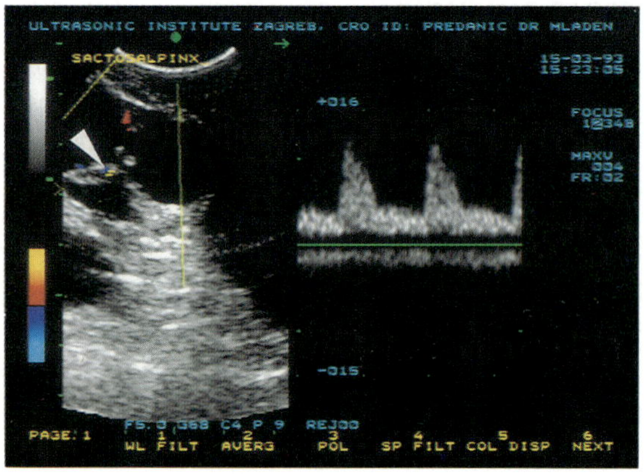

Figure 20 Same case as in Figure 19. Color Doppler shows subtle vascularization of the septa (arrow) in sactosalpinx. Pulsed Doppler sonogram shows high vascular impedance to blood flow in depicted vessel. These findings lead the sonographer to an accurate diagnosis of benign adnexal tumor

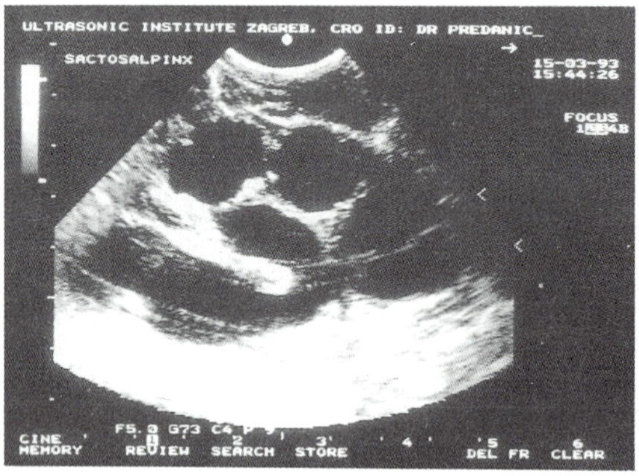

Figure 19 A case of sactosalpinx. This finding could easily be misinterpreted as ovarian malignancy. Irregular walls and thick septa are usually the cause of false-positive results in cases such as this

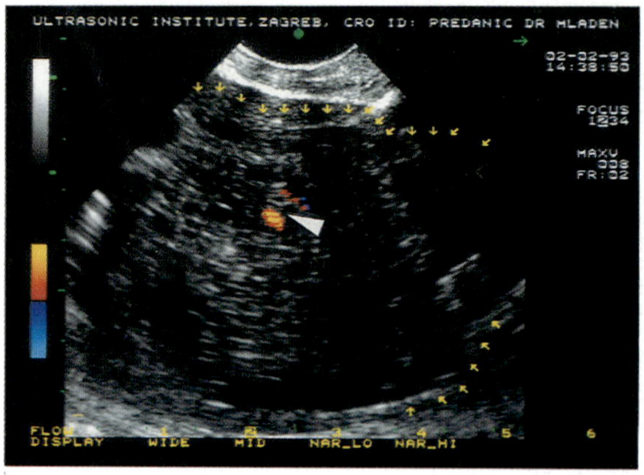

Figure 21 An example of central vascularization of malignant ovarian tumor. Blood vessels are located within the two inner thirds (arrow) of tumor cross-section

examined 1000 postmenopausal women with transvaginal color and pulsed Doppler ultrasound aiming to assess morphology as well as vascularity of normal and abnormal ovaries[66]. Seventy-four per cent were asymptomatic; the others were referred or self-referred for symptoms. There were 83 women with findings that resulted in surgery. Separation of the groups into benign and malignant did not reveal significant differences in age, duration of menopause or symptomatology. Thirty tumors were malignant with a prevalence rate of 36%. An ultrasound score was used to analyze the morphology of all tumors. The score was successful in separating benign from malignant with all indices of normality 90% or higher. Color flow was identified in 29 of 30 malignant tumors, and 64% of benign masses. A cut-off value in the Doppler RI of 0.40 in the feeder vessels, had a sensitivity and specificity of 93% and 98%, respectively, for separating benign from malignant tumors. Positive and negative predictive values were 97% and 96%.

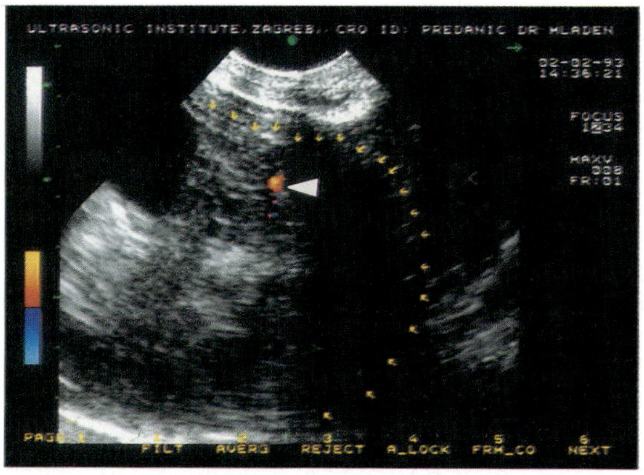

Figure 22 An example of peripheral vascularization of malignant ovarian tumor. Blood vessels (arrow) are located within the outer one third of malignant tumor cross-section

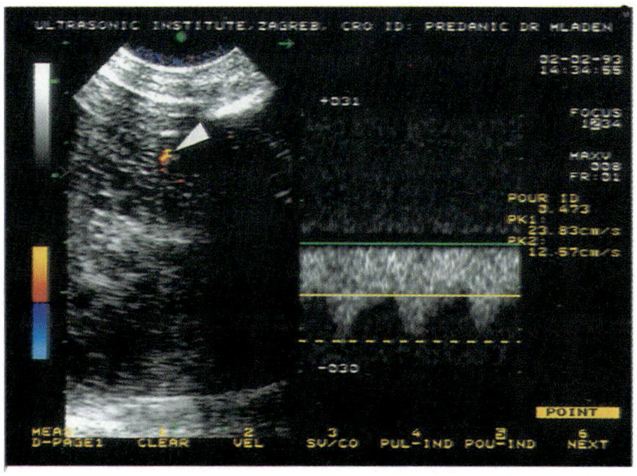

Figure 24 Another example of moderate vascular impedance to blood flow (resistance index = 0.47) in a case of malignant ovarian lesion. Blood vessels are located peripherally. Usually in malignant lesions, moderate to high vascular impedance can be found in peripherally located vessels. Neovascular signals (advancing tumor front) should be sought for accurate vascular assessment

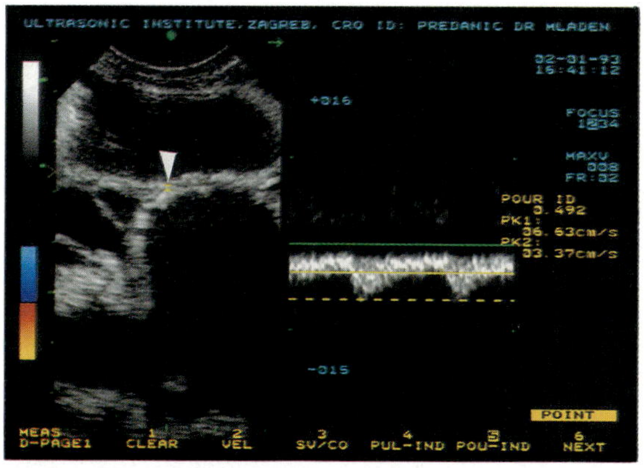

Figure 23 Malignant multilocular ovarian tumor, an example of a malignant tumor in which moderate vascular impedance to blood flow can be observed. Pulsed Doppler sonogram (right) shows vascular impedance of 0.49. If only this value was used in an assessment of tumor vascularization, a false-negative result would have been obtained

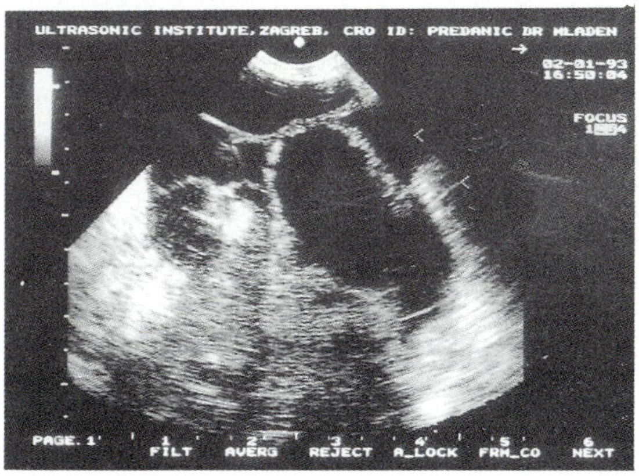

Figure 25 Large right ovarian mass with thick septa and papillary projections. Serous cystadenocarcinoma was diagnosed by histopathology

Detection of ovarian carcinoma at an early stage was considered as coincidence for a long time. Many methods of examination were introduced more or less successfully during the past decade, with the same aim to achieve a main goal – early ovarian malignancy detection, either in 'normal' or visibly altered ovarian tissue. But there are still many clinical problems in differentiating benign and malignant adnexal masses *in vivo*. Known features that characterize this difference (mitotic index and pleomorphism) cannot be detected with current imaging methods and procedures. Unfortunately, a preinvasive stage of ovarian cancer is still unknown. Therefore, the prognosis for ovarian cancer has remained unchanged for 30 years. Color flow imaging could be used to identify potentially malignant ovarian masses and help to elucidate the early stages of tumorigenesis. Bourne and associates[42] reported seven cases of primary ovarian carcinoma. In six

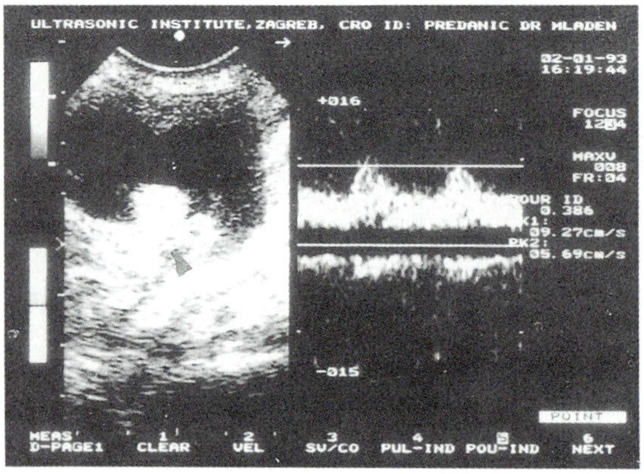

Figure 26 Same patient as in Figure 25, left ovary. Note large papillary projection at its upper wall. At the base of this papilla, pulsed Doppler signal showing low vascular impedance to blood flow (resistance index = 0.38) of detected vessel (arrow) was obtained

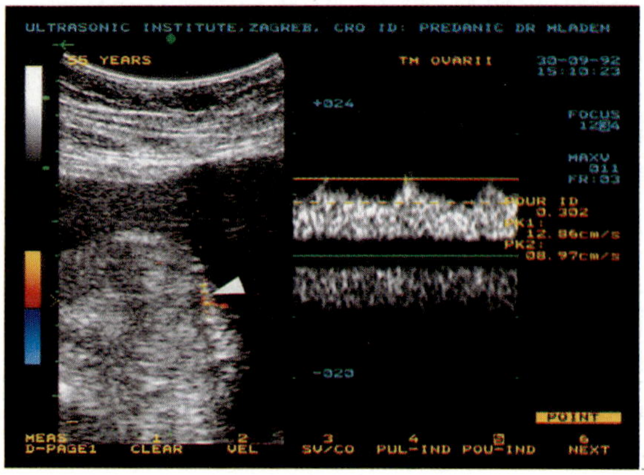

Figure 28 Pulsed Doppler sonogram (right) obtained from the vessel located at the periphery of solid adnexal tumor (arrow). Low vascular impedance to blood flow is observed (resistance index = 0.30), indicating characteristic blood flow pattern for tumor neovascularization

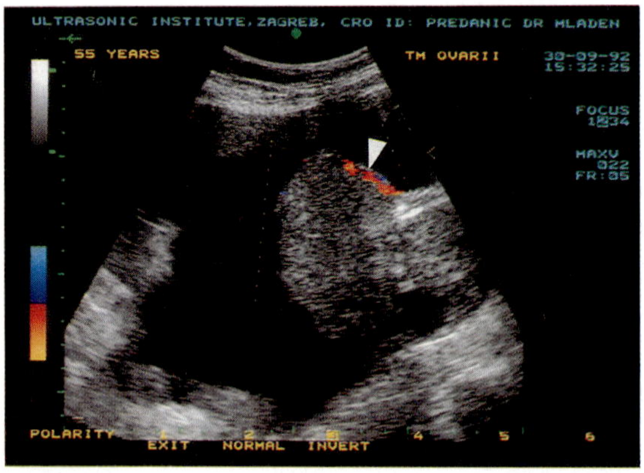

Figure 27 Transabdominal scan was performed to show the size of adnexal malignant lesion. Note abundant color Doppler signal at periphery of solid mass (arrow)

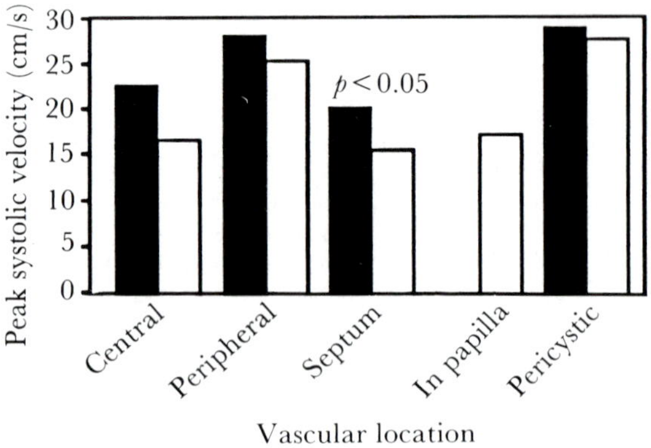

Figure 29 Comparison of peak systolic velocities between benign (white bars) and malignant (solid bars) ovarian lesions

cases, areas of neovascularization and low PI values were found. The false-negative result was obtained from an early borderline serous cystadenocarcinoma. The overall detection rate was 85.7%. The same authors were unable to define a cut-off value to separate the RI and PI of early ovarian cancer, corpora lutea and preovulatory follicles[67]. However, luteal and follicular blood flow could be excluded with examination in the proliferative menstrual phase, from the 3rd to the 10th menstrual day. In our recent study[68], 18 cases with ovarian carcinoma stage I (15 stage Ia and three stage Ib) were studied to evaluate the efficiency of transvaginal color Doppler sonography. Four patients were asymptomatic and were self-referred for their annual check up. Four asymptomatic women, two with morphologically normal ovaries and two with simple unilocular cysts, were picked up during the screening program (Table 4). Ovarian carcinoma stage I was detected in two normal-sized ovaries from only the color and pulsed Doppler signals, which represented tumor angiogenesis, and low impedance to blood flow. Fleischer and co-workers[60] published

Table 4 Sonographic patterns in stage I ovarian cancer found by Kurjak and colleagues[68]

Sonographic patterns	*n*
Normal morphology	2
Cystic: unilocular	2
multilocular	7
Cystic–solid	3
Solid	4
Total	18

data of nine stage I ovarian carcinomas where six had malignant morphology while three ovarian lesions had a benign appearance. The mean size was 13.4 cm with a range of 7–25 cm. The lowest mean PI was 0.9 (range 0.5–1.0) and vessels were mostly located in the central part of the tumor.

At the moment, morphology and color Doppler give predictive information which may aid in the proper use of medical resources and surgical approach, because size, complexity of ovarian mass and pulsed Doppler characteristics highly correlate with risk for malignancy[69]. For example, a postmenopausal woman with a mass greater than 5 cm and an RI below 0.50 had a malignancy risk of 66%, while a mass having an RI value of higher than 0.60 had only a risk of 1 in 41 (2.4%) of being malignant[69]. Interested readers can find more information from two recent review articles[70,71].

In conclusion, the findings presented in this chapter could have important clinical implications in morphologically normal and abnormal ovaries observed by transvaginal color Doppler sonography. Although at the present time, two opposite attitudes about its value are expressed, we strongly believe that this diagnostic tool is still the best available method for early detection of ovarian malignancy.

References

1. Miller, A. B., Chamberlain, J. and Day, N. E. (1990). Report on a workshop of the UICC project on evaluation of screening for cancer. *Int. J. Cancer*, **46**, 761–9
2. Kykes, P. W., Bradwell, A. R., Champan, C. E. and Vaugham, A. T. M. (1987). Radioimmunotherapy of cancer: clinical studies and limiting factors. *Cancer Treat. Rev.*, **14**, 87–96
3. Sharp, F. (1990). Screening for early ovarian cancer. In Sharp, F., Mason, W. P. and Leake, R. E. (eds.) *Ovarian Cancer: Biological and Therapeutic Challenges*, pp. 461–5. (London: Chapman and Hall Medical)
4. Einhorn, N., Nilsson, B. and Sjovall, K. (1985). Factors influencing survival in carcinomas of the ovary. *Cancer*, **55**, 2019–25
5. Yancik, R., Gloeckler, R. L. and Yates, J. W. (1986). Ovarian cancer in the elderly: an analysis of surveillance, epidemiology, and end results program data. *Am. J. Obstet. Gynecol.*, **154**, 639–47
6. Kurjak, A. and Zalud, I. (1991). Transvaginal color Doppler sonography. In Timor-Tritsch, I. E. and Rottem, S. (eds.) *Transvaginal Sonography*, 2nd edn., pp. 451–62. (New York: Elsevier)
7. Jain, R. K., Weissbrod, J. and Wei, J. (1980). Mass transfer in tumors: characterization and applications in chemotherapy. *Adv. Cancer Res.*, **33**, 251–5
8. Barber, H. R. K. (1984). Ovarian cancer: diagnosis and management. *Am. J. Obstet. Gynecol.*, **72**, 1103–8
9. Finkler, N. J., Benacerraf, B. and Lavin, P. T. (1988). Comparison of serum CA 125, clinical impression, and ultrasound in the preoperative evaluation of ovarian masses. *Obstet. Gynecol.*, **72**, 659–64
10. Sunden, B. (1964). On the diagnostic value of ultrasound in obstetrics and gynecology. *Acta Obstet. Gynecol. Scand.*, **43** (Suppl. 6), 46
11. Kratochwil, A. (1969). Ein neues vaginales Schnittbildverfahren. *Geburtshilfe Frauen heilkd.*, **29**, 379–85
12. Andolf, E., Svalenius, E. and Asted, B. (1986). Ultrasonography for early detection of ovarian carcinoma. *Br. J. Obstet. Gynaecol.*, **93**, 2386–9
13. Campbell, S., Royston, P. and Bhan, V. (1990). Novel screening strategies for early ovarian cancer by transabdominal ultrasonography. *Br. J. Obstet. Gynaecol.*, **96**, 304–11
14. Andolf, E. (1991). Sonography of the female pelvis with emphasis on ovarian tumors. *Acta Obstet. Gynecol. Scand.*, **70**, 89–90
15. Thaler, I., Bruck, A. and Ber-Yam, Y. (1988). The vaginal probe: physical consideration. In Timor-Tritsch, I. E. and Rottem, S. (eds.) *Transvaginal Sonography*, pp. 1–25. (New York: Elsevier)

16. Herrman, U. J. Jr, Locher, H. and Ovardi, J. (1987). Sonographic pattern of ovarian tumors: prediction of malignancy. *Obstet. Gynecol.*, **69**, 777–81
17. Andolf, E., Jorgensen, C. and Asted, B. (1990). Ultrasound examination for detection of ovarian carcinoma in risk groups. *Obstet. Gynecol.*, **75**, 106–9
18. Kurjak, A., Salihagic, A., Kupesic-Urek, S. and Predanic, A. (1992). Clinical value of the assessment of gynecological tumor angiogenesis by transvaginal color Doppler. *Ann. Med.*, **24**, 97–103
19. Goldstein, S. R. (1990). Incorporating endovaginal ultrasonography into the overall gynecologic examination. *Am. J. Obstet. Gynecol.*, **162**, 625–32
20. Kupfer, M. C., Schwimer, S. R. and Lebovic, J. (1992). Transvaginal sonographic appearance of endometriomata: spectrum of findings. *J. Ultrasound Med.*, **11**, 129–33
21. Rottem, S. and Timor-Tritsch, I. E. (1991). Ovarian pathology. In Timor-Tritsch, I. E. and Rottem, S. (eds.) *Transvaginal Sonography*, 2nd edn., pp. 145–73. (New York, Amsterdam, London: Elsevier)
22. Rottem, S., Levit, N., Thaler, I., Yoffe, N., Bronshtein, N., Manor, D. and Brandes, J. M. (1990). Classification of ovarian lesions by high frequency transvaginal sonography. *J. Clin. Ultrasound*, **18**, 359–63
23. Bourne, T., Campbell, S., Whitehead, M. I. and Collins, W. P. (1990). Transvaginal ultrasound screening for ovarian cancer in a high risk group. Presented at *The Third World Congress of Vaginosonography in Gynecology*, June 14–17, San Antonio, Texas
24. Granberg, S., Nosrom, A. and Wikland, M. (1990). Tumors in the lower pelvis as imaged by vaginal sonography. *Gynecol. Oncol.*, **37**, 224–9
25. Herrman, U. J. Jr, Locher, G. W. and Goldhirsch, A. (1987). Sonographic pattern of ovarian tumors: prediction of malignancy. *Obstet. Gynecol.*, **69**, 777–81
26. Sassone, A. M., Timor-Tritsch, I. E., Artner, A., Carolyn, W. and Warren, W. B. (1991). Transvaginal sonographic characterization of ovarian disease: evaluation of a new scoring system to predict ovarian malignancy. *Obstet. Gynecol.*, **78**, 70–6
27. Folkman, J., Melrel, E., Abernethy, C. and Williams, G. (1971). Isolation of a tumor factor responsible for angiogenesis. *J. Exp. Med.*, **133**, 275–88
28. Klagsbrun, M. and D'Amore, P. A. (1991). Regulators of angiogenesis. *Annu. Rev. Physiol.*, **53**, 217
29. Folkman, J. and Shing, J. (1992). Minireview. *J. Biol. Chem.*, **267**, 10931–4
30. Auerbach, R. (1981). Angiogenesis-inducing factors: a review. In Pick, E. (ed.) *Lymphokines*, pp. 69–88. (London: Academic Press)
31. Folkman, J. (1985). Tumor angiogenesis. *Adv. Cancer. Res.*, **43**, 175–80
32. Jain, R. K. and Ward-Harley, K. (1984). Tumor blood flow – characterization, modifications and role in hyperthermia. *Trans. Sonics Ultrasonics*, **31**, 504–9
33. Strickland, B. (1959). The value of arteriography in the diagnosis of bone tumors. *Br. J. Radiol.*, **32**, 705–9
34. Gammill, S. L., Shipkey, F. H., Himmelfarb, E. H., Parvey, L. S. and Rabinowits, J. G. (1976). Roentgenology–pathology correlation study of neovascularization. *Am. J. Radiol.*, **126**, 376–81
35. Wells, P. N. T., Halliwell, M., Skidmore, R., Webb, A. J. and Woodcock, J. P. (1977). Tumor detection by ultrasonic Doppler blood flow signals. *Ultrasonics*, **15**, 231–4
36. Burns, P. N., Halliwell, M., Wells, P. N. T. and Webb, A. J. (1982). Ultrasonic Doppler studies of the breast. *Ultrasound Med. Biol.*, **8**, 127–32
37. Minasian, M. and Bamber, J. C. (1982). A preliminary assessment of an ultrasonic Doppler method for the study of blood flow in human breast cancer. *Ultrasound Med. Biol.*, **8**, 357–62
38. Jellins, J., Kossoff, G., Boyd, J. and Reeve, T. S. (1983). The complementary role of Doppler to the B-mode examination of the breast. *J. Ultrasound Med.*, **59**, 89–93
39. Taylor, K. J. W., Ramos, I., Carter, D., Morse, S. S., Snower, D. and Fortune, K. (1988). Correlation of Doppler ultrasound tumor signals with neovascular morphologic features. *Radiology*, **166**, 57–61
40. Hata, H., Hata, K., Yamane, Y. and Kitao, M. (1988). Real-time two-dimensional and pulsed Doppler ultrasound detection of intrapelvic neoplastic tumor and abnormal pathogenic changes: preliminary report. *J. Cardiovasc. Ultrasonogr.*, **7**, 135–9
41. Kurjak, A., Zalud, I., Jurkovic, D., Alfirevic, Z. and Miljan, M. (1989). Transvaginal color Doppler for the assessment of pelvic circulation. *Acta Obstet. Gynecol. Scand.*, **68**, 131–5
42. Bourne, T., Campbell, S., Steer, C., Whitehead, M. I. and Collins, W. P. (1989). Transvaginal color flow imaging: a possible new screening technique for ovarian cancer. *Br. Med. J.*, **299**, 1367–70
43. Kurjak, A., Zalud, I. and Alfirevic, A. (1991). Evaluation of adnexal masses with transvaginal color ultrasound. *J. Ultrasound Med.*, **10**, 295–7
44. Hata, T., Hata, K., Senoh, D., Makihara, K., Aoki, S., Takamiya, O. and Kiato, M. (1989). Doppler ultrasound assessment of tumor vascularity in gynecologic disorders. *J. Ultrasound Med.*, **8**, 309–14
45. Hata, K., Makihara, K., Hata, T., Aoki, S. and Kitao, M. (1991). Transvaginal color Doppler imaging for hemodynamic assessment of reproductive tract tumors. *Int. J. Gynecol. Obstet.*, **36**, 301–8
46. Fleischer, A. C., Rodgers, W. H., Rao, B. K., Keppler, D. M., Worrel, J. A., Williams, L. and

Howard, W. J. (1991). Assessment of ovarian tumor vascularity with transvaginal color Doppler sonography. *J. Ultrasound Med.*, **10**, 563–8

47. Fleischer, A. C., Rodgers, W. H., Rao, B. K., Keppler, D. M. and Jones, H. W. (1991). Transvaginal color Doppler sonography of ovarian masses with pathological correlation. *Ultrasound Obstet. Gynecol.*, **1**, 275–8
48. Weiner, Z., Thaler, I., Beck, D., Rottem, S., Deutchs, M. and Brandes, J. M. (1992). Differentiating malignant from benign ovarian tumors with transvaginal color flow imaging. *Obstet. Gynecol.*, **79**, 159–62
49. Timor-Tritsch, I. E., Lerner, J., Monteagudo, A. and Santos, R. (1993). Transvaginal sonographic characterization of ovarian masses by means of color flow-directed Doppler measurements and a morphological scoring system. *Am. J. Obstet. Gynecol.*, **168**, 909–13
50. Kawai, M., Kano, T., Kikkawa, F., Maeda, O., Oguchi, H. and Tomoda, Y. (1992). Transvaginal Doppler ultrasound with color flow imaging in the diagnosis of ovarian cancer. *Obstet. Gynecol.*, **79**, 163–7
51. Locci, M., Nazzaro, G., De Placido, G., Di Renzo, C. G. and Montemagno, U. (1993). Transvaginal color Doppler in the study of utero-ovarian angiogenesis. Our experience during the last three years. *Ultrasound Obstet. Gynecol.*, **3** (Suppl. 1), 24
52. Reynolds, K., Bicknell, R., Harris, A. L., Bourne, T. H., Lawton, F., Collings, W. P. and Campbell, S. (1993). Expression of the angiogenic factor platelet-derived endothelial cell growth factor in ovarian tumors. *Ultrasound Obstet. Gynecol.*, **3** (Suppl. 1), 23
53. Tekay, A. and Jouppila, P. (1992). Validity of pulsatility and resistance indices in classification of adnexal tumors with transvaginal color Doppler ultrasound. *Ultrasound Obstet. Gynecol.*, **2**, 338–44
54. Hata, K., Hata, T., Manable, A., *et al.* (1992). A critical evaluation of transvaginal Doppler studies, transvaginal sonography, magnetic resonance imaging, and CA 125 in detecting ovarian cancer. *Obstet. Gynecol.*, **80**, 922–6
55. Valentin, L. and Sladkevicius, P. (1993). Limited contribution of Doppler velocimetry to the differential diagnosis of extrauterine pelvic tumors. *Ultrasound Obstet. Gynecol.*, **3** (Suppl. 1), 21
56. Zanneta, G., Della Vaille, C., Trio, D., Rangoni, G. and Pittelli, M. R. (1993). Usefulness of color Doppler ultrasound (CDU) in discriminating benign from malignant ovarian masses before surgery. *Ultrasound Obstet. Gynecol.*, **3** (Suppl. 1), 21
57. Kurjak, A., Schulman, H., Sosic, A., Zalud, I. and Shalan, H. (1992). Transvaginal ultrasound, color flow, and Doppler waveform of the postmenopausal adnexal mass. *Obstet. Gynecol.*, **80**, 917–21
58. Kurjak, A. and Predanic, M. (1992). New scoring system for prediction of ovarian malignancy based on transvaginal color Doppler. *J. Ultrasound Med.*, **11**, 631–8
59. Kurjak, A., Predanic, M., Kupesic, S. and Jukic, S. (1993). Transvaginal color and pulsed Doppler assessment of adnexal tumors vascularity. *Gynecol. Oncol.*, **50**, 3–9
60. Fleischer, A. C., Rodgers, W. H., Kepple, D. M., Williams, L. L. and Jones III, H. W. (1993). Color Doppler sonography of ovarian masses: a multiparameter analysis. *J. Ultrasound Med.*, **12**, 41–8
61. Bonilla-Musoles, F., Ballester, M. J., Simon, C., Serra, V. and Raga, F. (1993). Is avoidance of surgery possible in patients with perimenopausal ovarian tumors using transvaginal ultrasound and duplex color Doppler sonography? *J. Ultrasound Med.*, **12**, 33–9
62. Koonings, R. P., Campbell, S., Mishell, D. R. and Grimes, D. A. (1989). Relative frequency of primary ovarian neoplasms: a 10-year review. *Obstet. Gynecol.*, **74**, 359–73
63. Campbell, S., Bhan, V., Royston, P., Whitehead, M. and Collins, W., (1989). Transabdominal ultrasound screening for early ovarian cancer. *Br. Med. J.*, **299**, 1363–7
64. Duda, V. and Rude, G. (1990). Transvaginal sonography: pilot study for use in the ovarian screening program. *Geburtshilfe Frauenheilkd.*, **50**, 388–93
65. van Nagell, J. R., DePriest, P. D., Puls, L. E., Donaldson, E. G., Gallion, H. H. and Pavlik, J. (1991). Ovarian cancer screening in asymptomatic postmenopausal women by transvaginal sonography. *Cancer*, **68**, 458–62
66. Fleischer, A. C., McKee, M. S., Gordon, A. N., Page, D. L., Kepple, D. M., Worrell, J. A., Jones, H. W., Burnett, L. S. and James, A. E. (1990). Transvaginal sonography of postmenopausal ovaries with pathologic correlation. *J. Ultrasound Med.*, **9**, 637–44
67. Campbell, S., Bourne, T. H., Reynolds, K., Hampson, J., Royston, P., Whitehead, M. I. and Collins, W. P. (1992). Role of color Doppler in an ultrasound-based screening program. In Sharp, F., Mason, W. P. and Creasman, W. (eds.) *Ovarian Cancer 2: Biology, Diagnosis and Management*, pp. 237–47. (London: Chapman & Hall Medical)
68. Kurjak, A., Shalan, H., Matijevic, R. and Predanic, M. (1993). Stage I ovarian cancer by transvaginal color Doppler sonography: a report of 18 cases. *Ultrasound Obstet. Gynecol.*, **3**, 195–8
69. Crade, M., Patel, J. and Yiu-Chiu, V. (1993). Evaluation of 103 pelvic masses: correlation of surgical diagnosis with transvaginal ultrasound size, complexity scores and resistive index values. *Ultrasound Obstet. Gynecol.*, **3** (Suppl. 1), 23
70. Kurjak, A., Shalan, H., Kupesic, S., Predanic, M., Zalud, I., Breyer, B. and Jukic, S. (1993). Transva-

ginal color Doppler sonography in the assessment of pelvic tumor vascularity. *Ultrasound Obstet. Gynecol.*, **3**, 137–54

71. Zalud, I. and Kurjak, A. (1900). University of Zagreb program. In Fleischer, A. and Jones III, H. W. (eds.) *Early Detection of Ovarian Carcinoma with Transvaginal Sonography*, pp. 161–76. (New York: Raven Press)

The postmenopausal ovary 16

H. R. K. Barber

The ovary progresses through many changes, including puberty, pregnancy and menopause. Although the former have been well studied and described, the least attention has been given to the menopausal and postmenopausal ovary.

THE PREMENOPAUSAL AND POSTMENOPAUSAL OVARIES

Whereas the normal ovary measures 3.5 × 2.0 × 1.5 cm, the menopausal ovary tends to atrophy and shrink when the Graafian follicles and ova disappear. The tunica albuginea becomes dense and causes the surface of the ovary to become scarred and shrunken. The cortex is marked with increased thinning as well as numerous corpora fibrosa and corpora albuginea, with areas of dense fibrosis and hyalinization. The ovary shows varying degrees of avascularity[1].

Eventually, the ovary becomes an inert residue that consists of connective tissue, and it clings to the posterior leaf of the broad ligament. Its pink color becomes pure white. It shrinks to 2.0 × 1.5 × 0.5 cm, and in some instances it may be as small as 1.50 × 0.75 × 0.50 cm. Its wrinkled surface resembles the gyri and sulci of the cerebrum. At this point it cannot be palpated.

Although the ovary is often just a streak along the pelvic wall in the late postmenopausal and geriatric years, there are often different configurations of the postmenopausal ovary. The menopause is merely the patient's last menstrual period. It should not be confused with the climacteric. The menopause may be due to a decreased sensitivity of the hypothalamus-to-steroid feedback and alteration of ovarian sensitivity to follicle-stimulating hormone and luteinizing hormone, or simply to the absence of primordial cells in the ovary. It is possible that all three phenomena at some time play a role. However, ultrastructural data indicate that there is an occasional primordial follicle in a postmenopausal ovary. Although differentiating ovarian follicles are rare, both these follicles and their oocytes usually appear to be normal.

After menopause the ovaries are smaller and more fibrotic and usually exhibit pits on their surfaces. Besides the diminution of primary and differentiating follicles, ultrastructural studies indicate a great increase of fibroblasts and connective tissue throughout, especially in the cortex where germinal structures are largely absent. The advanced follicles, identified in postmenopausal ovaries, are usually undergoing atretic changes. Although there is a great increase in atretic follicles in postmenopausal ovaries, normal-appearing follicles are occasionally found; the granulosa cells, however, are smaller. Occasionally, the follicles can be found in a resting state in the advanced menopausal years. Generally the advanced follicles identified in postmenopausal ovaries are undergoing atretic changes, but they may contain small, cystic structures. Any observed corpus luteum is also undergoing atresia (corpora albicantia). Sometimes a small cyst may be present in the so-called 'burned out' corpus luteum or corpus albicans. However, the follicle or corpus luteum that may persist in women in this age group will be in a resting state.

Although the ovarian cortex becomes progressively more atrophic, the medullary region of interstitial cells is more abundant and usually active for a period of time. Groups of functional stromal cells may be found throughout the postmenopausal ovary, especially around the hilar region. On occasion, single cells or smaller clusters of very active cells are apparent near the atretic follicle or corpus luteum. It is difficult to differentiate these cells as either follicle cells, follicle cells differentiating into stromal cells, or stromal cells. The stromal cells show similarities to Leydig's cells of the testes. When cells atrophy they revert back to fibroblast-type cells. It has been shown that the stromal cells have the ability to synthesize androgens, and that there is an abundance of active stromal cells in the postmenopausal ovary, and these cells may be producing androgens. The length of time for which they are functioning is quite variable[2].

HORMONAL CHANGES IN THE MENOPAUSAL OVARY

It has been well documented that androgens enter the blood from the adrenal glands, the ovaries, and the peripheral tissues. The ovary can convert acetate to cholesterol, the obligatory precursor of all steroids, but low-density lipoprotein cholesterol is a precursor also. The steroid biosynthetic pathway in the ovary is from cholesterol to androgens and then estrogens. Thus, androgens are the immediate precursor of estrogens, and it can even be said that testosterone is a weak estrogen in some tissues.

During the climacteric, androgen production rates decline with the cessation of ovarian follicle development and the concomitant decrease in adrenal secretion.

The ovaries secrete less precursors but more active androgens than the adrenals. Estradiol, the principal estrogen secreted by the ovary, is formed by aromatization of testosterone. Estrone, formed from androstenedione, is also secreted by the ovary. However, another important source of estrone is extraglandular conversion of androstenedione in peripheral tissue. In ovulating women, 60% of mean estrogen formation during the menstrual cycle is in the form of estradiol, produced primarily by the ovaries, and the remainder is estrone, produced in part in extraglandular tissues. The steroid biosynthetic pathway in the ovary is from cholesterol to androgens and then estrogens.

The secretion of androgens by the adrenal gland is stimulated and regulated by adrenocorticotropic hormone (ACTH). The adrenals primarily secrete the androgen precursor, dehydroepiandrosterone sulfate (DHAS). Only small amounts of testosterone are released by the adrenals.

The premenopausal ovaries secrete androgen. The amount of androgen produced by the ovary is controlled primarily by luteinizing hormone (LH); secretion of androgen is also affected by the status of the ovarian follicles. Although the androgen secretion rate (of precursors and active androgens) is greater for the adrenal glands, the ovaries secrete less precursors but more active androgens than the adrenals. It appears that the ovaries secrete no DHAS and only small amounts of dehydroepiandrosterone (DHA), but mainly androstenedione and testosterone.

The amount of active androgen produced by peripheral tissue is determined by the amount of androgen precursors that the tissue extracts from the blood, and the ability of the tissue to convert a precursor to an active androgen. Among the peripheral tissues involved in androgen conversion are skin, muscle, adipose tissue, brain and kidney.

Production of androgens by the adrenals is higher in younger women than in postmenopausal women. The decrease in adrenal androgen production during the climacteric appears to be a function of age, similar to the phenomenon that occurs with aging in men. In women, a slight shift in the overall ratio of adrenal secretory products accompanies the decline in total adrenal androgen production.

During the menopause, overall ovarian secretion of androgens decreases markedly with the cessation of follicle development. During the menopause, androgen production rates decline, and this decrease is due in large part to the reduction of dehydroepiandrosterone and androstenedione secretion by the ovaries. The production rate of dehydroepiandrosterone decreases by as much as 75% and that of androstenedione by approximately 50%. In many postmenopausal women the levels of testosterone in the ovarian venous blood are higher than in the arterial blood, indicating that secretion of this androgen continues. Despite the fact that the ovaries continue to produce testosterone, the blood production rate of this androgen is reduced by 50% after the menopause because of the reduced availability of its precursors for peripheral tissue conversion[3]. Although the androgen production rate is greater than that of estrogen at all times in women, more attention has been paid to the loss of estrogen during menopause because the effects of estrogen loss are more apparent. The overall metabolism of androgens does not appear to be affected by age. However, a major change is seen in the peripheral aromatization of androgens in menopausal women. Such activity increases as much as twofold at the time of the menopause when ovarian function is declining. However, the increase in peripheral aromatization does not occur immediately in oophorectomized women[4].

The production of androgen by the menopausal ovary has relevance to clinical medicine. In women who are receiving estrogen replacement therapy in the menopause and postmenopausal years and who state that the symptoms are not relieved or helped by increasing the amount of estrogen, the addition of testosterone often alleviates the symptoms. It has been shown that androgens are psychotonic agents and that testosterone modulates the neurohormones of the brain and has an effect on anxiety, migrainoid headaches, and non-psychotic depression. Women often complain of loss of libido at this time and studies show that testosterone is the steroid primarily critical for maintaining sexual motivation or sexual interest in women. Androgens are not important for the physiological sexual response but they are critical for such sexual functioning as the woman's desire[5].

THE POSTMENOPAUSAL PALPABLE OVARY SYNDROME

In the postmenopausal palpable ovary syndrome, the finding of what is interpreted as a normal-sized ovary in the premenopausal patient represents an ovarian tumor in the patient who is at least 5 years after the menopause. This statement does not mean that anything that is palpated in the adnexa is abnormal[6]. It only refers to the size and consistency of the ovary. With advances in diagnostic imaging, small 1 cm cysts are often reported by the sonographer as being abnormal. This is not medically sound. Unfortunately, it is often referred to as the postmenopausal palpable ovary syndrome, adding to the confusion. The gynecologist should obtain the films of the sonogram and review them independently. If the cyst is 1 or 2 cm and looks like a coin lesion, and on inspection with magnification is clear, there is no need for alarm. Occasionally, follicles can be found in a resting state in the advanced menopausal years. Generally, the advanced follicles identified in postmenopausal ovaries are undergoing atretic changes, but they may contain small, cystic structures. Any observed corpus luteum is also undergoing atresia (corpora albicantia). Sometimes a small cyst may be present in the so-called 'burned out' corpus luteum or corpus albicans or in a follicle. However, either the follicle or the corpus luteum that may persist in patients in this age group will be in the resting state. When this report is received and the films reviewed by the gynecologist, the patient should be directed to take an enema and to return to the office for an examination. If the physician cannot palpate the structure in the adnexa that resembles a premenopausal-sized ovary, the patient should be re-evaluated in 6–8 weeks with another pelvic examination and sonogram. If the findings are the same (and almost certainly they will be), the patient does not require an exploratory laparotomy with removal of uterus, tubes and ovaries. However, she should be directed to return again in 6–8 weeks for a repeat examination and sonogram. If the findings are again the same and the tumor markers have remained within normal limits, the patient can be followed in 4–6 months[7]. Following this, she can be followed according to the judgment of the responsible gynecologist. With the advances in sonography, particularly transvaginal sonography, more and more of these small cysts will be picked up during a work-up by either the gynecologist or the internist and strong measures must be taken to establish a protocol for making the proper diagnosis. The gynecologist must communicate with the patient and advise her that the small cyst does not put her at jeopardy, but that the rest of the ovary is never too old to form a cancer, and the peak incidence for ovarian cancer is age 77. Therefore, the patient must be followed as any patient in this age group should, every 6 months, and the reasons for the follow-up must be carefully explained to the patient.

CONCLUSIONS

The postmenopausal ovary stops secreting estrogen after the last menstrual period when the follicles atrophy. However, the stroma continues to produce an androgenic substance for an indefinite time into the postmenopausal years.

The postmenopausal ovary shrinks to 2.0 × 1.5 × 0.5 cm and in some it may be as small as 1.50 × 0.75 × 0.50 cm. Its wrinkled surface resembles the gyri and sulci of the cerebrum. At this point it cannot be palpated. Later, it is often a small streak on the lateral pelvic wall. However, small benign cysts have been found in the ovary of patients in the very late postmenopausal years.

Since the stroma of the ovary secretes androgens for a period of time, the gynecologist must take this into account when he is treating the patient with estrogen replacement when the response is less than desirable. Androgens are psychotonic agents and testosterone modulates the neurohormones of the brain and has an effect on anxiety, migrainoid headaches, and non-psychotic depression. The addition of testosterone often alleviates these symptoms and it has been shown that the addition of testosterone in the postmenopausal years can improve the libido.

Although the ovary becomes too old to function, it is never too old to form a cancer and the peak age for the appearance of common epithelial ovarian cancer is age 77.

References

1. Barber, H. R. K. and Graber, E. A. (1971). The PMPO syndrome (postmenopausal palpable ovary syndrome). *Obstet. Gynecol.*, **38**, 921
2. Rice, B. F. and Savard, K. (1966). Steroid hormone formation in the human ovary: IV. Ovarian stromal compartment formation of radioactive steroid from acetate 1-14C and action of gonadotropins. *J. Clin. Endocrinol.*, **26**, 563
3. Guraya, S. S. (1972). Interstitial gland tissue of mammalian ovary. *Acta Endocrinol.*, **72** (Suppl. 171), 3–27
4. Longcope, C., Hunter, R. and Franz, C. (1980). Steroid secretion by the postmenopausal ovary. *Am. J. Obstet. Gynecol.*, **38**, 564
5. Sherwin, B. B. (1985). Changes in sexual behavior as a function of plasma sex steroid levels in postmenopausal women. *Maturitas*, **7**, 225
6. Barber, H. R. K. (1979). The postmenopausal palpable ovary syndrome. *Compr. Ther.*, **5**(9), 58
7. Barber, H. R. K. (1988). Editorial: A second look at the postmenopausal palpable ovary. *Fem. Patient*, **13**, 13–14

Screening for ovarian cancer

17

A. Prys Davies and D. Oram

INTRODUCTION

The ovary is the site of origin for a larger variety of primary cancers than any other organ[1]. The majority of primary ovarian cancers are, however, epithelial in origin[2], and this chapter represents a review of the literature on epithelial ovarian cancer with particular reference to its early detection.

The impact of ovarian cancer in Western society can be measured in terms of individual suffering, or more objectively, in national death rates. Progress against this disease, when assessed by long-term survival, has been poor. From the data, the 5-year survival rate for women with ovarian cancer has not changed significantly over the past 30 years. The most important prognostic factor remains the stage of disease at the time of diagnosis. Unfortunately, the anatomical position of the ovaries and absent or vague symptomatology in the early stages of the disease mean that the majority (75%) of women are diagnosed with stage III or IV disease, when treatments are usually palliative rather than curative. The 5-year survival figure for stage IV ovarian cancer is of the order of 4%[3] (Table 1).

To appreciate the impact of ovarian cancer on American or European societies, the causes of mortality in adult women must be examined. Data for 1986 from the American Cancer Society[4] shows cancer to be the most common cause of death in women aged 35–74 years. Analysis of all cancer deaths in women reveals ovarian cancer to be the fourth leading cause of cancer death (following lung, breast and colorectal cancers), accounting for one of 17 cancer deaths. Overall, ovarian cancer is responsible for approximately 2% of deaths in this age group. The data for the United Kingdom are similar[5]. In 1989, ovarian cancer accounted for 6% of all cancer deaths, with a death rate from ovarian cancer of 150 per million women (all ages). The lifetime risk of developing ovarian cancer is of the order of 1:70, compared to a 1:12 lifetime risk of developing breast cancer. Using official data from the World Health Organization data base, an analysis of trends in ovarian mortality in 25 European countries over the period 1955–89 showed the mortality from the disease to be on the increase in Ireland, Britain and Southern Europe. Trends, however, were more favorable in middle-aged and young women, among whom substantial declines, approaching 50%, were observed in Britain over the last decade[6].

At first glance, therefore, it might appear that ovarian cancer is not a major concern for Western societies. However, the next decades may well see deaths from ovarian cancer increasing as a proportion of all deaths, as health promotion programs (stop-smoking campaigns, healthier diets, exercise regimens and mammography) lead to a lowering in the individual risk of the other causes of death, whilst the trend towards an earlier menarche and smaller families may lead to an

Table 1 Five-year survival rates[3] by stage at presentation for epithelial ovarian cancer

Stage	*Incidence* (%)	*5-year survival* (%)
Ia	17.9	69.7
Ib	4.3	63.9
Ic	3.0	50.3
Total stage I	25.2	67.1
IIa	4.8	51.8
IIb + c	12.8	42.4
III	39.5	13.3
IV	17.7	4.1
Total stages III + IV	57.2	10.4
Total all stages	100.0	30.6

increase in the risk of developing ovarian cancer. Methods of preventing ovarian cancer are not currently available – although it is recognized that the combined contraceptive pill may lead to a 30% decrease in the incidence of ovarian cancer[7,8]. To perform prophylactic oophorectomies on the general female population, in order to prevent a 1:70 chance of developing a disease, might not be acceptable when one considers the risk involved of general anesthesia and the adverse effects of a premature menopause (heart disease, osteoporosis) should hormone replacement not be taken. Nevertheless, for individual women such surgery might be an acceptable option either as a primary procedure or at the time of pelvic surgery for benign disorders[9,10].

In order to improve the prognosis for epithelial ovarian cancer, the stress must therefore be upon early detection. It is reasonable to conclude that increasing the proportion of women diagnosed with cancer confined to the ovary (FIGO stage I) when 5-year survival may be as high as 95%, should lead to an improvement in mortality statistics[11].

SCREENING FOR OVARIAN CANCER

Rationale

The stated aim of a screening program is to identify in an apparently healthy population individuals at sufficient risk of a disorder to warrant subsequent investigations. In the case of cancer, it is argued that diagnosing cancer in its asymptomatic stage, with the ensuing earlier initiation of treatment, will lead to improved survival. However, establishing the efficacy of a screening program for a progressive disease such as cancer may not be straightforward, and may be confounded by both length and lead bias.

Slowly growing, indolent cancers, from which there is an inherent better survival rate, are more likely to be detected in a preclinical phase by an interval screening program. Therefore, in a group of cancers diagnosed early, there will be a disproportionate number of indolent cases, with good life expectancy (the length bias). Should the onset of death despite the earlier diagnosis and treatment not be delayed, any improvement in survival (i.e. the longer interval between diagnosis and death) would be apparent only (the lead bias).

The specificity and sensitivity of the test used will also determine the efficacy of a screening program.

Specificity

It was stated above that the aim of a screening program is to detect individuals at an apparent increased risk of a condition sufficient to warrant further investigation. In order to minimize unnecessary intervention and anxiety in healthy individuals who give a positive result on screening (false positives), it is important that the screening test is able to discriminate between unaffected and affected individuals (specificity). This is especially true when screening for ovarian cancer, when the definitive histological diagnosis may only be made following surgery under general anesthesia. In order to achieve an odds ratio of 1:10 for ovarian cancer at laparotomy, it has been calculated that the specificity of the screening test, when screening a population of women over 45 years of age in whom the annual incidence of ovarian cancer is 1 per 2500 should be 99.6%, assuming a test sensitivity of 100%.

Sensitivity

A high detection rate (sensitivity) is also a prerequisite of a screening test in order to minimize the false reassurance given to 'diseased' women who have provided a negative screen result, and also to maximize the benefits of a screening program.

Methods of screening

Over the past 20 years or so, various techniques for detecting ovarian cancer have been explored[12,13], and the majority have been found to be wanting as screening methods.

Malignant ovarian cells have been detected on Papanicolaou smears. However, in a study by Shapiro and Nunez[14] cytological examination was positive in only 30% of advanced cases of ovarian cancer, rendering cervical smears insufficiently sensitive as a method for screening for ovarian cancer. Peritoneal cytological examination has been proposed as a method for early detection, but it is too invasive a test to be acceptable as a means of population screening[15]. More recent imaging methods – immunoscintigraphy[16], CAT scans[17] and magnetic resonance imaging[18] – may detect small-volume ovarian cancer and have a role in the detection and monitoring of clinical disease. However, their invasiveness and expense precludes their use as primary screening tests for the general population.

Methods currently under evaluation as screening tests include:

(1) Bimanual pelvic examination;

(2) Ultrasound; and

(3) Tumor markers.

For an understanding of some of the problems encountered when using the first two techniques, it is important to have some knowledge of the morphological findings in normal and diseased ovaries.

Pathology

The average post-menopausal ovary measures 1.5 cm and has a volume of less than 2 cm^3. Multiparity, obesity and/or hormone replacement therapy may increase the volume. The ovaries of ovulating, menstruating women are larger and their volume and morphology change throughout the menstrual cycle.

Approximately 90% of cystic ovarian tumors are benign. Functional ovarian cysts are a common feature of normal ovarian activity. Such cysts are thin-walled, unilocular or multilocular with thin septations[19]. Serous cystadenomas may be unilocular or multilocular and may in addition have papillary growths into the cavity. A study by Russell[20] showed that 19% of benign serous ovarian tumors had a large stromal component and in 4.5%, papillary formations were documented inside the cyst wall. Mucinous cystadenomas are thin-walled and are mostly multilocular (65%) and unilateral (2.5% are bilateral). Papillary formations may be present, and 5% of mucinous ovarian cystadenomas have both cystic and solid areas[20].

Serous cystadenocarcinomas are the most common type of malignant ovarian tumor. Serous and mucinous cystadenocarcinomas are usually bilateral, with solid and cystic elements, and surface and intracavity papillary growths. Endometrioid carcinomas tend to be less cystic than serous or mucinous carcinomas. Solid areas often alternate with cysts or comprise the entire bulk of the tumor. Intracystic papillary projections are found in some tumors[19].

Bimanual pelvic examination, ultrasound and tumor markers will be considered in turn with respect to their suitability as a screening test.

Bimanual pelvic examination

There are obvious attractions for using pelvic examination as a screening method for ovarian cancer. It is relatively easy to perform and may be incorporated into an existing cervical screening program; it does not require specialized equipment and hence the overheads are low. However, neither the specificity nor the sensitivity of the test for early ovarian cancer is known. The maximum diameters of a normal postmenopausal ovary are $2 \times 1 \times 0.5$ cm, rendering it impalpable on bimanual examination. A tumor volume of 1 cm^3, which is probably the smallest mass detectable on clinical examination, contains about a billion cancer cells and may already be associated with widespread intra-abdominal seeding[21].

An early population-based study investigating the sensitivity of bimanual pelvic examination for ovarian cancer was that of MacFarlane and colleagues[22]. Over a 14-year period, a total of 18 753 pelvic examinations were performed on 1319 women aged 30–80 years, yielding six ovarian cancers.

Most studies evaluating bimanual pelvic examination as a means of detecting ovarian cancer have used women attending outpatient departments or undergoing laparotomy, and their significance for screening a healthy population is therefore unclear. Reeves and associates[23] compared pelvic examination with a preoperative pelvic ultrasound scan in 72 women undergoing a laparotomy for a pelvic mass. With respect to the accuracy of detection, estimation of size or determination of bilateral position of the pelvic mass, no significant difference was found between the two examinations. However, ultrasound was significantly more accurate in determining the solid or cystic nature of the mass – a feature which is considered to be important for differentiating benign from malignant ovarian masses. Four of the women had ovarian cancer (stage not determined). Thus, although Reeves and associates credited pelvic examination with accuracy of location of a pelvic mass, the ability of pelvic examination to distinguish benign from malignant disease and the sensitivity of detection in the general population remain unresolved.

A study by Andolf and co-workers[24] found bimanual examination to be defective in detecting ovarian cancer. The subjects for this study were 805 women aged between 40 and 70 years attending a gynecology outpatients' clinic. The person performing the scan was unaware of the examination findings, and in some instances up to 12 weeks had lapsed between the examination and the scan. In 12 cases the bimanual examination was considered to be abnormal, whilst the first scan (performed using the transabdominal route) was abnormal in 83 cases. For ten women, both examinations proved to be abnormal. Surgical exploration was performed on 39 women, including eight in whom the physical examination was considered to be abnormal. All eight cases were associated with benign ovarian pathologies. The pelvic examination of a woman diagnosed as having invasive ovarian cancer (stage III) and two women with borderline ovarian cancer (maximum diameters of 6 and 4 cm, respectively) had been passed as normal or as not suspicious of malignancy. Andolf and co-workers concluded that ultrasound was superior to bimanual pelvic examination in detecting ovarian cancer.

The unreliability of pelvic examination for detecting ovarian tumors has also been illustrating by Fleischer[25]. He has demonstrated ovarian tumors of over 30 cm in size ultrasonically that were not suspected clinically or on palpation.

In summary, although bimanual pelvic examination is currently the most common method of diagnosing clinical ovarian cancer, it is neither sufficiently sensitive nor sufficiently specific to be used for population screening.

Ultrasound

Over the past three decades, advances in pelvic ultrasound technology have resulted in a method of visualizing ovaries and documenting the morphological changes that occur under various physiological and pathological conditions. Initially, pelvic ultrasound examination was performed using the transabdominal route, with the full-bladder technique. With the advent of high-frequency vaginal transducers, the transvaginal route has been increasingly employed. The main advantage of the transvaginal route is the short scanning distance, so that the images obtained are more acute, making their interpretation easier. The demand for a full urinary bladder is also obviated. In experienced hands, the vaginal probe is easy and quick to use in connection with routine gynecological examination. The technique, however, does have its limitations. Postmenopausal vaginal atrophy may restrict access and or patient acceptability. The ultrasound frequencies used may improve resolution, but limit penetration to 10 cm. Thus ovaries that are situated high or laterally in the pelvis, or are greatly enlarged so that they are no longer in the pelvis, may not be seen on the scan. Similarly, the internal structure of an ovarian cyst greater than 10 cm in diameter cannot be reliably assessed using the transvaginal probe[26].

Most studies investigating the value of ultrasound in diagnosing ovarian tumors have used symptomatic women undergoing laparotomy for a suspected ovarian mass as subjects. They have documented a good accord between ultrasound assessment and surgical determination of the size and position of the ovaries and the characteristics of the ovarian tumors.

Many investigators have tried to use the ultrasound image to characterize benign and malignant ovarian tumors. However, no ultrasound criterion with 100% specificity for a malignant ovarian tumor has been described. The ultrasound findings indicative of ovarian cancer include semisolid, semicystic masses with thick septa and surface papillary growths, bilateral lesions, and ascites[27,28]. Using these features as indicators of malignancy, DeLand and co-workers[29] correctly identified 13 of 14 women who were diagnosed as having ovarian cancer from a total of 60 women undergoing a laparotomy for a pelvic mass. More than 70% of lesions with complex or solid patterns were malignant, although the stage of the disease was not specified. These characteristics, however, are not exclusive to ovarian cancer. A study by Herrmann and colleagues[28] of 404 women with suspicious pelvic masses or histories suggestive of ovarian cancer showed that 58% of benign ovarian tumors had some solid element. Beck and associates[30] described papillary growth on the outer ovarian surface of almost 50% of malignant ovarian tumors – and in approximately 10% of benign cases. Benacerraf and co-workers[31], in a study of 100 women undergoing a laparotomy for an ovarian mass within 8 weeks of an ultrasound scan, found the interpretation of the scan findings to be misleading in 15% of cases, with misreading of whether the lesions were benign or malignant.

It has also been suggested that tumor size may be a risk factor for malignancy – the larger the tumor, the greater the risk of malignancy. However, tumor size has not been found by all investigators to be a reliable indicator of malignancy, with Sassone and colleagues[32], for example, finding many large cysts (> 10 cm in diameter) to be benign.

Thus, although changes in ovarian morphology associated with malignancy have been well documented, the changes are not exclusive. The interpretation of ultrasound images is also subjective, adding to the uncertainty of the reliability of the diagnosis of malignancy. Fleischer[25] reported a twofold difference in the diagnosis of ovarian cancer between the initial ultrasound report and a review or expert interpretation of the ultrasound picture (i.e. an increase in sensitivity from 30% to 62%). With the dual aim of improving the discrimination between benign and malignant ovarian disease and standardizing the definition of a 'positive' scan, various scoring systems have been developed incorporating the ultrasound features of ovarian malignancy. The sensitivity and specificity of some ultrasound scoring systems are noted in Table 2.

Table 2 Sensitivity and specificity of ultrasound scoring systems for discrimination of benign from malignant ovarian disease, in women undergoing surgery for adnexal masses

Author	*Patients* (*n*)	*Sensitivity* (%)	*Specificity* (%)
Benacerraf *et al.*[31]	100	80	87
Finkler *et al.*[33]	102	62	95
Granberg *et al.*[34]	180	82	92
Hata *et al.*[35]	63	85	69
Herrmann *et al.*[28]	241	82	93
Kurjak *et al.*[36]	1000	48	98
Sassone *et al.*[32]	100	100	83
Weiner *et al.*[37]	53	94	69
Total	1839		
Mean		79	86

The studies referred to above have been based on women presenting with clinical disease, and the stage of the ovarian cancers, when noted, has shown a predominance of advanced disease. Both factors limit their application to screening a healthy population. The morphological changes associated with early ovarian disease may be more difficult to detect using ultrasound, and are based on the determination of ovarian volume and echogenicity. Some of the first work to establish criteria for normality came from King's College Hospital Medical School. In 1982, Campbell and colleagues[38] reported the pelvic findings of 31 postmenopausal women undergoing a transabdominal ultrasound examination. Both ovaries were identified in 26 patients, and the calculated ovarian volumes ranged from 1.47 to 10.43 cm^3 (mean 4.33 cm^3), and were confirmed at laparotomy. They also found that an ovary with a volume more than twice that of the overall mean and also more than twice that of its pair should be regarded with some suspicion. In 1988, having calculated ovarian volumes of 2221 women, the same group published a nomogram of mean ovarian volume according to years since menopause[39]. They concluded that a woman with a mean ovarian volume above the 99.5th centile should be considered at risk of having ovarian cancer, and subject to further investigation. Other features of a normal postmenopausal ovary included uniform echogenicity, an ovoid shape and a smooth echogenic outline[39].

Using the above as criteria for normality, Campbell and colleagues[40] screened 5479 self-selected volunteers (aged 18–78 years, mean age 52) for ovarian cancer. They were to undergo three annual transabdominal ultrasound scans, and 77% of the volunteers completed the program, giving a total of 15 977 scans. Women found to have an abnormality on scan were either referred for surgery or underwent a repeat examination 6 weeks later. Abnormal ultrasound findings indicating the need for surgical intervention were detected in 326 of the volunteers (5.9%). These included five patients with primary ovarian cancer (two stage Ia borderline, one stage Ib borderline, and two stage Ia) giving a positive predictive value for primary ovarian cancer of 1.5%. Two of the malignancies were detected in the course of the first screen and three at the second, implying that the lead time of ultrasound for malignancy may be short. Four other patients at laparotomy had metastatic ovarian cancer. Interestingly no case of advanced primary ovarian cancer was detected in the course of the prevalence screen. Other pathologies at laparotomy included benign ovarian cysts, endometrioid cysts, and sex-cord stromal and germ-cell tumors. No abnormality was detected in 26% of the volunteers who underwent surgery.

Methods have been proposed for improving the positive predictive value of an abnormal scan and include:

(1) Incorporating abnormal ovarian volume and a change in volume in addition to morphological abnormalities into a screening program (using volume change as the criterion for an abnormal scan, Campbell and associates[41] improved the odds ratio of finding ovarian cancer at laparotomy from 1:65 to 1:34);

(2) Restricting screening to women perceived to be at high risk, e.g. postmenopausal women and those with a family history of the disease[42]; and

(3) Using transvaginal ultrasound in conjunction with color-flow and Doppler studies[36,42–44].

Van Nagell and associates[45] have screened 1300 asymptomatic postmenopausal women using annual transvaginal ultrasonography. Persistent ovarian abnormalities were detected in 33 women (2.5%), and 27 were referred for surgical exploration. Two cases of ovarian cancer were detected (FIGO Stage I), one in the wake of the prevalence screen, and the second at the third annual screen. The other 25 women had benign pathologies, giving a specificity for ovarian cancer of 98%. The apparent sensitivity of the screening program was 100%.

Kurjak[44] performed a transvaginal scan on 1000 postmenopausal women, of whom 76% had presented for screening. Eighty-three women were referred for surgery, and in the group of women who had presented for screening, four cases of primary ovarian cancer were diagnosed. They found the sensitivity of their morphological score in distinguishing benign from malignant disease to be 48% with a specificity of 98%.

Doppler Whilst ultrasound imaging has provided a non-invasive method of studying ovarian morphology, pulsed Doppler combined with real-time ultrasound (duplex) has the potential to examine patterns of blood flow and hence to identify functional changes. The normal postmenopausal ovary has poor blood flow and a high resistance to flow. The blood flow in ovulating woman changes during the menstrual cycle – the artery supplying the ovary containing the dominant follicle or corpus luteum shows a lower pulsatility index (PI) than its pair, implying increased blood flow[46].

Malignant tumors may be associated with changes in vascularization. In animal experiments, pulsed Doppler has been used to identify tumors on finding high peak velocities, increased mean velocities and a low PI in supplying vessels[47]. It has recently been possible to obtain color Doppler signals using the transvaginal probe, and this technique has been used to investigate the possibility of improving the discrimination between benign and malignant ovaries.

Kurjak and colleagues[36] have used this technique as a secondary test in an ovarian cancer-screening program. A thousand postmenopausal women underwent transvaginal sonography (26% referred because of symptoms, 74% self-referred). The ovarian morphology was classified

Table 3 Sensitivity and specificity of Doppler ultrasound criteria for discrimination of benign from malignant ovarian disease

Author	*Patients*		*Criterion*	*Sensitivity* (%)	*Specificity* (%)
	n	*Description*			
Bourne *et al.*[42]	18	7 premenopausal 11 postmenopausal	PI < 1	88	91
Hata *et al.*[35]	63	35 premenopausal 28 postmenopausal	RI < 0.72	93	53
Kawai *et al.*[48]	24	ages 24–90 years	PI > 0.8	89	100
Kurjak *et al.*[36]	83	all postmenopausal	RI < 0.41	96	95
Weiner *et al.*[37]	52	ages 20–69 years	PI < 1	94	97
Mean				92	87

PI, pulsatility index; RI, resistance index

using a scoring system. Color flow was imposed upon any ovarian mass in order to detect neovascularization. A Doppler cursor was placed upon the flashing signal of each vessel and a flow velocity waveform obtained, from which a resistance index (RI) was calculated. Abnormal flow was defined as an RI below 0.41.

Eighty-three women were referred for surgery, and 29 malignant ovarian cancers were diagnosed. Compared with 35% of the 54 benign tumors, all but two malignant tumors exhibited color flow. Using an RI of >0.41 as a cut-off for normal, 26 of the malignant masses had abnormal flow. The investigators concluded that whilst ovarian morphology alone (as assessed by transvaginal sonography) was a 'poor discriminator' between benign and malignant disease, the use of color flow and Doppler waveform improved the predictive value of an abnormal test.

Others have also assessed color flow and Doppler for discriminating benign from malignant disease in the preoperative assessment of ovarian masses, and the tests' performance in terms of sensitivity and specificity are noted in Table 3. False-positive results may be obtained from dermoid cysts, serous cystadenomas, ovarian endometrial cysts and developing corpora lutea. Although these results are encouraging, they continue to show that the specificity may be less than the 99.6% needed to achieve a positive predictive value for malignancy of 10% (on screening a population with an incidence of ovarian cancer of 4:10 000).

Despite these problems, it is probable that transvaginal color Doppler may help overcome some of the difficulties related to the early diagnosis of ovarian carcinoma using ultrasound alone. However, it is yet to be shown that its use as a secondary test, having found a pelvic abnormality in a postmenopausal woman participating in an ovarian cancer-screening program, will lead to a significant reduction in the surgical intervention rate, for the technique does depend on the prior detection of abnormal morphology. Many gynecologists, and patients themselves, may feel uneasy leaving an ovarian mass or cyst in a postmenopausal woman. However, information from such flow studies may modify both the type and place of surgery. Women perceived to be at high risk of malignancy may be referred to a gynecologist with an interest in oncology[49,50], whilst those perceived to be at very low risk of malignancy undergo cyst aspiration under ultrasound control (with cytological examination of the cyst fluid)[51,52].

Ultrasound screening for women with a family history of ovarian cancer In 1990, Andolf and co-workers[53] published the results of a study of screening 801 high-risk women for ovarian cancer using transabdominal ultrasonography. Participants were perceived to be at high risk in view of their family history of the disease, a family or personal history of breast or endometrial cancer or nulliparity. Women with unspecified abdominal complaints were also included. In 638 cases, the ultrasound scan was considered to be normal (79%). The ultrasound findings were persistently abnormal, leading to surgical exploration in 62 cases (9.7%), and three gynecological malignancies were diagnosed. Two women had endometrial cancer and the third had bilateral ovarian tumors of borderline malignancy. The latter had presented with abdominal pain. The two women with endometrial cancer also complained of symptoms – postmenopausal bleeding. The fact that the cancers detected were symptomatic, that one in five of the participants needed follow-up scans or other investigations, and the low yield of ovarian cancers, led Andolf and co-workers to conclude that ultrasound screening for ovarian cancer should not be recommended, even for high-risk groups. However, it is probably premature to reach such a conclusion. With respect to the yield of cancers, the authors commented that the incidence of ovarian cancer in the age groups scanned was 40–130 per 100 000. In view of the study size, it was notable that a case of ovarian cancer was detected.

Transvaginal ultrasound with Doppler studies has also been investigated as a means of screening asymptomatic women who have had close relatives develop the disease[42]. The screening test was ideally performed on days 3–8 of the menstrual cycle in order to decrease the number of false-positive results due to physiological changes. Abnormal ovarian volume or morphology were indications for a repeat scan. This was performed between 3 and 7 weeks later in order to assess whether the abnormality was persistent and whether there had been an increase in ovarian size. Women who were screen-positive at this second examination were then referred for surgery.

Having screened 1601 self-referred women, the investigators detected six cases of primary ovarian cancer (five stage Ia, one stage III). Overall, 3.8% of the participants had a positive screen result and were referred for surgery, giving a positive predictive value of a positive result of 9.8% and a specificity of 96.6%. These odds were higher in women[54] with a pedigree consistent with site-specific ovarian cancer (autosomal dominant inheritance) or Lynch type II cancer family syndrome[55].

In a retrospective analysis, the authors calculated, for each detected mass, a score using a weighted morphology index (incorporating features such as the number of cysts or locules, the presence of papillary projections, the echogenicity of the cyst fluid, and irregularity in outline)[42]. Operating only upon those women with a score of 5 or above would have reduced the number of false-positive results by 89%, from 55 to six. However, one case of borderline ovarian cancer would have been missed, giving a sensitivity (up to 18 months following screening) of 83%.

The value of Doppler was also assessed on this population. In a retrospective analysis, a PI of < 1.0 in a persistent ovarian lesion was taken as an index of cancer, and an indication for surgical referral. Using this definition, one case of borderline ovarian cancer would have been missed (one case of borderline cancer was not assessed using Doppler), with a reduction in the number of false-positive cases from 55 to 13. The sensitivity of this screening algorithm would therefore have been 80% with a specificity of 99.2%.

Had the screening program required that any persistent ovarian lesion have a morphological score of > 5 and a PI of < 1.0 before surgery was indicated, two cases of cancer would have been missed, giving a sensitivity of 66%. The false-positive rate would also have fallen, increasing the specificity to 99.8%. Using either a PI of < 1.0 or a morphology index of > 5 as the criterion for cancer, would have given a specificity of only 99.1%, but a sensitivity (at 1 year) of 100%.

With longer follow-up, three interval cases of primary ovarian cancer have been diagnosed in the study population (and two cases of disseminated intra-abdominal carcinomatosis) giving an overall sensitivity of the program for primary ovarian cancer of 66.6%.

This study illustrates the benefits of a secondary screening test (either a morphology score or Doppler studies) in decreasing the false-positive rate of ultrasound. Using such tests, the specificity of the screening program was increased from 96.6% to 99.6% and 99.2%, respectively. This increase in specificity was achieved at a loss of sensitivity (at 18 months) from 100% to 80%.

In conclusion, ultrasound has a place in the detection of asymptomatic ovarian cancer in defined high-risk groups; the apparent sensitivity of the test within the confines of the available data

Table 4 Ultrasound screening studies for epithelial ovarian cancer. Overall specificity, 94.9%; specificity of transvaginal studies, 96.7%

Author	*Patients* (*n*)	*Route*	*Ovarian cancer*	*Stage*	*Other operations*	*Comment*
Campbell *et al.*[40]	5479	T/A	2	Ia (b/l)	321	self-referred
			1	Ib (b/l)		
			2	Ia		
Andolf *et al.*[53]	801	T/A	1	Ib (b/l)	61	family history symptomatic
Kurjak *et al.*[36]	704	T/V	3	I	40*	postmenopausal self-referred
			1	III		
Van Nagell *et al.*[45]	1300	T/V	2	Ia	25	postmenopausal
Bourne *et al.*[42]	1601	T/V	2	I	55	family history
			3	I (b/l)		
			1	III		
Total	9885		18		502	

*Estimate (74% of 54 operations performed in the entire study of 1000 women); T/A, transabdominal; T/V, transvaginal; b/l, borderline

is probably high. Over 9000 women have been screened using this method, with the detection of 18 cases of ovarian cancer, and the vast majority have been diagnosed with the malignancy confined to the ovary (Table 4). The limitations of the method, however, are:

(1) The poor specificity when used in isolation. However, the addition of flow studies or a morphology index may lead to an improvement in the test performance. The choice of secondary test may be determined by the facilities available and by the age of the population under study. Whilst Kurjak and colleagues[36] found abnormal flow to be the more reliable indicator of malignancy, a morphology index provided better specificity in the study by Bourne and co-workers[42]. However, the populations under study were different. Whilst Kurjak and colleagues looked at postmenopausal women, the Bourne study contained about twice as many premenopausal as postmenopausal women. It is recognized that the false-positive rate of neovascularization is higher in premenopausal women with conditions such as endometriosis, teratomas and functional cysts giving positive results;

(2) The need for expensive equipment and trained staff; and

(3) The apparent short lead time of the diagnosis by ultrasound screening over 'clinical' diagnosis, leading to the requirement for a short inter-screen interval[56].

Tumor markers

Quantitative and qualitative changes in numerous circulating substances have been associated with epithelial ovarian cancer. These may reflect a 'general' response to the malignant process, or an alteration in ovarian function or surface molecular structure[12,57]. The anatomical site of the ovaries may render them inaccessible to direct examination, but may make ovarian cancer particularly suitable for detection by a serum marker. Antigen produced by ovarian cancer may reach the general circulation by two routes. Antigen in cystic or solid areas of the tumor may diffuse into the lymphatics or blood vessels in the well-vascularized ovarian stroma whilst antigen shed into the peritoneal cavity may enter the venous circulation via the diaphragmatic lymphatics and the thoracic duct.

Changes in serum levels of enzymes (placental alkaline phosphatase[58,59,60], amylase[61], galactosyl transferase[62], lactate dehydrogenase[63], 5′ nucleotidase[64]), hormones (human placental lactogen[58], progesterone[65], estrogen[66]), oncofetal proteins (human chorionic gonadotropin, α-fetoprotein[67], carcinoembryonic antigen[68]), metabolic products (ferritin, fibrin degradation products[69], circulating immune complexes[70,71]) have all been identified in women with ovarian cancer. Apart from the association of α-fetoprotein with germ cell ovarian cancer (in particular endodermal sinus and embryonal tumors[72]) and human chorionic gonadotropin with choriocarcinoma[73], these markers used in isolation are yet to show sufficient sensitivity or specificity for early epithelial ovarian cancer to be of value as screening tests.

Advances in the technology of antigen purification and radioimmunoassay development during the 1960s and 1970s led to the production of polyclonal antisera against a number of antigens which have been evaluated in relation to ovarian cancer, e.g. HMFG1, HMFG2[16], CA 19–9[74] and DUPAN-2[75]. However, an antigen expressed uniquely by ovarian malignancy is yet to be defined. All antigens described to date have been tumor-associated rather than tumor-specific and are expressed by other normal and diseased cells. This lack of specificity does not of necessity imply that antigen detection has no role in diagnosing ovarian cancer. Tumor-associated antigens, with a satisfactory sensitivity for early-stage disease, may be of value in the early detection of ovarian cancer, if:

(1) There is little or no overlap between the serum levels in diseased and healthy individuals; and/or

(2) A secondary test can be applied that will differentiate between those individuals with raised serum levels that have ovarian cancer and those that do not.

Amongst the first ovarian cancer antigens to be detected were OCC and OCA[76–78]. OCA levels were reported to be raised in 70% of women with stage I and II epithelial cancer, and in 10% of healthy individuals. In 1983, Bast and colleagues[79] described the CA 125 antigen, which has come to be the most extensively studied epithelial ovarian cancer tumor-associated antigen.

CA 125 CA 125 is an antigenic determinant on a high-molecular-weight glycoprotein recognized by a monoclonal antibody (OC 125) which was raised using an ovarian cancer cell line as an immunogen. Immunohistochemical studies have demonstrated CA 125 expression to be a feature of cells derived from the embryonal celomic epithelium and Müllerian duct[80] and both benign and malignant pathologies affecting tissues with these embryological origins have been associated with increased CA 125 expression[81]. The original observation that benign, serous and most malignant serous ovarian tumors expressed CA 125[80], whilst neither the normal fetal nor adult ovarian surface epithelium expressed CA 125, was interpreted as evidence of a distinct differentiation pathway of ovarian surface epithelium in ovarian malignancy. However, there have been subsequent reports of CA 125 expression in some sections of normal ovarian epithelium[82].

Using radioimmunoassay, the CA 125 antigen may be detected in serum, and serum levels are greater than 35 U/ml in over 80% of women with ovarian cancer[79,83]. Bast and colleagues[79] have also shown that only 1% of healthy female blood donors have serum CA 125 levels of >35 U/ml. Elevated levels may also be found in association with benign gynecological pathologies, e.g. endometriosis and pelvic inflammatory disease, or in the first trimester of pregnancy. This overlap with benign conditions has led some authors to suggest that the specificity of a raised serum CA 125 level for ovarian cancer would be poor, precluding it as a method of screening for ovarian cancer[84]. However, the incidence of these benign conditions in postmenopausal women – the largest at-risk group for ovarian cancer – is low, reducing the impact on specificity.

Much of the work addressing the sensitivity of serum CA 125 for ovarian cancer has used women with adnexal masses as subjects. Many studies have reported preoperative serum CA 125 in women undergoing surgery for ovarian cancer[79,85,86]. These indicate that 80–85% of cases are associated with elevated levels. Closer analysis, however, shows this to be stage-dependent. Disease disseminated outside the ovary is associated with elevation of serum CA 125 levels in over 90% of cases (i.e. stages I, II and IV). With the tumor confined to ovarian tissue, serum CA 125 levels are elevated in 50% of cases only. This has obvious implications for a screening program using serum CA 125 levels as the primary screening method.

Zurawski and associates[87] showed that it was possible to detect elevated levels of CA 125 in serum, months (even years) prior to the diagnosis of ovarian cancer. A retrospective analysis of CA 125 levels was undertaken, using sera obtained from a serum bank. The study population consisted of 105 women who had donated serum to the bank, who were subsequently diagnosed as having ovarian cancer. Sera from 323 apparently healthy matched controls were also assayed. They found that the distribution of serum CA 125 levels was very different between the case and control populations over the entire collection to diagnosis interval (range 1–143 months). Cases had a higher median serum CA 125 concentration than controls (18 U/ml compared with 10 U/ml), but this is probably of little practical significance. However, serum CA 125 levels of >35 U/ml were measured in 50% of cases within 18 months of diagnosis and a third of cases had serum CA 125 levels >65 U/ml within 18 months of diagnosis. The implication from this study therefore is that it might be possible to screen for preclinical disease by measuring serum CA 125.

CA 125 and screening for ovarian cancer In view of the high specificity demanded of a prospective ovarian cancer screening program and the association of CA 125 with pathologies other than ovarian cancer, the positive predictive value of a single raised serum CA 125 level for the disease would be too low for serum CA 125, in isolation, to be acceptable as a screening test. Specificity may be rendered acceptable by combining CA 125 estimation with ultrasound[88].

At the Royal London Hospital, a screening program for ovarian cancer, using apparently healthy postmenopausal women as subjects, has been in operation since 1985. The study incorporates the use of serum CA 125 and ultrasound in a stepwise or sequential manner (see Figure 1). Approximately 22 000 women have undergone the screening program. In accordance with the

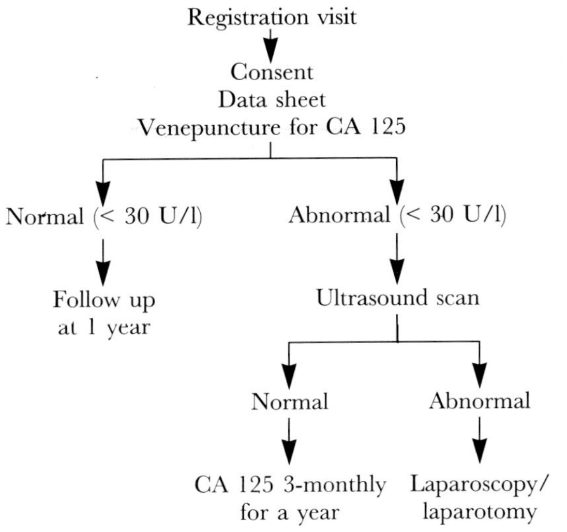

Figure 1 The Royal London Hospital multimodal screening program for ovarian cancer – study design

study protocol, all volunteers had their serum CA 125 measured using a commercially available radioimmunoassay. When the serum CA 125 level was greater than 30 U/ml, an ultrasound scan was performed. (In the first years of the study, the transabdominal route was employed; latterly the transvaginal route has also been used.)

Ultrasound findings were considered to be normal, if:

(1) After the ovaries had been visualized and measured in three dimensions,
   (a) the ovarian volume was ⩽8.8 ml;
   (b) the ovaries were of uniform echogenicity;
   (c) the ovarian outline was smooth; or
(2) Despite the ovaries not being identified, no pelvic abnormality was detected.

Ultrasound findings were considered to be equivocal when the ovarian volume was ⩽8.8 ml but the ovarian morphology was abnormal. If the result of the ultrasound scan was abnormal, arrangements were made either for repeating the scan at a later date or for surgery.

Women with normal ultrasound findings were followed up with 3-monthly serum CA 125 estimations for a year. During this follow-up phase, volunteers could be recalled for subsequent ultra-

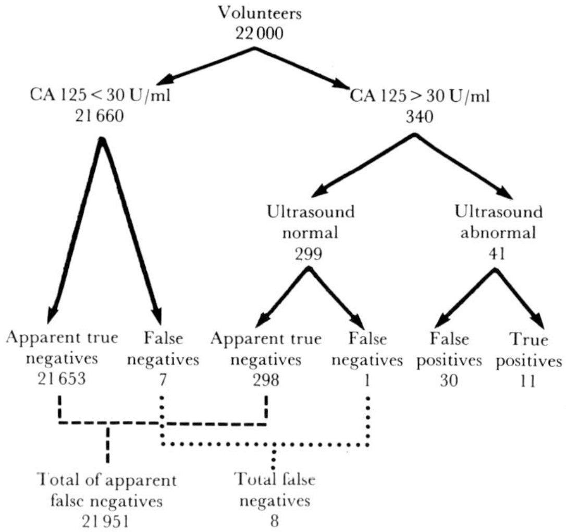

Figure 2 The Royal London Hospital multimodal screening program for ovarian cancer – results of the prevalence screen

Table 5 Histology and serum CA 125 levels in the 11 ovarian cancers detected by the prevalence screen of the Royal London Hospital multimodal screening program

FIGO stage	*Histology*	*Serum CA 125* (U/ml)
Ia	clear cell cystadenocarcinoma	32
Ia	clear cell cystadenocarcinoma	33
Ib	serous cystadenocarcinoma	80
IIa	serous cystadenocarcinoma	119
III	serous cystadenocarcinoma	68
III	serous cystadenocarcinoma	78
III	mucinous cystadenocarcinoma	66
III	poorly differentiated cystadenocarcinoma	360
III	poorly differentiated cystadenocarcinoma	54
IV	poorly differentiated cystadenocarcinoma	436
IV	serous cystadenocarcinoma	400

sound examinations in response to the serum CA 125 level – e.g. a doubling in the serum CA 125 level between two consecutive samples or a level remaining greater than 100 U/ml in two consecutive samples.

Women with an equivocal ultrasound scan attended at 3-monthly intervals for a repeat ultrasound scan and serum CA 125 estimation for a 12-month period. If, during follow-up, the repeat ultrasound scan was classified as normal or abnormal, further management was as described above for volunteers with an initially normal or abnormal scan.

The results are shown in Figure 2. Approximately 2% of the screened population were recalled for an ultrasound examination, following which 42 operations were performed. Eleven women were diagnosed as having primary ovarian cancer, and three cases of cancer of the Fallopian tube were diagnosed. The remaining 28 women had benign pathologies, including epithelial cysts, endometriosis, adhesions and ovarian thecomas. Three women had no abnormality detected at laparotomy. During the year of follow-up, three cases of ovarian cancer were diagnosed in women who were allocated to the screen-negative group – false negatives. The results of this prevalence screen show the specificity of the screening program for ovarian cancer to be 99.8%, with a detection rate of 78% at 1 year following screening and a positive predictive value of 33.3%[89]. With longer follow-up, further cases of ovarian cancer have been diagnosed in screen-negative women, reducing the sensitivity of the screening program to approximately 50%.

Of the 11 ovarian cancers detected by the screening program, only four were 'early', FIGO stage I or II (Table 5). This, however, is what might be expected from a prevalence screen (especially for a condition such as ovarian cancer which is notorious for late symptomatology), and the sensitivity of the screening test for early stage disease cannot be calculated from the study. It is postulated that should screening with serum CA 125 and ultrasound be an effective method of early diagnosis, follow-up interval screening of the study population should detect a larger proportion of early cancers than was the case during the prevalence screen. In order to address this, a randomized, controlled study of annual screening, using the original volunteers to the program as subjects, has been ongoing since 1990/91. The results of the first interval screen, although preliminary, are encouraging. The high specificity of the screening program has been confirmed. Further cases of cancer are needed before any

Table 6 Comparison of multimodal screening program[89], using CA 125 measurements as a preliminary test, followed by ultrasound ($n = 22\,000$) with ultrasound-only screening program[42] ($n = 1601$)

Screening tests	Sensitivity At 1 year (%)	Sensitivity Overall (%)	Specificity (%)
(1) CA 125 > 30 U/ml[89] (2) Abnormal scan	78 86†	57.9*	99.8
(1) Abnormal scan[42] (2) Abnormal scan	100	66	96.6
(1) Abnormal scan‡[42] (2) MI > 5	83	55.5	99.6
(1) Abnormal scan‡[42] (2) PI < 1	80	50	99.2
(1) Abnormal scan‡[42] (2) MI > 5 *and* PI < 1	66	37	99.8
(1) Abnormal scan‡[42] (2) MI > 5 *or* PI < 1	100	66	99.1

*Incomplete follow up (probably lower); †all women with a raised CA 125 attended for a scan; ‡calculated retrospectively; MI, morphology index; PI, pulsatility index

statement on stage distribution at diagnosis and survival benefit can be made.

The results of The Royal London Hospital multimodal screening program for ovarian cancer are compared with the results of an ultrasound-only screening program in Table 6.

Einhorn and colleagues[90], having screened 5550 apparently healthy women using serum CA 125 as an initial test, came to the conclusion that in postmenopausal women (> 50 years of age) the specificity of a raised serum CA 125 level for ovarian cancer was adequate, and sufficiently good to justify a larger study with mortality as an end point. They obtained, in this group of women, specificities of 97% and 98.5% for cut-offs in serum CA 125 levels of 30 U/ml and 35 U/ml, respectively. Not surprisingly, the specificities for younger women were lower.

Nine ovarian cancers were diagnosed in this study population – six occurred in women over 50 years, and three in women under 50 years. All six in the older group were detected through the screening program as a result of finding elevated serum CA 125 levels (range 73–593 U/ml). The three cases of cancer occurring in younger women were 'missed' by the screening program as serum CA 125 levels in all three cases were less than 35 U/ml, at 5.9, 34.4 and 10.5 U/ml.

These two studies illustrate that the sensitivity of a screening program employing serum CA 125 levels as a preliminary test will probably be no greater than 50%. Methods of improving the detection rate of serum screening are being assessed, and include temporal changes in marker concentrations and the use of a panel of markers.

Temporal changes in serum CA 125 Having determined serum CA 125 concentrations in 1082 women (over 40 years), Zurawski and associates[91] found that 3.3% had levels of > 35 U/ml. Follow-up CA 125 levels were obtained from the 36 women with raised serum CA 125 concentrations at 24 months, and a significant fall in mean CA 125 levels was found. In only two instances was a doubling in the serum CA 125 level observed, and in only one of these cases was the increase sustained. This woman, following intensive clinical investigation, was later diagnosed as having ovarian cancer (stage III). Interestingly, pelvic ultrasound examinations both at 10 and 4.5 months prior to the surgical diagnosis were considered as not being suggestive of ovarian malignancy. The diagnosis was made 21 months after the initial elevated serum CA 125 measurement and 15 months after the first measured doubling. No other case of ovarian cancer was diagnosed in the study population. Zurawski and co-workers claimed a specificity of 99.9% using the doubling of an initially elevated value as the criterion for determining positivity and 100% using as the criterion a sustained increase in level for those with initially elevated levels that doubled.

It is postulated that the CA 125 antigen enters the circulation because of a disruption in the blood/tissue barrier; and in association with malignancy, this may represent invasive destruction of the basement membrane with metastatic spread. Serial serum CA 125 measurements have become an increasingly employed means of monitoring clinical ovarian cancer, where persistently rising serum CA 125 levels are associated with disease progression, and a doubling of CA 125 is seen as a reliable indicator of recurrent disease. Although there is less known about changes in serum CA 125 levels and disease progression prior to the diagnosis of ovarian cancer, rapid and sustained increases in preoperative serum CA 125 levels probably represent tumor dissemination with implications for the resectability of the cancer, and morbidity and mortality from the disease. Although Cruickshank and colleagues[92] found no correlation between preoperative serum CA 125 levels and disease outcome in 41 patients over a follow-up period of 3–18 months, this was not the finding of a collaborative study by the Gynaecological Tumour Marker Group[93]. Having monitored 202 patients over a median of 73 months, they found that survival for women with preoperative serum CA 125 levels of <65 U/ml was significantly better than those with a level of >65 U/ml.

Multiple tumor markers Employing a panel of tumor markers may lead to an improvement in the sensitivity of serological screening for ovarian cancer. Dhokia and co-workers[94] measured HMFG1, HMFG2 and CA 125 in sera from 85 patients with histologically proven epithelial ovarian cancer. Sera from five patients with negative HMFG1 (<0.13 OD), HMFG2 (<0.13 OD) and CA 125 (<35 U/ml) levels were further tested for serum placental alkaline phosphatase levels. Approximately 85% of patients with active tumor had elevated levels (>35 U/ml) of CA 125. Using a panel of HMFG1 and HMFG2 with CA 125, the sensitivity was increased to 95%, without loss of specificity. Three of the five patients who had normal CA 125, HMFG1 and HMFG2 levels had elevated serum placental alkaline phosphatase concentrations. The sensitivity, using all four markers, was 98.8%. Ward and associates[95] also found that combining CA 125 with HMGF2 and placental alkaline phosphatase resulted in a statistically significant improvement, from 18% to 69%, in the detection rate of ovarian cancer. In 37 patients the antigens were assayed before operation and 41 patients were monitored following treatment.

It has been suggested that the urinary fragment of a metabolite of the beta subunit of human chorionic gonadotropin (hCG), beta core, may, in conjunction with serum CA 125, be of value in distinguishing benign from malignant ovarian disease. The combined test gave a sensitivity of 88%, which was higher than the sensitivity of either test alone[96]. The work is being repeated.

Serum M-CSF and OVX1 may also be complementary to CA 125. Woolas and colleagues[97] measured levels of these three markers in the sera of 46 patients with clinical stage I ovarian cancer. Elevated levels of CA 125 (>30 U/ml), M-CSF (>3 ng/ml) and OVX1 (12 U/ml) were detected in 65%, 52% and 48%, respectively. The corresponding figures for 204 apparently healthy postmenopausal women were 2%, 3% and 6%. In the cancer group, at least one marker was elevated in 98% of cases and two markers in 54%, compared to 11% and 0% in the controls. In order to assess the sensitivity of the tumor marker panel for preclinical ovarian cancer, stored serum samples from the Royal London Hospital Ovarian Cancer Screening Study were analyzed. M-CSF or OVX1 levels were elevated in 8/18 of women who developed ovarian cancer within 2 years of an initial CA 125 level of <30 U/ml. These results suggest that the sensitivity of screening for ovarian cancer may be increased by the use of a panel of markers. The consequent loss of specificity may be overcome by the use of ultrasound as a secondary test.

In summary, serum CA 125 measurements, with ultrasound as a secondary test, may have a place in the early detection of ovarian cancer. Di-Xia and co-workers[98] reported detecting CA 125 in saliva. The sensitivities of the saliva and serum CA 125 assays in 16 patients with epithelial ovarian cancer were 81.3% and 93.8%, respectively (using a level of >65 U/ml for the serum assay and 3000 U/ml for the saliva assay). The collection of saliva is simple, and may pave the way for a 'home screening kit'.

In conclusion, the main limitation of screening using CA 125 is the poor sensitivity of the test which is probably of the order of 50% for early-stage disease. Improvements in sensitivity may be achieved by the use of a panel of markers. However, this will be achieved at the expense of specificity and simplicity, and at increased financial cost. Current evidence suggests that the mean length of time from CA 125 elevation to clinical presentation in cases which become CA 125-positive is 1.9–3 years[54].

Mortality

A large randomized controlled study is needed in order to assess the impact of screening for ovarian cancer on mortality from the disease, as was the recommendation of the report of the UK CCCR[99]. As mortality rates from ovarian cancer are approximately a third those of breast cancer, the randomized trials of ovarian cancer screening would need to be three times as large if the same degree of effect were to be detected. However, this would be expensive, and, as the screening tests themselves are still under investigation, has not to date been performed. In the interim, some answers may be obtained using a mathematical model based on the perceived benefits of screening using currently available data from screening trials. Skates and Singer[100] have produced such a mathematical model for the annual screening of 1 000 000 women aged 50–70 over a 30-year period using an elevation in serum CA 125 levels as the screening test. In their simulated model, almost three-fifths (59.2%) of all cases were detected by the screening program, and 75% of screen-detected cases were detected in an earlier stage. The earlier initiation of treatment following the detection of ovarian cancer by screening extended the life of 45% of the detected cases by an average of 7.75 years. In some instances, 30 years of life were saved by the earlier detection. Averaged over all cases, the years of life saved were 3.42 ± 0.10. There was a shift to the right with respect to the calculated age at death from 69.7 in the not-screened population to 73.1 years in the screened population. Whilst stage shifts from III–I contribute the most years of life saved, there may also be benefits from detecting advanced disease earlier. These, however, are more difficult to quantify, and must include the morbidity associated with the adjuvant chemotherapy prescribed to women with disseminated ovarian cancer.

The question remains of the cost effectiveness of a screening program. Cost effectiveness is influenced by several factors including the cost of the screening test, the cost of the diagnostic test and the saving achieved by treating early- instead of late-stage disease. Although the cost of these expenses are fixed, the ratio of expenditure to saving will be influenced by the specificity and sensitivity of the test employed and the incidence of the disease in the screened population. Cost effectiveness is therefore another reason for selecting a population with a relatively high incidence of ovarian cancer and for which the test employed has a high specificity.

Basing their calculations on the protocol and results of the Royal London Hospital Ovarian Cancer Screening program, Scott and associates[101] have estimated the cost of screening as £15 per woman screened per year – the same as it costs their health region to screen for cervical cancer, a disease which has half the mortality of ovarian cancer.

Whether the health benefit is sufficient to merit the cost of screening is a wider issue, involving health service priorities and political issues. Nevertheless, there is a broad consensus that, in the absence of effective treatment for established disease, the quest for early diagnosis is of urgent importance.

ACKNOWLEDGEMENTS

The work of Ann Prys Davies was funded by a grant from Birthright. The work of The Ovarian Cancer Screening Unit at The Royal London Hospital was funded by The Gynaecology Cancer Research Fund.

References

1. Serov, S. F., Scully, R. E. and Sobin, L. H. (1973). Histological typing of ovarian tumours. *International Classification of Tumours No 9*. (Geneva: World Health Organisation)
2. Fox, H. and Langley, F. A. (1976). *Tumours of the Ovary*. (London: Heinemann)

3. Kottmeier, H. (ed.) (1982). *Annual Report on the Results of Treatment in Gynaecological Cancer*, 18. (Stockholm: FIGO)
4. American Cancer Society (1990). *Cancer Statistics*, **40**, 9–26
5. OPCS, Registrations (1989). *Causes of Diagnosed Cancer Registered in England and Wales*. (London: HMSO)
6. La Vecchia, C., Levi, F., Lucchini, F., Negri, E. and Franceshi, S. (1992). Descriptive epidemiology of ovarian cancer in Europe. *Gynecol. Oncol.*, **46**, 208–15
7. Villard-Mackintosh, L., Vessey, M. P. and Jones, L. (1989). The effects of oral contraceptives and parity on ovarian cancer trends in women under 55 years of age. *Br. J. Obstet. Gynaecol.*, **96**, 783–8
8. Hankinson, S. E., Colditz, G. A., Hunter, D. J., Spencer, T. L., Rosner, B. and Stampfer, M. J. (1992). A quantitative assessment of oral contraceptive use and risk of ovarian cancer. *Obstet. Gynecol.*, **80**, 708–14
9. Jacobs, I. J. and Oram, D. H. (1988). Oophorectomy and prevention of ovarian cancer. In Chamberlain, G. (ed.) *Contemporary Obstetrics and Gynaecology*, pp. 397–408. (London: Butterworths)
10. Kerlikowske, K., Brown, J. and Grady, D. G. (1992). Should women with familial ovarian cancer undergo prophylactic oophorectomy. *Obstet. Gynaecol.*, **80**, 700–7
11. Dembo, A. J., Davy, M., Stenwig, A. E., Berle, E. J., Bush, R. S. and Kjorstad, K. (1990). Prognostic factors in patients with stage I epithelial ovarian cancer. *Obstet. Gynecol.*, **75**, 263–73
12. Smith, L. H. and Ol, R. H. (1984). Detection of malignant ovarian neoplasms: a review of the literature II. Laboratory detection. *Obstet. Gynecol. Surv.*, **39**, 329–45
13. Prys Davies, A. and Oram, D. (1991). Screening for ovarian cancer. In Studd, J. (ed.) *Progress in Obstetrics and Gynaecology*, pp. 349–74. (London: Churchill Livingstone)
14. Shapiro, S. P. and Nunez, C. (1983). Psammoma bodies in the cervicovaginal smear in association with a papillary tumour of the peritoneum. *Obstet. Gynecol.*, **61**, 130–4
15. Keetel, W. C., Pixley, E. E. and Buchsbaum, H. J. (1974). Experience with peritoneal cytology in the management of gynecologic malignancies. *Am. J. Obstet. Gynecol.*, **120**, 174–82
16. Epenetos, A. A., Britton, K. E., Mather, S., Shepherd, J., Granowska, M. and Taylor-Papadimitriou, J. (1982). Targeting of iodine-123-labelled tumour-associated monoclonal antibodies to ovarian, breast and gastrointestinal tumours. *Lancet*, **2**, 999–1005
17. Brenner, D. E., Grosh, W. W. and Jones, H. W. (1983). An evaluation of the accuracy of computed tomography in patients with ovarian carcinoma prior to second look laparotomy. *Am. Soc. Clin. Oncol. Proc.*, **2**, 149
18. Powell, M. C., Worthington, B. S. and Symonds, E. M. (1987). The application of magnetic resonance imaging (M.R.I.) to ovarian carcinoma. In Sharp, F. and Souther, W. P. (eds.) *Ovarian Cancer – the Way Ahead*, pp. 141–58. (London: Royal College of Obstetricians and Gynaecologists)
19. Copplesson, M. (1981). *Gynecologic Oncology*, Vol. 2, pp. 644–50. (Melbourne, New York: Churchill Livingstone)
20. Russell, P. (1979). The pathological assessment of ovarian neoplasms. I. Introduction to the common epithelial tumours and analysis of benign epithelial tumours. *Pathology*, **2**, 5–23
21. Barber, H. R. K. (1979). Ovarian cancer, Part I. *CA – Cancer J. Clin.*, **29**, 341–51
22. MacFarlane, C., Sturgis, M. C. and Fetterman, F. S. (1955). Results of an experiment in the control of cancer of the female pelvic organs and report of a fifteen year research. *Am. J. Obstet. Gynecol.*, **69**, 294–9
23. Reeves, D., Drake, T. S. and O'Brien, I. F. (1980). Ultrasonographic versus clinical evaluation of a pelvic mass. *Obstet. Gynecol.*, **55**, 551–4
24. Andolf, E., Svalenius, E. and Åstedt, B. (1986). Ultrasonography for early detection of ovarian carcinoma. *Br. J. Obstet. Gynecol.*, **93**, 1286–9
25. Fleischer, A. C. (1988). Transvaginal sonography helps find ovarian cancer. *Diagn. Imaging*, **10**, 124–8
26. Granberg, S. and Wikland, M. (1988). A comparison between ultrasound and gynecologic examination for detection of enlarged ovaries in a group of women at risk of ovarian carcinoma. *J. Ultrasound Med.*, **7**, 59–64
27. Moyle, J. W., Rochester, D., Sider, L., Shrock, K. and Krause, P. (1983). Sonography of ovarian tumors: predictability of tumour type. *Am. J. Radiol.*, **141**, 985–91
28. Herrmann, U. J., Locher, G. W. and Goldhirsch, A. (1987). Sonographic patterns of ovarian tumors: prediction of malignancy. *Obstet. Gynecol.*, **69**, 777–81
29. DeLand, M., Fried, A., van Nagell, J. R. and Donaldson, E. S. (1979). Ultrasonography in the diagnosis of tumours of the ovary. *Surg. Gynecol. Obstet.*, **148**, 346–8
30. Beck, D., Deutsch, M. and Bronshtein, M. (1988). The ovary. In Timor-Tritsch, I. E. and Rottem, S. (eds.) *Transvaginal Sonography*, pp. 59–86. (London: Heinemann Medical Books)
31. Benacerraf, B. R., Finkler, N. J., Wojciechowski, C. and Knapp, R. C. (1990). Sonographic accuracy in the diagnosis of ovarian masses. *J. Reprod. Med.*, **35**, 491–5
32. Sassone, A. M., Timor-Tritsch, I. E., Artner, A., Westhoff, C. and Warren, W. B. (1991). Transva-

ginal sonographic characterization of ovarian disease: evaluation of a new scoring system to predict ovarian malignancy. *Obstet. Gynecol.*, **78**, 70–6

33. Finkler, N. J., Benacerraf, B., Lavin, P. T., Wojciechowski, C. and Knapp, R. C. (1988). Comparison of serum CA 125, clinical impression and ultrasound in the preoperative evaluation of ovarian masses. *Obstet. Gynecol.*, **72**, 659–64
34. Granberg, S., Norsrom, A. and Wikland, M. (1990). Tumors in the lower pelvis as imaged by vaginal sonography. *Gynecol. Oncol.*, **37**, 224–9
35. Hata, K., Hata, T., Manabe, A., Sugimura, K. and Kitao, M. (1992). A critical evaluation of transvaginal Doppler studies, transvaginal sonography, magnetic resonance imaging, and CA 125 in detecting ovarian cancer. *Obstet. Gynecol.*, **80**, 922–6
36. Kurjak, A., Schulmann, H., Sosic, A., Zalud, I. and Shalan, H. (1992). Transvaginal ultrasound, colour flow and Doppler waveform of the postmenopausal adnexal mass. *Obstet. Gynecol.*, **80**, 917–21
37. Weiner, Z., Thaler, I., Beck, D., Rottem, S., Dentsh, M. and Brandes, J. M. (1992). Differentiating malignant from benign ovarian tumors with transvaginal colour flow imaging. *Obstet. Gynecol.*, **79**, 159–62
38. Campbell, S., Goessens, L., Goswamy, R. and Whitehead, M. (1982). Real-time ultrasonography for determination of ovarian morphology and volume. *Lancet*, **1**, 425–6
39. Goswamy, R. K., Campbell, S., Royston, J. P., Bhan, V., Battersby, R. H., Hall, V. J., Whitehead, M. I. and Collins, W. P. (1988). Ovarian size in post-menopausal women. *Br. J. Obstet. Gynaecol.*, **95**, 795–801
40. Campbell, S., Bhan, V., Royston, P., Whitehead, M. I. and Collins, W. (1989). Transabdominal ultrasound screening for early ovarian cancer. *Br. Med. J.*, **299**, 1363–7
41. Campbell, S., Royston, P., Bhan, V., Whitehead, M. I. and Collins, W. P. (1990). Novel screening strategies for early ovarian cancer by transabdominal ultrasonography. *Br. J. Obstet. Gynecol.*, **97**, 304–11
42. Bourne, T. H., Campbell, S., Reynolds, K. M., Whitehead, M. I., Hampson, J., Royston, P., Crayford, T. J. B. and Collins, W. P. (1993). Screening for early familial ovarian cancer with transvaginal ultrasonography and colour flow imaging. *Br. Med. J.*, **306**, 1025–9
43. Bourne, T., Campbell, S., Steer, C., Whitehead, M. I. and Collins, W. P. (1989). Transvaginal colour flow imaging; a possible new screening technique for ovarian cancer. *Br. Med. J.*, **299**, 1367–70
44. Kurjak, A. (1991). Adnexal masses. In Kurjak, A. (ed.) *Tranvaginal Color Doppler*, pp. 118–19. (Carnforth, UK: Parthenon Publishing)
45. Van Nagell, J. R., De Priest, P. D., Puls, L. E., Donaldson, E. S., Gallion, H. H., Pavlik, E. J., Powell, D. E. and Kryscio, R. J. (1991). Ovarian cancer screening in asymptomatic postmenopausal women by transvaginal sonography. *Cancer*, **68**, 458–62
46. Taylor, K. J. W., Burns, P. N., Wells, P. N. T., Conway, D. I. and Hull, M. G. R. (1985). Ultrasound Doppler flow studies of the ovarian and uterine arteries. *Br. J. Obstet. Gynecol.*, **92**, 240–6
47. Rubin, J. M., Carson, P. L., Zlotecki, R. A. and Ensminger, W. D. (1987). Visualization of tumor vascularity in a rabbit VX2 carcinoma by Doppler flow mapping. *J. Ultrasound Med.*, **6**, 113–20
48. Kawai, M., Kano, T., Kikkawa, F., Maeda, O., Ognchi, H. and Tomoda, Y. (1992). Transvaginal Doppler ultrasound with color flow imaging in the diagnosis of ovarian cancer. *Obstet. Gynecol.*, **79**, 163–7
49. Mayer, A. R., Setsuko, K. C., Graves, E., Holm, C., Tseng, P. C., Nelson, B. E. and Schwartz, P. E. (1992). Ovarian cancer staging: does it require a gynecologic oncologist? *Gynecol. Oncol.*, **47**, 223–7
50. Eisenkop, S. M., Spirtos, N. M., Montag, T. W., Nalick, R. H. and Wang, H. (1992). The impact of subspeciality training on the management of advanced ovarian cancer. *Gynecol. Oncol.*, **47**, 203–9
51. De Crespigny, L. C. L., Robinson, H. P., Davoren, R. A. M. and Fortune, D. (1989). The 'simple' ovarian cyst: aspirate or operate? *Br. J. Obstet. Gynecol.*, **96**, 1035–9
52. Diernaes, E., Rasmussen, J., Soerensen, T. and Hasch, E. (1987). Ovarian cysts: management by puncture? *Lancet*, **1**, 1084
53. Andolf, E., Jorgensen, C. and Astedt, B. (1990). Ultrasound examination for detection of ovarian carcinoma in risk groups. *Obstet. Gynecol.*, **75**, 106–9
54. Collins, W. P., Bourne, T. H. and Reynolds, K. (1992). Ultrasound for early cancer screening. In Sharp, F., Mason, W. P. and Creaseman, W. (eds.) *Ovarian Cancer 2: Biology, Diagnosis and Management*, pp. 225–36. (London: Chapman and Hall)
55. Lynch, H. T., Albano, W., Black, L., Lynch, J. F., Recabaren, J. and Pierseon, R. (1981). Familial excess of cancer of the ovary and other anatomic sites. *J. Am. Med. Assoc.*, **245**, 261–4
56. Jacobs, I., Prys Davies, A. and Oram, D. (1992). Early detection of ovarian cancer: a rational and realistic objective? *Diagn. Oncol.*, **2**, 24–43
57. Bast, R. C. and Knapp, R. C. (1987). Humoral markers for epithelial ovarian carcinoma. In

Piver, M. S. (ed.) *Ovarian Malignancies. Diagnostic and Therapeutic Advances*, pp. 11–25. (Edinburgh: Churchill Livingstone)

58. Crowther, M., Grudzinskas, J. G, Poulton, T. A. *et al.* (1979). Trophoblastic proteins in ovarian carcinoma. *Obstet. Gynecol.*, **53**, 59–61
59. Doellgast, G. J. and Homesley, H. D. (1984). Placental-type alkaline phosphatase in ovarian cancer fluids and tissues. *Obstet. Gynecol.*, **63**, 324–9
60. Nouwen, E. J., Pollet, D. E., Schelstraete, J. B., Eerketens, M. W., Hansch, C., van de Voorge, A. and de Broe, M. E. (1985). Human placental alkaline phosphatase in benign and malignant ovarian neoplasia. *Cancer Res.*, **45**, 892–902
61. Sirsart, A. V., Talavdekar, R. V., Suraiya, J. N and Kullkami, J. N. (1982). Studies on serum amylases in ovarian, prostatic and colonic cancer. *Ind. J. Can.*, **19**, 204–6
62. Bhattacharya, M., Chatterjee, S. K. and Barlow, J. J. (1976). Uridine 5-diphosphate galactose glycoprotein galactosyltransferase activity in the ovarian cancer patient. *Cancer Res.*, **36**, 2096–9
63. Awais, G. M. (1978). Carcinoma of the ovary and serum lactic dehydrogenase levels. *Surg. Gynecol. Obstet.*, **146**, 893–5
64. Chatterjee, S. K., Bhattacharya, M. and Barlow, J. J. (1981). Evaluation of 5-nucleotidase as an enzyme marker in ovarian carcinoma. *Cancer Res.*, **47**, 2648–53
65. Heinonen, P. K., Tuimala, R., Pyykko, K. and Pystynen, P. (1982). Peripheral venous concentrations of oestrogens in postmenopausal women with ovarian cancer. *Br. J. Obstet. Gynaecol.*, **89**, 84–6
66. Backstrom, T., Mahlck, E. G. and Kjellgren, O. (1983). Progesterone as a possible tumour marker for 'nonendocrine' ovarian malignant tumours. *Gynecol. Oncol.*, **16**, 129–38
67. Donaldson, E. S., van Nagell, J. R., Pursell, S., Guy, E. C., Meeker, N. R., Kushmiri, R. and van de Voorde, J. (1980). Multiple biochemical markers in patients with gynecologic malignancies. *Cancer*, **45**, 943–53
68. Stall, K. E. and Martin, E. W. (1981). Plasma carcino-embryonic antigen levels in ovarian cancer patients. A chart review and survey of published data. *J. Reprod. Med.*, **26**, 75–9
69. Hafter, R., Schrock, R., von Hugo, R. and Graeff, H. (1985). Measurement of cross linked fibrin derivatives in plasma and ascitic fluid with monoclonal antibodies against D dimer using EIA and latex test. *Scand. J. Clin. Lab. Invest.*, **45**, 137–44
70. Dodd, J., Tyler, J. P. P., Crandon, A. J., Blumenthal, N. J., Fay, R. A. and Baird, P. J. (1985). The value of the monoclonal antibody (cancer antigen 125) in serial monitoring of ovarian cancer: a comparison with circulating immune complexes. *Br. J. Obstet. Gynaecol.*, **92**, 1054–60
71. Lukomska, B., Olszewski, W. L. and Engeset, A. (1981). Acute phase reactive proteins and complement components and inhibitors in patients with ovarian cancer. *Gynecol. Oncol.*, **11**, 288–98
72. Gallion, H., van Nagell, J. R. and Donaldson, E. S. (1983). Immature teratoma of the ovary. *Am. J. Obstet. Gynecol.*, **146**, 361–5
73. Bagshawe, K. D. (1976). Risk and prognostic factors in trophoblastic neoplasia. *Cancer*, **38**, 1373–85
74. Charpin, C., Bhan, A. K. and Zurawski, V. (1982). Carcinoembryonic antigen (CEA) and carbohydrate determinant 19–9 (CA 19–9) localization in 121 primary and metastatic ovarian tumors; an immunohistochemical study with the use of monochonal antibodies. *Int. J. Gynecol. Pathol.*, **1**, 231–45
75. Metzgar, R. S., Gaillard, M. T., Levine, S. J., Tuck, F. L., Bozzen, E. H. and Borowitz, M. J. (1982). Antigens of human pancreatic adenocarcinoma cells defined by murine monoclonal antibodies. *Cancer Res.*, **42**, 601–8
76. Bhattacharya, M. and Barlow, J. J. (1973). Immunologic studies of human serous cystadenocarcinoma of ovary. Demonstration of tumor-associated antigens. *Cancer*, **31**, 588–95
77. Bhattacharya, M. and Barlow, J. J. (1978). Ovarian tumour antigens. *Cancer*, **42**, 1616–20
78. Knauf, S. and Urbach, G. I. (1980). A study of ovarian cancer patients using a radioimmunoassay for human ovarian tumor-associated antigen OCA. *Am. J. Obstet. Gynecol.*, **138**, 1222–3
79. Bast, R. C., Klug, T. L., St John, E., Jenison, E., Niloff, J. M., Lazarus, H., Berkowitz, R. S., Leavitt, T., Griffiths, C. T., Parker, L., Zurawski, V. R. and Knapp, R. C. (1983). A radioimmunoassay using a monoclonal antibody to monitor the course of epithelial ovarian cancer. *N. Engl. J. Med.*, **309**, 883–7
80. Kabawat, S. E., Bast, R. C., Welch, W. R., Knapp, R. C. and Colvin, R. B. (1983). Immunopathologic characterization of a monoclonal antibody that recognizes common surface antigens of human ovarian tumours of serous, endometrioid and clear cell types. *Am. J. Clin. Pathol.*, **79**, 98–104
81. Niloff, J. M., Knapp, R. C., Schaetzl, E., Reynolds, C. and Bast, R. C. (1984). CA 125 antigen levels in obstetric and gynecologic patients. *Obstet. Gynecol.*, **64**, 703–7
82. Nouwen, E. J., Hendrix, P. G., Danwe, S., Eerdekens, M. W. and De Broe, M. E. (1987). Tumor markers in the human ovary and its neoplasms. *Am. J. Pathol.*, **126**, 230–42
83. Hawkins, R. E., Roberts, K., Wiltshaw, E., Munday, J. and McCready, V. R. (1989). The clinical correlates of serum CA 125 in 169 patients

with epithelial ovarian carcinoma. *Br. J. Cancer*, **60**, 634–7

84. Schilthuis, M. S., Aalders, J. G., Bouma, J., Kooi, H., Fleuren, G. J., Willemse, P. H. B. and De Bruijn, H. W. A. (1987). Serum CA 125 levels in epithelial ovarian cancer: relation with findings at second-look operations and their role in the detection of tumour recurrence. *Br. J. Obstet. Gynaecol.* **94**, 202–7
85. Fuith, L. C., Daxenbichler, G. and Dapunt, O. (1987). CA 125 in the serum and tissue of patients with gynecological disease. *Arch. Gynecol. Obstet.*, **241**, 157–64
86. Zurawski, V. R., Orjaseter, H., Andersen, A. and Jellum, E. (1988). Elevated serum CA 125 levels prior to diagnosis of ovarian neoplasia: relevance for early detection of ovarian cancer. *Int. J. Cancer*, **42**, 677–80
87. Zurawski, V. R., Knapp, R. C., Einhorn, N., Kenemans, P., Mortel, R., Ohmi, K., Bast, R. C., Ritts, R. E. and Malkasian, G. (1988). An initial analysis of preoperative serum CA 125 levels in patients with early stage ovarian carcinoma. *Gynecol. Oncol.*, **30**, 7–14
88. Jacobs, I., Stabile, I., Bridges, J., Kemsley, P., Reynolds, C., Grudzinskas, J. G. and Oram, D. H. (1988). Multimodal approach to screening for ovarian cancer. *Lancet*, **1**, 268–71
89. Jacobs, I., Prys Davies, A., Bridges, J., Stabile, I., Fay, T., Lower, A., Grudzinskas, J. G. and Oram, D. (1993). Prevalence screening for ovarian cancer in postmenopausal women by CA 125 measurement and ultrasonography. *Br. Med. J.*, **306**, 1030–3
90. Einhorn, N., Sjovall, K., Knapp, R. C., Hall, P., Scully, R. E., Bast, R. C. Jr and Zurawski, V. R. Jr (1992). Prospective evaluation of serum CA 125 levels for early detection of ovarian cancer. *Obstet. Gynecol.*, **80**, 14–18
91. Zurawski, V. R., Sjovall, K., Schoenfeld, D. A., Brodrick, S. F., Hall, P., Bast, R. C., Eklund, G., Mattsson, B., Connor, R. J., Prorok, P. C., Knapp, R. C. and Einhorn, N. (1990). Prospective evaluation of serum CA 125 levels in a normal population, phase I: the specificities of single and serial determinations in testing for ovarian cancer. *Gynecol. Oncol.*, **36**, 299–305
92. Cruickshank, D. J., Fullerton, W. T. and Klopper, A. (1987). The clinical significance of preoperative serum CA 125 in ovarian cancer. *Br. J. Obstet. Gynaecol.*, **94**, 692–5
93. Kaesemann, H., Caffier, H., Hoffmann, F. J., Crombach, G., Wurz, H., Kreienberg, R., Mobus, V., Schmidt-Rhode, P. and Sturm, G. (1986). Monoklonale Antikorper in Diagnostik und Verlaufskontrolle de Ovarialkarzinoms. CA 125 als Tumormarker. *Klin. Wochenschr.*, **64**, 781–6
94. Dhokia, B., Canney, P. A., Pectasides, D., Munro, A. J., Moore, M., Wilkinson, P. M., Self, C. and Epenetos, A. A. (1986). A new immunoassay using monoclonal antibodies HMFG1 and HMFG2 together with an existing marker CA 125 for the serological detection and management of epithelial ovarian cancer. *Br. J. Cancer*, **54**, 891–5
95. Ward, B. G., Cruickshank, D. J., Tucker, D. P. and Love, S. (1987). Independent expression in serum of three tumour-associated antigens: CA 125, placental alkaline phosphatase and HMFG2 in ovarian carcinoma. *Br. J. Obstet. Gynaecol.*, **94**, 696–8
96. Cole, L. A., Joo-Lyun, N., Chambers, S. T. and Schwartz, P. E. (1990). Urinary gonadotrophin fragment, and new tumor marker II. Differentiating a benign from a malignant pelvic mass. *Gynecol. Oncol.*, **36**, 391–4
97. Woolas, R., Jacobs, I. J., Xu, F., Oram, D. H. and Bast, R. C. (1993). Serum levels of CA 125, M-CSF and OVX1 in stage I and preclinical ovarian cancer. Presented at *British Gynaecology Cancer Society*, London
98. Di-Xia, C., Schwartz, P. E. and Li, F. Q. (1990). Saliva and serum CA 125 assays for detecting malignant ovarian tumors. *Obstet. Gynecol.*, **75**, 701–4
99. U.K. Co-ordinating Committee in Cancer Research (1989). *Ovarian Cancer Screening*. (London)
100. Skates, S. J. and Singer, D. E. (1991). Quantifying the potential benefit of CA 125 screening for ovarian cancer. *J. Clin. Epidemiol.*, **44**, 365–80
101. Scott, I. V., Milford Ward, A., Selby, C., Whitehead, S. and Wilcox, M. (1990). Development of population-based studies of ovarian cancer screening. In Sharp, F., Mason, W. P. and Leake, R. E. (eds.) *Ovarian Cancer. Biological and Therapeutic Challenges*, pp. 245–58. (London: Chapman & Hall Medical)

Ethical and legal aspects 18

F. A. Chervenak and L. B. McCullough

The purpose of this chapter is to provide the reader with a clinically applicable ethical framework for informed consent for ultrasound examination of the ovary and the management of ovarian disorders. This framework is consistent with legal approaches to informed consent. We begin with a brief introduction to ethics in medicine, in which we define 'ethics' and describe two fundamental ethical principles, beneficence and respect for autonomy, and the beneficence and autonomy models of moral responsibility in medicine. On this basis, we provide an account of informed consent that incorporates and puts into clinical practice the beneficence and autonomy models.

ETHICS DEFINED

Ethics involves the disciplined study of morality. Morality concerns moral character, as well as right and wrong conduct. Moral character concerns the virtues that ought to be cultivated and the vices that ought to be avoided, while right and wrong conduct concerns what one ought or ought not to do. Ethics, as the disciplined study of morality, asks, 'What ought morality to be?'

It is important to distinguish between theological and philosophical ethics. Theological ethics studies morality on the basis of a particular faith tradition and its commitments about what morality ought to be. The intellectual and practical legitimacy and authority of theological ethics therefore depend on whether one can be expected to accept that particular faith tradition and accepts, generally, religious convictions about what morality ought to be.

Philosophical ethics does not start with a set of shared commitments about what morality ought to be. It requires, instead, a general commitment to the process of rational discourse and its results. Philosophical ethics requires rational arguments about what morality ought to be. As a consequence, there are no unargued, concrete assumptions about what correct conduct and moral character should involve. Philosophical ethics is better suited for understanding the ethics of medicine, because medicine, as a health care profession, is secular in nature, and because the society it serves is increasingly pluralistic. In such a society medical ethics must be able to bridge gaps and include individuals, groups, and institutions of widely varying moral commitments, and philosophical ethics provides the basis for doing so[1].

ETHICS AND THE PLURALISTIC SOURCES OF MORALITY

Physicians should not confuse ethics with the many sources of morality in a pluralistic society. These include, but are not limited to, law, our political heritage, religions, ethnic and cultural traditions, families, the traditions and practices of medicine, and personal experience. These sources of morality are useful beginning points for ethical enquiry. None, however, can be the basis of ethics in medicine in a pluralistic society[1].

The traditions and practices of medicine, including education and training, constitute an obvious and basic source of morality for health care professionals. This is because the very notion of a professional encompasses the view that the professional understands the difference between the right and the wrong use of special knowledge and skills. The traditions and practices of medicine underscore the centrality of the obligation to protect and promote the interests of the patient. This obligation states what morality in medicine ought to be, but in very general, abstract terms. Providing a more definite, clinically applicable account of that obligation is the central task of ethics in medicine.

CRITERIA FOR ETHICS IN MEDICINE

The task of philosophical ethics applied to medicine, in response to these pluralistic sources of morality, is to develop accounts that are clear, consistent, coherent, and applicable to medical practice. Meeting the test of these criteria leads to reasoned and therefore reliable accounts. As in clinical judgement, the rigor of ethical reasoning is the basis of its reliability, because certainty rarely can be achieved.

Two fundamental ethical principles

To make clinically applicable the general obligation of protecting and promoting the interests of the patient, ethics in medicine focuses on the question of 'How *ought* physicians to conduct themselves with patients?' The relevant tools of ethics for answering this question are ethical principles, because they help the physician to interpret and implement his or her moral obligation to protect and promote the interests of the patient, which has been the traditional moral foundation of the patient–physician relationship[2].

The principle of beneficence requires the physician to act in a way that is expected reliably to produce the greater balance of benefit over harm for patients[2]. To put this principle into clinical practice requires a reliable account of what benefit and harm are relevant to the care of the patients, and of how this benefit and harm should be reasonably balanced against each other when choices have to be made in particular situations.

In addition to the principle of beneficence, there has been increasing emphasis in the literature of ethics in medicine on the principle of respect for autonomy[2]. This principle requires the physician to acknowledge and carry out the value-based preferences of the patient, irrespective of what the physician may think the consequences for the patient might be.

Neither beneficence nor respect for autonomy in and of itself should be viewed as a 'trump', to borrow a metaphor from the card games of bridge and whist. That is, beneficence does not always override respect for autonomy, and vice versa. Instead, both principles should be understood as theoretically equally weighted and thus potentially in conflict in actual clinical practice. In clinical practice the competing demands of both principles must be balanced and negotiated to determine what protects and promotes the patient's interests[2].

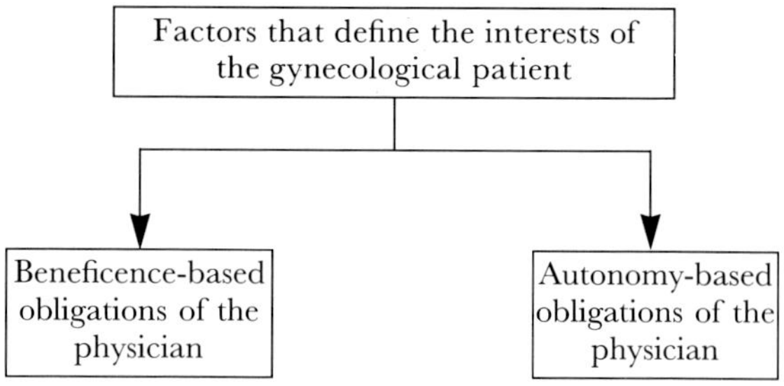

Figure 1 Two fundamental ethical principles

Two models of the moral responsibilities of physicians

The ethical principles of beneficence and respect for autonomy generate two models of moral responsibility that together create an ethical framework that directs and guides the conduct of the physician by generating beneficence-based and autonomy-based obligations on the part of the physician[3]. Both models find their beginning point in the moral obligation of the physician to protect and promote the interests of the patient (Figure 1).

The beneficence model of responsibility

The most ancient and, until the 20th century, the dominant model of the moral responsibilities of the physician has been the beneficence model[2,3]. The beneficence model makes a peculiar claim: to interpret reliably the interests of the patient from the perspective of medicine. This perspective is provided by the accumulated scientific research, clinical experience, and reasoned responses to uncertainty. It is thus not a perspective peculiar or idiosyncratic to any individual physician and requires clinical judgement to meet the criteria for ethics in medicine.

The beneficence model identifies the benefits relevant to the application of the principle of beneficence in clinical practice based on the competencies of medicine. The benefits that medicine is competent to seek for patients are the prevention, cure, or at least the amelioration of disease, injury, handicap, and unnecessary pain and suffering. Pain and suffering become unnecessary when they do not result in achieving the other benefits of medical care.

Physicians need to be aware that there is an inherent risk of paternalism in this model. By this we mean that the beneficence model, if it is, mistakenly, considered to be the sole source of moral responsibility and therefore moral authority in medical care, invites the unwary physician to conclude that beneficence-based judgments can be imposed on patients in violation of their autonomy[3]. Paternalism is perhaps one of the most dehumanizing responses to patients, and therefore should be systematically avoided in the practice of ultrasound examination of the ovary. For example, not disclosing a diagnosis of ovarian cancer would be egregiously paternalistic.

The antidote to this inherent paternalism is for the physician to explain the diagnostic, therapeutic, and prognostic reasoning that leads to his or her clinical judgement about what is in the interest of the patient so that the patient can assess that judgement for herself. The physician should disclose and explain to the patient the major factors of this reasoning process, including matters of uncertainty. (Note that this does not require that the patient be provided with a complete medical education.) The physician should then explain how and why other clinicians might differ from his or her clinical judgement, especially where ultrasound images have been difficult to obtain or are difficult to interpret. The physician should then present a well-reasoned response to this critique. The outcome of this process is that beneficence-based clinical judgements take on a rigor that they often lack and that the process of their formulation includes explaining them to the patient.

Such a process enhances the patient's ability to understand and deal effectively with the technical aspects of ultrasound examination, an important consideration in this area of gynecological practice. Recent data suggest the need for such enhancement. The Louis Harris survey[4], prepared for the President's Commission on Ethics in Medicine, presents an important finding.

> The vast majority of physicians report that they address most aspects of the condition and treatment with their patients as a matter of course. This is substantiated by the large majority of the public who report that their physicians usually discuss these matters with them.

This survey also reports a 'large and reliable difference of approximately 15 to 25 percentage points' between the proportion of physicians who report themselves as discussing some aspects of medical care and the proportion of the public who report that their physicians discuss such matters as diagnosis and prognosis, nature and purpose of treatment, pros and cons of the treatment, and side effects[4]. The process of disclosure described above, if adopted as a standard of care, could well close these significant gaps in the care of patients with gynecological problems and concerns.

One advantage for physicians in carrying out this approach to communicating with patients would be to increase the likelihood of compliance, e.g. with follow-up examinations or referral to specialists. Another advantage would be to provide the patient with a better-informed opportunity to make a decision about whether to seek a second opinion. The approach outlined above should make such a decision less threatening to the physician, who has already shared with the patient the limitations on clinical judgement. A final advantage may be a reduction of the percentage (20%) of physicians who reportedly dismiss patients who disagree with them and the high percentage (36%) of patients who report that they have changed physicians who disagree with them[4].

The autonomy model of moral responsibility

The gynecological patient increasingly brings to her medical care her own perspective on what is in her best interests. The principle of respect for autonomy translates this fact into a second model of the moral responsibilities of physicians: the autonomy model[3].

This model finds its roots in the law of malpractice, dating from the second decade of the

20th century, and then in ethics, dating from the 1960s. Because each patient's perspective on her interests is a function of her values and beliefs, it is impossible to specify the benefit and harm of the model in advance. Indeed, it would be inappropriate to do so, because the definition of benefit and harm and their balancing are matters for the gynecological patient to determine. Not surprisingly, this model is strongly antipaternalistic in nature.

To understand the moral demands of this model, we first require an operationalized concept of autonomy, to make it relevant to clinical practice. To do so, we identify three sequential autonomy-related behaviors on the part of the patient:

(1) Absorbing and retaining information about ovarian disease and dysfunction and alternative diagnostic and therapeutic responses to it;

(2) Understanding that information, that is, evaluating and rank-ordering those responses; and

(3) Expressing a value-based preference for a particular response.

The physician has a role to play in each of these. They are, respectively,

(1) To recognize the capacity of each patient to deal with medical information (and not to underestimate that capacity), including basic technological information about ultrasound and its limits, and recognize the validity of the values and beliefs of the patient;

(2) Not to interfere with but, when necessary, to assist the patient in her evaluation and ranking of diagnostic and therapeutic alternative responses to ovarian disease and dysfunction; and

(3) To elicit and implement the patient's value-based preference[5].

The first requirement recognizes that the patient relies to a considerable extent on her physician for accurate and complete information. At the same time, it underscores the patient's independent ability to seek out information, including technical information, on her own, for example by reading journals or textbooks on gynecological ultrasound. The second requirement places the physician in the counselling, not deciding, role, with the goal being the thoughtful exercise of autonomy by the patient. The demands of this role are more than those of the expert adviser who simply imparts information to the patient. The counsellor helps the patient, when necessary, to interpret and evaluate information, according to the patient's need or request for assistance in doing so[2]. The counsellor is also as non-directive as possible, for example by disclosing influential biases in the management decisions so that the patient can take these subtle factors of clinical judgement into account. The third requirement aims at the explicit exercise of resolution–autonomy by the patient, so that her preferences can be noted in her chart.

INFORMED CONSENT

Taken together, the beneficence and autonomy models provide the components for a clear, consistent, coherent, and applicable general ethical framework for the process of informed consent. The standard account of informed consent in the bioethics literature describes three elements in the process. They are:

(1) The disclosure of an adequate amount of information by the physician to the patient;

(2) The understanding of that information by the patient; and

(3) The voluntary choice by the patient for or against treatment[6].

The 'standard account' suffers from at least two inadequacies. First, it assumes that there is no role for beneficence-based moral responsibilities on the part of the physician. Instead, the physician is understood simply, and incorrectly, as a technically knowledgeable purveyor of information, not as a professional committed to the interests of the patient. Failing to appreciate this is a serious pitfall in the 'high tech' environment of gynecological ultrasound. Second, it assumes that all of us, when we become patients, are fully capable of participating at all times in this process, possessing

Table 1 Clinical applications of the informed consent process[5]

(1) The physician starts the process by finding out how much the patient knows about her condition, its diagnosis, available alternatives, and the prognosis of each alternative.

(2) The physician corrects factual errors in the patient's fund of knowledge.

(3) The physician provides and explains his or her clinical judgement about the patient's condition and all available management strategies (including doing nothing) in a way that provides an antidote to the inherent paternalism of the beneficence model.

(4) The physician works with the patient to develop as complete a picture as possible of her condition and available alternatives.

(5) The physician helps the patient, as needed or requested, to identify her relevant values and beliefs.

(6) The physician helps the patient evaluate her alternatives in terms of those values and beliefs with the goal of the patient's expression of autonomy.

(7) The physician makes a recommendation, based on the beneficence-based clinical judgement already expressed in Step 3.

(8) If there is a disagreement between the physician and the patient about the patient's management, the physician and the patient should negotiate, focusing first on the values and beliefs of the patient and how each one interprets the patient's best interests, then, on that basis, identifying a common ground among those values and beliefs, and then, on that basis, formulating a management plan.

(9) A mutual decision is reached, and it is implemented.

an autonomy that requires no assistance or empowerment by the physician.

The authors propose an alternative account of informed consent, one that avoids these deficiencies and is expressed in terms that can be translated directly into clinical practice in nine steps (Table 1).

This process could be usefully strengthened in a number of ways. Physicians could provide written and audiovisual materials for patients, and patients could be encouraged to seek out information from reliable publicly available sources, including medical libraries[7]. For chronic ovarian diseases in particular (e.g. ovarian cancers and infertility), physicians could provide the patient with a list of questions she eventually should have answers to – answers that make sense to her and form a basis for mutual decision making. This would help to structure the patient's learning process, especially by focusing attention on key technical aspects of ultrasound examination, and it would also help the patient measure her progress in self-education. Given the increasing institutionalization of health care into large-scale delivery mechanisms, non-physician health care professionals should be available who could play an important role in this communication process. Finally, this process need not be accomplished in a single visit for chronic conditions and should not require excessive amounts of time. As the President's Commission has noted, appropriate communication should be 'regarded as a necessary part of good patient care' and a 'separate reimbursable category of information-giving' need not be created[7].

A particularly important dimension of informed consent in gynecological practice involves what have come to be known as 'advance directives', especially for terminal or ultimately terminal ovarian diseases. Spurred by the famous case of Karen Quinlan in New Jersey in 1976, more than 40 state legislatures have enacted 'living will' legislation and, in many states, there is legislative or common-law authority for durable power of attorney for health care.

The basic idea of an advance directive is that a patient, when competent, may make decisions regarding her medical management in advance of a time during which she may become incompetent, either as a result of the natural history of disease or injury or as a result of iatrogenic disease or injury. The ethical dimensions of autonomy that are relevant here are the following:

(1) A patient may exercise her autonomy now, when competent;

(2) Autonomy exercised in the past in the form of explicit preferences or statements of values[8] and left unchanged remains in effect for any future time during which the patient becomes incompetent;

(3) Past preferences and statements of values should therefore translate into treatment plans at the time the patient becomes incompetent; and

(4) Autonomy exercised in the form of refusal of life-prolonging medical intervention, in particular, should translate into the withholding or withdrawal of such interventions, when the patient is no longer competent.

The living will is an instrument that permits the patient to make a direct decision to refuse life-prolonging medical intervention in the future. The living will becomes effective when the patient is a 'qualified patient', usually terminally or irreversibly ill, and is also incompetent. (Obviously, competent terminally or irreversibly ill patients retain their autonomy to make their own decisions, according to the informed consent process described above.) Some states prescribe the wording of this document, while others do not. The reader should become familiar with the legal requirements in any particular jurisdiction. Living wills, to be useful and effective, should be as explicit as possible. Thus, some have proposed addenda, such as the 'medical directive'[9,10] or the 'values history'[8]. The legal basis for the living will is the legal right of self-determination, the right of any competent adult to determine what shall be done to her body. A number of state courts have made it clear that this right extends to the refusal of both hydration and nutrition. The recent US Supreme Court ruling in the famous Cruzan case is ambiguous about whether there is such a right based in the US Constitution[11]. As a consequence, hospitals and other health care institutions have begun to reconsider the refusal of hydration and nutrition based on a living will.

The concept of a durable power of attorney is that any competent adult, in the event that he or she later becomes incompetent, can assign his or her decision making authority to another person. The advantage of the durable power of attorney for health care is that it applies only when the patient becomes incompetent. It does not, as does the living will, require that the patient also be terminally or irreversibly ill. However, unlike the living will, the durable power of attorney does not provide explicit direction, only the explicit assignment of decision-making authority. Obviously, any patient who assigns durable power of attorney for health care to someone should communicate her values, beliefs, and preferences to that person. The physician can play a facilitating role in this process. Indeed, in order to protect the patient's autonomy, the physician should play an active role in encouraging this communication process, so that there will be minimal doubt about whether the person holding durable power of attorney is faithfully representing the wishes of the patient. Again, the physician should be aware of his or her hospital policies under the Patient Self-Determination Act.

The main virtues of these two forms of advance directives are that they encourage patients to think carefully in advance about the refusal of medical intervention and that these directives, therefore, help to prevent ethical crises in the management of incompetent patients and incompetent and terminally or irreversibly ill patients. Unfortunately, the use of advance directives is not as widespread as it should be. The reader is encouraged to think of advance directives as powerful, practical strategies for preventive ethics and to encourage patients to consider them carefully, especially patients with ovarian diseases – particularly ovarian cancers – that are now or could be life threatening.

CONCLUSION

Ethics is an important, but sometimes insufficiently appreciated, dimension of the clinical management of patients with gynecological problems and concerns. While ethics in the practice of ovarian ultrasound relies on the discipline of philosophy as one of its bases, it is clinically oriented and applicable. Ethics is thus not some 'ivory tower' undertaking, but an essential clinical skill in the clinical practice of ultrasound examination of the ovary and the management of ovarian disorders[12].

References

1. Engelhardt, H. T. Jr. (1986). *The Foundations of Bioethics.* (New York: Oxford University Press)
2. McCullough, L. B. and Chervenak, F. A. (1994). *Ethics in Obstetrics and Gynecology.* (New York: Oxford University Press)
3. Beauchamp, T. L. and McCullough, L. B. (1984). *Medical Ethics: The Moral Responsibilities of Physicians.* (Englewood Cliffs: Prentice-Hall)
4. Louis Harris and Associates (1982). Views on informed consent and decisionmaking: parallel surveys of physicians and the public. In *Making Health Care Decisions*, vol. 2, *Appendices: Empirical Studies of Informed Consent*, pp. 17–316. (Washington, DC: US Government Printing Office)
5. McCullough, L. B. (1988). An ethical model for improving the patient–physician relationship. *Inquiry*, **25**, 454–68
6. Faden, R. R. and Beauchamp, T. L. (1986). *A History and Theory of Informed Consent.* (New York: Oxford University Press)
7. President's Commission for the Study of Ethical Problems in Medicine and Biomedical and Behavioral Research (1982). A review of empirical studies of informed consent and decisionmaking. In *Making Health Care Decisions*, vol. 2, *Appendices: Empirical Studies of Informed Consent*, pp. 1–5. (Washington, DC: US Government Printing Office)
8. Doukas, D. J. and McCullough, L. B. (1994). The values history: the evaluation of the patient's values and advance directives. *J. Fam. Prac.*, in press
9. Emanuel, L. and Emanuel, E. J. (1989). The medical directive: a new comprehensive advance care document. *J. Am. Med. Assoc.*, **261**, 3288–93
10. Emanuel, E. J. and Emanuel, L. (1990). Living wills: past, present, and future. *J. Clin. Ethics*, **1**, 9–19
11. Annas, G. J. (1990). Nancy Cruzan and the right to die. *N. Engl. J. Med.*, **323**, 670–3
12. Chervenak, F. A. and McCullough, L. B. (1993). Identification and management of ethical conflict in this patient–gynecologist relationship. *J. Reprod. Med.*, **38**, 553–7

Index